TOWARD A 21st CENTURY
HEALTH SYSTEM

Toward a 21st Century Health System

The Contributions and Promise of Prepaid Group Practice

Alain C. Enthoven
Laura A. Tollen

Editors

Foreword by William L. Roper

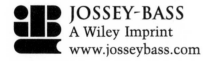

JOSSEY-BASS
A Wiley Imprint
www.josseybass.com

Published by Jossey-Bass
A Wiley Imprint
989 Market Street, San Francisco, CA 94103-1741   www.josseybass.com

Jossey-Bass books and products are available through most bookstores. To contact Jossey-Bass directly
call our Customer Care Department within the U.S. at 800-956-7739, outside the U.S. at 317-572-
399386 or fax 317-572-4002.

Jossey-Bass also publishes its books in a variety of electronic formats. Some content that appears in print
may not be available in electronic books.

Epigraph reprinted with permission from *Crossing the Quality Chasm* (2001, pp. 1, 4) by the National
Academy of Sciences, courtesy of the National Academies Press, Washington, D.C.

Library of Congress Cataloging-in-Publication Data
Toward a 21st century health system : the contributions and promise of
prepaid group practice / Alain C. Enthoven, Laura A. Tollen, editors ;
foreword by William L. Roper.—1st ed.
     p. ; cm.
   Includes bibliographical references and index.
   ISBN 0-7879-7309-2 (alk. paper)
  1. Health maintenance organizations—United States.   2. Managed care plans
(Medical care)—United States.
     [DNLM: 1. Group Practice, Prepaid—trends—United States.   2. Delivery of
Health Care—United States.   3. Group Practice, Prepaid—economics—United States.
     4. Health Policy—United States.   5. Quality of Health Care—United States. W 92 T737 2004]
I. Enthoven, Alain C., 1930—II. Tollen, Laura A.
   RA413.5.U5T69 2004
   362.1'042584—dc22   2003027932

Printed in the United States of America
FIRST EDITION
HB Printing 10 9 8 7 6 5 4 3 2 1

CONTENTS

TABLES AND EXHIBITS

Tables

Exhibits

ACKNOWLEDGMENTS

The editors would like to acknowledge the help and support of many people without whom this project could not have been completed. Robert M. Crane, director of the Kaiser Permanente Institute for Health Policy, welcomed the proposal for this book, secured financial support, and generally provided encouragement and wise counsel. Jon Stewart of the Permanente Federation, which encompasses all of the Permanente Medical Groups, provided skillful editorial advice and editing. Jennifer Neisner, of the Kaiser Permanente Institute for Health Policy, provided the editors and many of the authors with valuable research assistance and access to experts and data within the organization. Amalia Martino and Tova Wolking, also of the Institute for Health Policy, provided highly competent and skilled project management and editing assistance, respectively. Finally, we want to thank all of our coauthors for the brilliance with which they thought and wrote, the faithfulness with which they met deadlines, and their general support, cooperation, and valuable advice.

"The American health care delivery system is in need of fundamental change. . . . The current care systems cannot do the job. Trying harder will not work. Changing systems of care will."

Institute of Medicine, *Crossing the Quality Chasm: A New Health System for the 21st Century* (Washington, D.C.: National Academy Press, 2001), pp. 1, 4.

THE CONTRIBUTORS

George Avery, M.P.A., is a doctoral candidate with the Division of Health Services Research and Policy at the University of Minnesota School of Public Health and holds an adjunct faculty appointment with the Department of Psychology at the University of Minnesota-Duluth. He served for ten years with the Division of Public Health Laboratories, Arkansas Department of Health, and holds a master's degree in public administration.

Robert A. Berenson, M.D., is Senior Fellow at the Urban Institute and an adjunct professor at the University of North Carolina School of Public Health and the Fuqua School of Business at Duke University. For the last three years of the Clinton administration, he was a senior political appointee in the Centers for Medicare and Medicaid Services, responsible for Medicare payment policy and managed care contracting. He is a board-certified internist who practiced for twelve years in a Washington, D.C., group practice and has served on many medical panels and committees, including the Health and Public Policy Committee of the American College of Physicians. He was chair of the Managed Care Panel on Health Care Quality of the Institute of Medicine and has served on numerous IOM study panels. Prior to starting his medical practice, Berenson spent three years on President Carter's White House Domestic Policy staff, working on national health policy issues, including hospital cost containment and national health insurance. In 1993, he cochaired two working groups as part of President Clinton's

White House Task Force on Health Care Reform. He earned his bachelor's degree at Brandeis University and his medical degree at the Mount Sinai University School of Medicine. He is a Fellow of the American College of Physicians.

Donald M. Berwick, M.D., M.P.P., is president and chief executive officer of the Institute for Healthcare Improvement (IHI). Based in Boston, Massachusetts, IHI is a nonprofit organization dedicated to improving the quality of health care systems through education, research, and demonstration projects and through fostering collaboration among health care organizations and their leaders. Berwick is clinical professor of pediatrics and health care policy at Harvard Medical School. He is also a pediatrician, an associate in pediatrics at Boston's Children's Hospital, and a consultant in pediatrics at Massachusetts General Hospital.

William H. Campbell, Ph.D., is professor in the School of Pharmacy at the University of North Carolina (UNC). He also served as Dean at the UNC School of Pharmacy from 1992 to 2003. Prior to his UNC appointment he served as Dean of the School of Pharmacy at Auburn University (1988–1992) and Chair of the Department of Pharmacy at the University of Washington (1975–1988). His research and teaching interests have focused on managed health care, first as a research environment for conducting epidemiologic assessments of drug safety and effectiveness, later on systems design and assessment for delivering pharmaceutical services and products, and more recently on managed care policy issues with particular emphasis on pharmaceutical benefits and pharmacy manpower and education. His experience has included appointments as senior investigator for the Kaiser Foundation Center for Health Services Research (Northwest Region) from 1971 to 1977 and research associate with Group Health Cooperative of Puget Sound, Center for Health Research (Seattle), from 1975 to 1988. He has been actively involved in national and local organizations, including the American Pharmaceutical Association, the American Society of Health Systems Pharmacists, the Academy of Managed Care Pharmacy, the American Public Health Association, and the Association of Health Services Research. He is a former president of the American Association of Colleges of Pharmacy and a member of the board of trustees of the United States Pharmacopoeia, and he serves as a consultant to numerous organizations.

Jon B. Christianson, Ph.D., is an economist with extensive research and teaching experience in the financing and delivery of medical care. He has published seven books and more than one hundred articles in the areas of managed care, rural health care, mental health care, and care process improvement and has collaborated with health care providers in a variety of practice settings to evaluate new treatment approaches. He earned his Ph.D. at the University of Wisconsin-Madison and is currently on the faculty of the Carlson School of Management at the University of Minnesota, where he is the James A. Hamilton Chair in Health Policy and Management. Christianson serves on a number of editorial boards and scientific advisory panels and directs the Center for the Study of Healthcare Management in the Department of Healthcare Management at the Carlson School.

Kenneth H. Chuang, M.D., is Veterans Affairs Quality Scholar at the San Francisco Veterans Affairs Medical Center. His research interests include developing improved measures of quality of care, translating evidence into practice, and spreading best practices between institutions. Chuang received his medical degree from the University of Texas at Southwestern in 1997. He is board certified in internal medicine.

Francis J. Crosson, M.D., is the executive director of The Permanente Federation, the national organization of the Permanente Medical Groups, which is the physician component of Kaiser Permanente. He serves as cochair of the Kaiser Permanente Partnership Group (the Kaiser Permanente joint management body) and as CEO and president of the Permanente Company, which carries out the federation's business functions. He is a member of the California Medical Association board of trustees and the governing board of the American Medical Group Association. He is a graduate of the Kaiser Permanente Executive Program at Stanford Business School. Crosson received an undergraduate degree in political science and, in 1970, a medical degree from Georgetown University. He completed a residency in pediatrics at the New England Medical Center Hospitals and a fellowship in infectious diseases at the Johns Hopkins University Medical School. He is certified by the American Board of Pediatrics.

Helen Darling, M.A., is president of the National Business Group on Health (NBGH) (formerly the Washington Business Group on Health), an organization that fosters innovative health benefits decision making among corporate purchasers and helps them share best practices and new solutions to their business problems. A Capitol Hill veteran, Darling works with Congress to advance the understanding of corporate health care issues. She is also president of the Institute on Health Care Costs and Solutions, an organization within NBGH, founded to focus entirely on solutions to the health care cost crisis from a business perspective. In addition, she currently serves as cochair of the National Committee on Quality Assurance's Committee on Performance Measurement. She is a member of the Medical Advisory Panel, Technology Evaluation Center of the Blue Cross Blue Shield

Association; the Institute of Medicine's Board on Health Promotion and Disease Prevention; the Council on Health Care Economics and Policy; and the board of Gaylord Rehabilitation Hospital. She is also a member of the National Advisory Committees of two of The Robert Wood Johnson Foundation's grant programs, Pursuing Perfection and Rewarding Results. Darling received her master's degree in demography and sociology and her bachelor of science degree in history and English, cum laude, from the University of Memphis.

R. Adams Dudley, M.D., M.B.A., is associate professor in the Institute for Health Policy Studies, the Department of Medicine, and the Department of Epidemiology and Biostatistics at the University of California, San Francisco (UCSF). His research interests include developing improved measures of quality of care, improving techniques to adjust for the financial risk that health plans and providers face based on the prevalence and severity of illness among their enrollees, and assessing the feasibility of changing the relative weights put on quality versus price by participants in the health care market. He has authored and coauthored numerous articles in scientific journals. Dudley received his master's degree in business administration from Stanford University's Graduate School of Business in 1990 and his medical degree from Duke University in 1991. He is board certified in internal medicine and pulmonary medicine. He was a Pew Fellow in Health Policy at UCSF from 1995 to 1997 before joining the UCSF faculty.

David M. Eddy, M.D., Ph.D., is an internationally recognized authority on such topics as practice guidelines, technology assessment, outcomes, mathematical modeling, quality measurement, cost effectiveness, and priority setting. The author of five books, more than one hundred articles, and a series of essays for the *Journal of the American Medical Association,* his writings span from technical mathematical theories to broad health policy topics. A collection of his policy essays has recently been published by *JAMA.* Eddy is widely recognized as one of the founders of evidence-based medicine. He has received top national and international awards in several fields, including applied mathematics, health technology assessment, health care quality, and outcomes research. He has been elected or appointed to more than forty national and international boards and commissions, including Consumers Union, the National Board of Mathematics, the World Health Organization Panel of Experts, and the National Committee for Quality Assurance, and is a member of the Institute of Medicine, of the National Academies. He was a professor of engineering and medicine at Stanford and then the J. Alexander McMahon Professor of Health Policy and Management at Duke University before resigning to become an independent researcher and writer.

Alain C. Enthoven, Ph.D., is a Senior Fellow in the Center for Health Policy, Institute of International Relations, at Stanford University and the Marriner S. Eccles Professor of Public and Private Management (emeritus) in the Graduate School of Business at Stanford University. He holds degrees in economics from Stanford, Oxford, and the Massachusetts Institute of Technology. The positions he has held include economist with the RAND Corporation, Assistant United States Secretary of Defense, and president of Litton Medical Products. In 1963, he received the President's Award for Distinguished Federal Civilian Service from John F. Kennedy. In 1977, while serving as a consultant to Department of Health and Human Services Secretary Joseph Califano and the Carter administration, he designed and proposed Consumer Choice Health Plan, a plan for universal health insurance based on managed competition in the private sector. Enthoven is a member of the Institute of Medicine, of the National Academies, and a fellow of the American Academy of Arts and Sciences. He is a consultant to Kaiser Permanente; the former chair of the Health Benefits Advisory Council for CalPERS, the California state employees' medical and hospital care plans; and former chair of Stanford's University Committee on Faculty and Staff Benefits. He has been a director of the Jackson Hole Group, PCS, Caresoft Inc., and eBenX Inc. He is now a director of Rx Intelligence. He was the 1994 winner of the Baxter Prize for Health Services Research and also the 1995 Board of Directors Award given by the Healthcare Financial Management Association. In 1997, Governor Pete Wilson appointed him chair of the California Managed Health Care Improvement Task Force. Commissioned by the state legislature, the task force addressed health care issues raised by managed care. In 1998–1999, he was the Rock Carling Fellow of the Nuffield Trust of London and also visiting professor at the London School of Hygiene and Tropical Medicine. He has recently written the Rock Carling Lecture *In Pursuit of an Improving National Health Service* recommending the introduction of market forces in the National Health Service.

Raymond Fink, Ph.D., was associate director and then director of research and vice president of the Health Insurance Plan of Greater New York from 1962 through 1978. The studies he directed include evaluations of the insurability of mental health care and of primary care physicians' role in that care and tests on the viability of enrolling Medicaid recipients and other poor persons in established prepaid group practices. He also directed the social science aspects of research in breast cancer and other medical screening programs. From 1978 through 2000, Fink was professor of community and preventive medicine at New York Medical College and founded the Program in Health Policy and Management in its new graduate school. He is a member of the board of directors of the Medical and Health Research Association of New York City and was its chair for twenty-six years, during which time it became a major provider of health services to disadvantaged New Yorkers and a nationally recognized center for research.

Merwyn (Mitch) R. Greenlick, Ph.D., is professor emeritus and past chair of the Department of Public Health and Preventive Medicine in the Medical School of Oregon Health and Science University. He also directs the Oregon Health Policy Institute. Until July 1995, he was director of the Kaiser Permanente Center for Health Research and vice president for research for Kaiser Foundation Hospitals. He received his doctorate in medical care organization from the University of Michigan. He has served as research adviser on many projects throughout the country and as an adviser to several foreign government research and medical care institutions. He was elected in 2002 to the Oregon House of Representatives, where he served on the House committees on transportation and on environment and land use. He also sat with the House Ways and Means Audit Subcommittee charged with restructuring the Oregon Health Plan. Greenlick was elected to the National Academies' Institute of Medicine in 1971 and has served on and chaired a number of NAS study committees. He has published more than two hundred books, articles, and papers. He is a Distinguished Fellow of the Academy for Health Services Research and Health Policy (now AcademyHealth) and in 1994 received the Academy's President's Award for his lifetime contributions to the field of health services research.

George C. Halvorson was named chairman and chief executive officer of Kaiser Foundation Health Plan and Kaiser Foundation Hospitals in March 2002. Kaiser Permanente, which comprises Kaiser Foundation Health Plan, Kaiser Foundation Hospitals, and the Permanente Medical Groups, is America's leading integrated health care organization. Founded in 1945, it is a nonprofit health plan serving more than 8.3 million members in nine states and the District of Columbia. Halvorson also serves on a number of boards, including those of the American Association of Health Plans, the Alliance of Community Health Plans, and the International Federation of Health Plans. He has more than thirty years of health care management experience. He was formerly president and chief executive officer of HealthPartners in Minneapolis. Prior to joining HealthPartners in 1986, he held several senior management positions with Blue Cross and Blue Shield of Minnesota. He was also president of Senior Health Plan and of Health Accord International, an international HMO management company. Halvorson is the author of several books on health care, including *Strong Medicine,* published by Random House, and *Epidemic of Care,* published by Jossey-Bass.

Richard E. Johnson, Ph.D., R.Ph., senior investigator emeritus, Center for Health Research, Kaiser Permanente, Northwest Region, received his pharmacy degree from Ohio Northern University in 1952 and his doctorate in pharmaceutical economics from the University of Pittsburgh in 1964. He joined the faculty at Oregon State University School of Pharmacy in 1965 and left in 1973 to join the Center for Health Research, Kaiser Permanente, Northwest Region. He retired from the center in 1998.

Sharon L. Levine, M.D., has been a pediatrician with The Permanente Medical Group since 1977. She has held many leadership roles within the medical group, including chief of pediatrics for the Fremont Medical Center, chief of quality, and physician in charge of the Fremont Medical Center. She has served as associate executive director for physician and professional services for the group since 1991. She currently has responsibility for human resources (recruitment, compensation, clinical and management training, and leadership development), government and community relations, health policy and external affairs, and pharmacy issues including drug use management. She is certified by the American Board of Pediatrics and is a member of the American College of Physician Executives, the California Medical Association, the American Medical Women's Association, and the American Medical Association. She is a member of the board of directors of the Integrated Healthcare Association and its chair for 2002–2003. She is a frequent speaker on issues of health policy and drug use management. Levine received her undergraduate degree from Radcliffe College at Harvard University and her medical degree from Tufts University School of Medicine.

Harold S. Luft, Ph.D., is Caldwell B. Esselstyn Professor of Health Policy and Health Economics and director of the Institute for Health Policy Studies at the University of California, San Francisco. His research and teaching have covered a wide range of areas, including medical care utilization, health maintenance organizations, hospital market competition, quality and outcomes of hospital care, risk assessment and risk adjustment, and health care market reforms in various states and communities. He is a member of the Institute of Medicine and served six years on the IOM Council. He chaired and was a member of the National Advisory Council of the Agency for Health Care Policy and Research (now the Agency for Healthcare Research and Quality). He serves on the board of AcademyHealth and is a coeditor of the journal *Health Services Research*. He has authored or coauthored and edited a number of books and has published numerous articles in scientific journals. Luft earned his A.B., M.A., and Ph.D. degrees in economics (specializing in health sector economics and public finance) at Harvard University.

Sachin H. Jain is a joint M.D. and M.P.P. degree candidate at Harvard Medical School and the John F. Kennedy School of Government and a magna cum laude graduate of Harvard College. He has researched health care policy at the Institute for Healthcare Improvement, the Alpha Center, and the Radcliffe Institute for Public Policy in addition to serving in an advisory capacity for a Massachusetts state legislator. He is a recipient of the John Kenneth Galbraith Scholarship in Social Policy and Inequality, a Herman M. Somers Long-Term Care Fellowship, and the Albert P. Schweitzer Fellowship and is an associate of the National Academy for Social Insurance.

James C. Robinson, Ph.D., is professor of health economics and chair of the Division of Health Policy and Management at the University of California, Berkeley, School of Public Health. His current research projects analyze the reinvention of health insurance in the consumer era, the role of financial markets in the consolidation of the hospital and health insurance sectors, the financial solvency and clinical processes of community clinics serving the Medicaid program, and the payment incentives implemented by physician organizations. Robinson grew up in southern California, where he was surprised to learn during his adolescence that not everyone belongs to Kaiser Permanente. An expert in health economics and organization, Robinson has found himself unable to explain to his children or his students why American physicians do not form large medical groups and thereby come to own the hospitals that serve them and the insurers that finance them.

William L. Roper, M.D., M.P.H., is dean of the School of Public Health at the University of North Carolina at Chapel Hill (UNC). He is also professor of health policy and administration in the School of Public Health and professor of pediatrics in the School of Medicine at UNC. Before joining UNC in July 1997, Dr. Roper was senior vice president of Prudential HealthCare. He joined Prudential in 1993 as president of the Prudential Center for Health Care Research. Before coming to Prudential, Dr. Roper was director of the Centers for Disease Control and Prevention (CDC), served on the senior White House staff, and was administrator of the Health Care Financing Administration (now the Centers for Medicare and Medicaid Services). Earlier, he was a White House Fellow. He received his medical degree from the University of Alabama School of Medicine and his M.P.H. from the University of Alabama at Birmingham School of Public Health. He completed his residency in pediatrics at the University of Colorado Medical Center. Dr. Roper is a member of the Institute of Medicine of the National Academies and serves on the Institute of Medicine governing council. He is vice chairman of the board of both the Partnership for Prevention and the National Quality Forum.

Julie Schmittdiel, M.A., received her bachelor's degree in mathematics from the Massachusetts Institute of Technology and her master's degree in biostatistics from the University of California, Berkeley, where she is currently a doctoral candidate in health services and policy analysis. Her primary research interests are examining the organizational determinants of the use of care management practices and the effect of primary health care practices on chronic illness care.

Stephen M. Shortell, Ph.D., is the Blue Cross of California Distinguished Professor of Health Policy and Management and professor of organizational behavior at the School of Public Health and Haas School of Business at the University of California, Berkeley. He is also dean of the university's School of Public Health and holds appointments in the Department of Sociology at UC Berkeley and at the Institute for Health Policy Research, UC San Francisco. A leading health care scholar, Shortell has been the recipient of many awards, including the distinguished Baxter-Allegiance Prize for his contributions to health services research. He is an elected member of the Institute of Medicine of the National Academies, where he serves on the executive committee of the governing council. He is currently conducting research on the evaluation of quality improvement initiatives and on the implementation of evidence-based medicine practices in physician organizations.

Jon A. Stewart, M.A., is communications director of The Permanente Federation, the national umbrella organization of the regional Permanente medical groups. He has held that position since 1997, when he transitioned from a twenty-year career in magazine and newspaper journalism. As a reporter, editor, and editorial writer, he covered a wide variety of issues, including health care, the environment, national security, and foreign policy. He holds a bachelor's degree in literature from Northern Michigan University and a master's degree in literature from the State University of New York (Binghamton).

Laura A. Tollen, M.P.H., is senior policy consultant with the Kaiser Permanente Institute for Health Policy, working on issues related to insurance market structure and functioning. Her recent work has focused on benefit design and the implications of the trend toward increased consumer cost sharing. Other areas of expertise include small group insurance markets, health care purchasing pools, risk adjustment, and delivery system organization. Prior to joining the institute, Tollen was senior analyst and project director at the Institute for Health Policy Solutions, a Washington, D.C.–based think tank. In that position, she provided technical assistance to states seeking to use Medicaid or SCHIP funds to buy into employer-based health insurance. Tollen's other experience includes work as a policy analyst in the Colorado Department of Health Care Policy and Financing. She earned a bachelor's degree in anthropology and a master's of public health with an emphasis in health policy at the University of California, Berkeley.

Allan J. Weiland, M.D., has served as president of Northwest Permanente, P.C., and regional medical director of Kaiser Permanente Northwest since January 1, 1993. Prior to this, he served as vice president and area medical director of Northwest Permanente and chief of staff of Bess Kaiser Medical Center in Portland from 1988 to 1992. Earlier, Weiland had been physician-in-charge of the Vancouver Medical Office and assistant area medical director at Bess Kaiser, during which time he served as both chair of the Quality Assurance Committee and later as regional director of quality assurance. Weiland joined Kaiser Permanente as an obstetrics-gynecology physician in 1977. He was a clinical instructor in the Department of Obstetrics-Gynecology at Oregon Health Sciences University School of Medicine until 1993. He is a fellow of the American College of Obstetrics and Gynecology and a member of the Oregon Obstetrics Gynecology Society and the American Uro-Gynecological Society. He received his undergraduate degree from the University of Washington in 1969 and his medical degree from Northwestern Medical School in 1972. He completed a rotating internship at Illinois Masonic Medical Center and an obstetrics-gynecology residency at Mercy Hospital in San Diego in 1977, receiving his board certification in 1980. He is certified by the American Board of Medical Specialties.

Jonathan P. Weiner, Dr. P.H., is professor of health policy and management at the Johns Hopkins Bloomberg School of Public Health and also holds a joint appointment at the Johns Hopkins School of Medicine. He is also deputy director of the Johns Hopkins Health Services Research and Development Center, where he is the principal investigator for many large research studies. Weiner is an internationally known health services researcher, health policy analyst, and lecturer. His areas of expertise include managed care, primary care, case mix and risk adjustment, and health workforce planning. He has extensive consulting experience with a variety of state, local, federal, and foreign government units, including the health reform task force of both the Clinton and Bush administrations. He is coauthor of the best-selling book *The New Medical Marketplace: The Physician's Guide to the Health Care System in the 1990s* (Johns Hopkins University Press, 1993). He holds a doctorate of public health in health services research from the Johns Hopkins University School of Public Health. He also holds a master's degree in health administration from the University of Massachusetts and a bachelor of arts degree in human biology from the University of Pennsylvania.

FOREWORD

William L. Roper

Over the past thirty years, we in the United States have had several rounds of discussion and debate about health care reform, and various proposals for more organized systems of care have played a key role in each of those debates.

After a widespread and serious push toward implementation of what Alain Enthoven calls "delivery system health maintenance organizations" in the 1970s, 1980s, and early 1990s, our country has now spent the past several years moving away from that model, in the interest of giving consumers greater choice of providers.

It is not at all clear that our "back to the future" movement to fee-for-service health care can deal with the continuing concern over health care costs. Furthermore, we have learned much over the past few years about our deplorable lack of consistently good quality and patient safety. An unorganized nonsystem of health care delivery is ill-equipped to provide the focus and mechanisms for quality improvement.

Prepaid group practices (PGPs) have remained the health reform prescription of choice of many in the health policy community, across the political

I have learned a great deal about organized care systems from Glenn Hackbarth, who has dealt with these issues in policy debates and in practical health care operations as he sought to work out the details in real-world applications. I appreciate his suggestions for this foreword.

spectrum, and I proudly put myself among them. Along the way, I have gained much from Alain Enthoven and from many of the other writers in this volume.

My first encounter with Enthoven and his health policy recommendations was in 1982. As a White House Fellow and very junior member of the White House domestic policy staff, I read and attempted to use his detailed and elegant reform proposals. Professor Enthoven was bold and comprehensive in his prescription for new ways of organizing the financing and delivery of health care services. His work has had an impact on every administration's health proposals before and since, over a period of three decades.

Despite the efforts of many of us promoting greater reliance on PGPs, it is clear that the American people have not been buying what we have been selling. This has been repeatedly brought home to me, quite literally, as my wife has vociferously protested the notion of our family enrolling in such care arrangements ourselves.

I believe that the potential of PGPs remains great, although it is surely not fully realized. That potential lies in four areas:

- Culture—the fact that clinicians seeking employment in such groups tend be different, which makes it easier to foster and maintain a quality-focused, parsimonious culture
- Infrastructure—investment in clinical information systems, patient education and support systems, and the like
- Compensation and reward systems—with incentives for cost restraint and quality
- Close collaborative relationships—with clinical partners such as hospitals and health plans

In addition, to realize their full potential, PGPs must have strong clinical leadership, a scarce resource. Excellent clinicians are not necessarily excellent leaders. Different mind-sets and even different personality traits are required for the roles. To be an excellent clinical leader, however, it really helps to be regarded by your colleagues as an excellent clinician. So we're searching for "twofers," a fairly rare combination.

Managed care came to a fork in the road in the early 1990s, and many leading organizations took the wrong road. For a variety of reasons, employers began reducing the number of plans offered and forcing all of their employees into "managed care." Instead of a consumer-choice-oriented system, they began to move toward one more actively managed by employers.

Two bad things happened as a result. First, because managed care was being forced on people who did not voluntarily choose it, the seeds of a backlash were sown. Second, health plans organized around PGPs were put at a disadvantage relative to big-network plans. If an employer was going to offer only one or two plans instead of six, it usually wanted plans offering lots of "choice," which is to say the ability for people to stay with their current doctor. To meet this demand by employers, many delivery system HMOs merged with or invested in developing IPA-type networks. Instead of investing time, energy, and resources in improving care, these plans focused on mergers, claims systems, marketing, and other non-health-related concerns.

It is tempting to blame employers, but that isn't completely fair. The path they followed looked attractive because PGPs were not performing to their potential; their quality and cost performance was not sufficiently better than other types of practice. Once it happened, however, it became much more difficult to attract new patients to PGPs embedded in the big networks. Consumers could stay with their current physician for the same price (premiums and copay) as switching to a PGP. In other words, the inertia became even greater.

Looking to the future, three things must happen for PGPs to flourish: (1) throughout the health care system, we must improve our ability to document performance (quality and cost); (2) PGPs must then establish a clear and conse-quential performance advantage; and then (3) employers and other payers must reward switching or leaving the security of an existing physician relationship for something new and different. None of these steps is easy.

A major question for those of us who have advocated for PGP-style health reform is whether such an agenda is possible at this point in our health care sys-tem's evolution. That is an arguable point, and it surely will be debated. But even if it is not possible, we have much to learn from the past efforts toward PGPs, and the various parts of the model give us real guidance for our work ahead.

From this point on, most proposals for health care reform will involve sub-stantial organizational change. In its recent report *Crossing the Quality Chasm,* the Institute of Medicine laid out a challenging agenda for improving health care in America. Here, as in many such proposals, the recommendations call for entities that have many of the characteristics of PGPs.

As Americans look critically at the structure and financing of health care in our nation, and as we try to improve the results we get for the vast resources used in the health care process, the issues and elements discussed by the authors in this volume are very worthy of our continued attention.

PREFACE

This book exists because the authors believe that the quality and affordability of the health care provided to Americans has been and must continue to be enhanced by the availability of alternatives to the "free-choice," fee-for-service, solo-practice financing and delivery system that has dominated American health care. Those alternatives must include financing and delivery models that stimulate competition based on value (defined as clinical and service quality plus affordability) and are known to promote more efficient use of increasingly costly health care resources. This book presents information on the potential and the actual performance of one such alternative—prepaid group practice—as envisioned and experienced by some of the nation's premier health care organizations over the past half-century.

This examination of prepaid group practice is undertaken within the context of widespread and growing discontent with the nation's mainstream health care system. Health expenditures are at historic highs and have been rising at unsustainable double-digit rates. Average employer premiums rose nearly 15 percent in 2002.[1] In 2003, the average annual cost per employee for health benefits is approaching $6,500, and family premiums of $10,000 are not unusual. In mid-2003, one firm projected that 2004 HMO premiums would increase 17.7 percent over 2003.[2]

Health expenditures are straining public finances at every level of government—local, county, state, and federal—crowding out other important social programs. The annual increases in employer-paid health insurance premiums are exceeding affordable increases in total compensation, forcing employers to shift health care costs to employees or even abandon health insurance altogether.

Rising premiums are also driving up the number of uninsured.[3] This leads to numerous and serious problems.[4] Some forty million Americans lack health insurance altogether,[5] and these people receive less care in total, and less preventive and disease management services, than their insured counterparts. Yet much of the care they do receive is provided in the most expensive setting—emergency rooms. Most of the uninsured cannot pay their bills, resulting in personal financial hardships and a growing burden on health care institutions.

That is the economic view of the situation. Health care quality advocates see additional problems. While we like to say that "the United States has the world's best health care," the reality is less reassuring. The Institute of Medicine finds that American medicine suffers from major quality deficits, including tens of thousands of deaths each year from avoidable medical errors.[6]

There are many causes for the multiple ills that beset American health care—political, legal, technological, and social—but surely one of the chief contributors must be our strong attachment to the traditional way health care has been organized, financed, and delivered in this country. Whatever name it goes by—traditional fee-for-service or the more contemporary "preferred provider organization" (PPO)—it is filled with inflationary incentives and almost devoid of incentives to organize, coordinate, or systematically improve care and enhance affordability. Combined with employer- and tax-subsidized insurance that shields consumers from the real cost of health care, this model has contributed to a cost explosion that by the early 1990s had put health care at the very top of the nation's political agenda.

In the wake of the Clinton administration's failure to deal effectively with the issue, American employers rushed to so-called managed care to control costs, often imposing it on employees with little or no choice. This heavy-handed approach, combined with the restrictive utilization policies of some managed care organizations, led to a "managed care backlash," attended by sensationalized media stories and a rash of politically inspired legislation and regulation that did little more than drive costs even higher.

By the turn of the twenty-first century, employers were responding to disgruntled employees by turning away from managed care organizations to the less restrictive but more costly PPOs and traditional insurers. But PPOs are also proving to be ineffective at controlling expenditure growth. For like the traditional fee-for-service model, the cost-consciousness of consumers is attenuated by employer- and government-subsidized insurance, and PPO providers are rewarded with more revenue for doing more, whether or not more is necessary or beneficial to the patient. In this model, providers lack accountability for quality or cost, and they generally lack the information systems and tools for improving them. This model is proving itself to be untenable in the long run.

Meanwhile, some eleven million Americans have been receiving health care through an alternative system—a real system—designed to promote quality improvement and affordability. By integrating the financing and delivery of care (in effect eliminating the third-party payer), prepaid group practice achieves greater accountability for the quality and cost of care in a system in which physicians actually manage care and resource use. In prepaid group practice, physicians work to maximize the health of the populations they serve within the resources their members are able and willing to provide. If encouraged and allowed to compete on a level playing field with the mainstream model, prepaid group practice could make a major contribution to solving the problems of quality and cost that plague American health care.

What Is Prepaid Group Practice?

Exactly what do we mean by "prepaid group practice"? In principle, a prepaid group practice (PGP) is an integrated entity that includes both a health care delivery system (doctors, other clinicians, laboratories, clinics, and hospitals) and an insurance function (financing arrangements, benefit plans, marketing, and customer service systems) "under one roof." Critical components of the PGP include the following:

- A multispecialty group practice—that is, a group of clinicians, including primary care generalists, nonphysician providers such as nurse practitioners, and specialist physicians, sharing finances, facilities, equipment, and responsibility for all enrolled members and committed to the team practice of medicine
- Any hospitals or other facilities owned by or affiliated with the multispecialty group practice
- A voluntarily enrolled population that contracts with the PGP through a sponsor (employer or public program) or as individuals
- Comprehensive health care services provided or arranged for by the PGP
- Per capita prepayment
- Accountability for the quality and cost of the care that is delivered
- A relationship (usually, but not necessarily, a mutually exclusive arrangement) between the delivery system and the insurance entity

Further explanation is needed regarding this last element of the definition of PGP: the relationship between the delivery system and the insurance entity. While a mutually exclusive relationship between the two is an important part of what it means to be a PGP, it is not the only type of relationship that can support quality and efficiency goals. Mutual exclusivity has advantages and disadvantages. Among the advantages are the ability of the medical group and the insurance entity to plan membership and facilities together, physician participation in coverage decisions, reduced complexity for physicians because they deal with only one insurer, and a partnership instead of an arm's-length, if not hostile, relationship. The profits of the insurance entity can be returned to the whole organization to finance expansion or costly improvements, such as clinical information systems. But as James Robinson notes in Chapter Ten, there are also disadvantages. "Contractual promiscuity," as he calls it, allows a medical group to contract with the best insurance carrier or with different carriers to reach different market segments or offer different insurance products. For example, a multispecialty group practice that wants to offer a "point-of-service" product can partner with an insurance carrier that has a wide network of participating providers.

In practice, few actual organizations, with the notable exception of Kaiser Permanente in some of its regions, fully comply with all of our definition's terms all of the time. Consequently, this book addresses a somewhat broader set of organizations that are based on multispecialty group practice, deliver or arrange comprehensive services through a close association with a single insurer or a small number of insurers, and receive the majority of their resources through per capita prepayment. In addition, they organize their patient care around a unitary, comprehensive medical record for each patient—often an electronic medical record, as discussed in the Epilogue—which allows every physician serving every patient to practice with the full knowledge of the patient's medical history. This seemingly simple, single feature helps avoid unnecessary duplication of diagnostic tests, facilitates collaboration and coordination of care, makes possible the study of practice patterns and variations, and allows monitoring of compliance with the group's practice guidelines.

PGPs' Limitations

This is not to suggest, however, that prepaid group practice, or any other model, is best for everybody or that it alone can solve America's problems of health care quality and expenditure growth. There are several good reasons that prepaid group practice will not work for all patients or all physicians. For instance, prepaid group practices are difficult to develop and slow to grow because organized delivery systems require careful planning. Furthermore, there are legitimate concerns about whether per capita prepayment motivates underuse of medical services (in other words, withholding of services that would benefit the patient). Also, there have been concerns among PGPs about customer service and responsiveness.

There are also geographical limitations on the appropriateness of prepaid group practice as a model. To reach the critical mass required to realize the economies gained from bringing most secondary specialist services into an integrated group, a PGP needs to serve roughly 120,000 members.[7] In practical terms, this means that PGPs are not a solution for most rural areas, though some multi-specialty groups with primary care outposts do bring high-quality care to rural areas.

Beyond these limitations, there are other powerful forces bearing on the health care system that work against all efforts to create more rational models. Viable health care systems are first of all human systems, and they require wise, if not visionary, leadership, which has been relatively rare in American health care in recent years—a subject that Drs. Francis Crosson, Allan Weiland, and Robert Berenson address in Chapter Nine. Another factor challenging all models of care is the rapid diffusion of new technologies, many of which confer great benefits for patients. However, the explosion of costly technologies is driven by open-ended insurance contracts that pay for them even when there is little or no evidence that they affect health outcomes—a subject that David Eddy addresses in Chapter Five.

Another challenge is an out-of-control tort system that motivates costly defensive medicine and defensive utilization management. Government purchasers and employers add to the problems by persisting in the use of inflationary models for paying for health care. Medicare, for instance, is still dominated by fee-for-service payment, and so far the government has not been able to find a way to let less costly systems compete for Medicare patients on equal terms. Most private employers do not offer their employees alternatives that include less costly PGPs or other types of health maintenance organizations (HMOs). Those that do offer them, for the most part, systematically pay more on behalf of employees who choose the more costly systems of care, thus removing incentives for employees to make responsible economic choices. If purchasers follow such inflationary policies, the whole system will experience inflation.

Yet even if the limitations and barriers working against PGPs and other value-enhancing systems prevent them from ever becoming the dominant model, their value to the overall system remains vital. At the least, PGPs can serve as incubators of innovations that enhance quality and efficient resource use, including their vital role in reducing inpatient hospital use and their demonstrated effectiveness in disease prevention, chronic disease management, and use of health care teams. PGPs also continue to play a critically important role as valuable research platforms for population-based health care, generating the kinds of clinical data on defined populations that are difficult or impossible to obtain anywhere else. In short, the existence of the PGP model in a pluralistic health care environment will reverberate in positive ways throughout the entire system. Their innovations in quality and efficiency can serve as models for the transformed twenty-first century health system that is called for by the Institute of Medicine in *Crossing the Quality Chasm.*

To better understand the advantages and limitations of the PGP model, it should be examined against the backdrop of the rapidly evolving mainstream models of financing and delivery, including independent practice associations, other HMO models, and the discounted fee-for-service variant known as preferred provider organizations.

The Evolving Mainstream

In the early 1970s, there was growing recognition in the federal government that the traditional fee-for-service model provided the wrong incentives to control costs and improve the quality of care. As a result, Congress, impressed by the cost containment achievements of PGPs such as Kaiser Permanente, Group Health Cooperative of Puget Sound, Group Health of Saint Paul, and the Health Insurance Plan of New York (HIP), passed the Health Maintenance Organization (HMO) Act of 1973. The act defined HMOs, provided grants and loans for the start-up of nonprofit HMOs, and required all employers of twenty-five or more employees to offer at least one PGP and one IPA-based HMO as health insurance options wherever they were available and requested to be offered. This requirement was a big boost to the development of HMOs, including PGPs, in the 1970s.

Independent Practice Associations

Physicians committed to the traditional fee-for-service, solo-practice model felt competitive pressures from PGPs in some communities, and their county medical societies responded by forming independent practice associations, which sought to offer patients the financial equivalent of a PGP (that is, comprehensive services at affordable prices) but with almost no restrictions on choice of physician. Today, most IPAs are simply financial associations of solo-practice doctors that collectively negotiate payment for professional services on a per capita, prepayment basis with various insurance companies. The insurers, in turn, contract with multiple medical groups and other IPAs for professional services. The original IPAs shared the following essential characteristics:

- The physician continues independent practice in his or her own office on a fee-for-service basis.
- At the same time, the association agrees to provide or arrange for comprehensive health care services on a per capita prepayment basis.
- To reconcile fee-for-service with the per capita prepayment, the physicians agree to various insurer controls, such as a fee schedule, peer review of the appropriateness of service, refusal to pay for inappropriate services, and preadmission certification.
- The physician bears some degree of financial risk through mechanisms such as a pool of funds withheld from fees ("withholds"), which is paid out only if there is enough money at the end of the year.

In recent years, IPAs have experimented with a variety of incentive payment arrangements in an effort to improve efficiency of practice and referral patterns.[8] Some primary care physicians are paid on a capitation basis for their own services, and some have experimented with "referral-based capitation" for specialists.

One notable feature of the IPA is that doctors might belong to two or more of them, as well as contracting with multiple insurance carriers. This reduces the likelihood that a doctor will develop loyalty and commitment to any single IPA, which complicates the efforts of some IPAs to encourage physicians to use practice protocols or pharmacy formularies aimed at quality improvement or efficient resource use. The lack of a close relationship between the associations and the participating physicians also increases the likelihood that doctors will come to view them as "just one more insurance carrier."

Nonetheless, due to their ability to partially bridge the gap between solo practice and true group practice, some IPAs have become effective competitors for PGPs. At their best, they represent an important transitional stage in the evolution toward a better-organized delivery system, and they deserve close attention from a health policy perspective.

Carrier and Delivery System HMOs

The health maintenance organization (of which PGPs are a subset) is an insurance organization that receives a premium to cover a comprehensive set of services for an enrolled population and accepts the obligation to deliver or arrange and purchase all medically necessary services, either directly or through contracts with providers. The term *HMO*, as many use it, has become synonymous with the ill-defined term "managed care organization." For others, "managed care" means anything other than traditional fee-for-service, including PPOs and similar arrangements.

Today, there are two types of HMOs, and there are important distinctions between them. Prepaid group practices, which we sometimes refer to as "delivery system HMOs," are built on the chassis of a multispecialty group practice. Typically, though not always, they have mutually exclusive health plan partners to handle enrollment, marketing, and insurance issues. In contrast, what we call "the carrier HMO" is built on the chassis of an insurance company, not a delivery system. The carrier HMO often (but not always) assumes the risk of the cost of care for comprehensive services and contracts with providers who may be otherwise unaffiliated with the insurer and with each other and who contract with other insurance carriers.

Carrier HMOs, in turn, can be divided into two types, the "delegated model" and the "nondelegated model." In the nondelegated model, which is predominant in most of the country, the providers bear little or no responsibility for the total cost of the care they deliver. The carrier alone seeks to manage costs through a variety of methods, including a negotiated fee schedule, risk sharing with providers, practice guidelines, utilization review, and prior authorization for costly services, though many have abandoned prior authorization as too controversial or not worth its cost.[9] Some carrier HMOs do business with self-insured employers. Physicians often see these carrier HMOs as adversaries, not partners, and litigation has not been uncommon.[10]

In the delegated model, the insurance carrier usually contracts with medical groups or IPAs for professional services on a per capita prepayment basis, with some risk sharing for institutional (hospital) services to enrolled members. An important advantage of the delegated model is that it enlists medical groups in the effort to manage costs. The delegated model is the predominant carrier HMO model in California, which has many multispecialty group practices, primary care groups that subcontract care to specialists, and IPAs. It is less prevalent in other states that have fewer multispecialty group practices.

Preferred Provider Organizations

The appellation "preferred provider organization" is a misnomer because there is no "organization" to speak of. We prefer the term "preferred provider insurance," because this model is primarily an insurance arrangement in which a carrier contracts with participating solo and small single-specialty group practice physicians and independent hospitals who agree to accept a negotiated, discounted fee when caring for patients covered by the plan. The providers may also agree to some utilization management methods, such as prior authorization for costly or elective hospitalizations. The insurer (which may be an insurance company, employer, or trust fund) then offers a contract in which enrollees are covered more fully if they receive their care "in network" than if they go to more costly "out of network" providers, whose fees remain unrestrained. Thus consumers have an incentive to use in-plan providers, which in turn gives the providers an incentive to accept the PPO's negotiated terms.

The PPO is a much more flexible arrangement than the prepaid group practice. Employers who self-insure with PPOs are exempt from costly state benefit mandates and have great freedom to cover whatever services they and their employees want. Since participating providers have no long-term relationship with the insurer, they can be added or deleted at the stroke of a pen, which means they can be concentrated wherever they are needed, not only where the provider organization's clinics or hospitals happen to be. And the PPO is much more compatible than the PGP with substantial cost sharing, including coinsurance and deductibles. In fact, along with provider discounts, such consumer incentives at the point of service are one of PPOs' primary tools for controlling costs.

However, reliance on consumer incentives at the point of service is not an effective mechanism for making health care economical. Health care expenses are very concentrated in a few people. Typically, 80 percent or more of the costs are associated with only 20 percent of enrollees.[11] Thus most spending is likely to be beyond the deductible amount, possibly even beyond the consumer's out-of-pocket limits. Most patients lack information on complex medical issues and depend on their doctors for advice on what is necessary. Also, patients are not likely to be in an economizing frame of mind when they are sick and in need of care. The RAND Health Insurance Experiment found that once patients are admitted to the hospital, variations in levels of coinsurance do not significantly affect expenditures.[12]

Using premiums as a way of comparing costs between PPOs and other systems is problematic because a PPO premium can be set very low simply by raising consumer cost sharing, including the limits on out-of-pocket outlays. But typically, PPO premiums are substantially higher than PGP premiums, especially when the sponsors choose to offer fairly comprehensive coverage in the PPO format.[13] Also, the total of premium and consumer out-of-pocket cost is most likely to be higher in a PPO than in a PGP if both plans cover populations with the same health risks.

In principle, a PPO could be effective in motivating providers to improve economic performance if the PPO could be selective and limit participation to providers capable of demonstrating high quality and efficiency. In practice, however, most employers use the PPO as a single source of coverage, which leads them to demand all-inclusive networks so that all their employees' favorite doctors are included, whether they are efficient and of high quality or not. Once the providers know that they must be included in the network, they can drive very hard bargains on compensation.[14] In effect, employers have reinvented the costly "any willing provider" principle they fought so hard to overturn in the 1980s.

In terms of quality improvement, PPOs are not cohesive organizations capable of studying practice patterns, reducing inappropriate practice variations, or creating best practice guidelines and implementing them. This is largely because doctors participate in so many PPOs that they have allegiance to none.

The relative merits of these different systems and styles of care ought to be sorted out in a marketplace based on informed, responsible consumer choice and competition to deliver value for money.

Can PGPs Improve Quality and Affordability?

The foregoing overview of the key strengths and weaknesses of the main health care financing and delivery models suggests several reasons that the traditional, solo-practice, fee-for-service model has been unable to control costs or to make significant headway in reducing inappropriate practice variation and improving overall quality of care. In contrast, today's prepaid group practices stake their claim to a level playing field on their reputed ability to deliver high-quality medical care at substantially less cost than the mainstream models. Why should the PGP model be superior in terms of affordability and quality (including both clinical and service quality), and is it?

The Cost Containment Record

In 1978, Harold Luft published a review of the literature to date, concluding, "Total costs (premium and out of pocket) for enrollees [in PGP and IPA health maintenance organizations] are 10 to 40 percent lower than those for comparable people with health insurance. . . . Most of the cost differences are attributable to hospitalization rates about 30 percent lower than those of conventionally insured populations."[15] In the case of prepaid group practices, hospitalization rates were 25 to 45 percent lower. However, as Luft noted, these studies were not randomized controlled trials, and there was always the possibility that the lower costs were attributable to favorable risk selection or enrollment of a healthier population.

The risk selection issue was addressed in the RAND Health Insurance Experiment. A study population in Seattle was randomly assigned to Group

Health Cooperative (a PGP) or to the traditional fee-for-service system. The result, published in 1984, was that Group Health Cooperative enrollees were hospitalized about 40 percent less, and their total resource use was about 25 percent less than that of fee-for-service enrollees.[16] The researchers concluded that "the lower rate of use that we observed, along with comparable reductions found in non-controlled studies by others, suggests that the style of medicine at prepaid group practices is markedly less 'hospital intensive' and, consequently, less expensive."[17]

It is noteworthy that Group Health Cooperative achieved this result in the absence of competition from another PGP and in a market environment that for the most part did not reward economical care. Joseph Newhouse subsequently reported, "In numerous comparisons of physiologic outcomes for the average person at the HMO and in the free fee-for-service plan, no strong evidence was found favoring one system over the other."[18]

Of course, that was twenty years ago. In the 1990s, the new carrier HMOs achieved significant cost savings by emulating the PGPs' reduction in hospital use. Other prospective payment methods, implemented in the 1980s by Medicare, have stimulated reductions in the hospital system as a whole, but what the U.S. health care system needs is not a mere one-time reduction in costs. Rather, the system needs a process of *continuous improvement* in quality and value for money—a transformation as called for by the Institute of Medicine's quality reports, comparable to what has happened in competitive industries elsewhere in the economy. *If market conditions favored competition on the basis of quality and price, could PGPs once again provide the cutting edge?*

There are many things that PGPs can do and are doing to cut costs without cutting the quality of care and in many cases improving the quality of care. Most of these are things that are facilitated by unique characteristics of the PGP model that would be more difficult, if not impossible, to achieve in the traditional model. A few examples follow:

- Organize continuous quality improvement teams, as discussed by Donald Berwick and Sachin Jain in Chapter Two. Doing it right the first time saves money.
- Focus on chronic disease management by multidisciplinary teams to reduce the need for hospitalization for acute exacerbations and the long-term disabilities brought on by chronic disease, thus improving quality of life for patients.
- Finance and deploy state-of-the-art electronic medical records technology and use it to improve chronic care management, to disseminate best practice guidelines, and to reduce unwanted variations, as discussed by George Halvorson in the Epilogue.

- Deploy new technologies efficiently—the right types in the right amounts, as discussed by David Eddy in Chapter Five.
- Concentrate costly and complex procedures in high-volume regional "centers of excellence" to gain the advantages of economies of experience.[19]
- Promote and practice disease prevention.
- Organize and implement cost-effective pharmacy benefit management through physician education and close integration of the medical group and the pharmacy and therapeutics committee, as discussed by William Campbell, Richard Johnson, and Sharon Levine in Chapter Six.
- Promote and institutionalize efficient use of medical personnel, as discussed by Jonathan Weiner in Chapter Seven.

Can PGPs Cross the Quality Chasm?

In its report *Crossing the Quality Chasm,* the Institute of Medicine (IOM) calls for a higher-quality, safer, and more integrated twenty-first century health care delivery system, one in which "clinicians and institutions . . . collaborate and communicate to ensure an appropriate exchange of information and coordination of care."[20]

PGPs are excellent examples of the type of "integrated delivery systems" called for by the IOM. They integrate across virtually every dimension, including the following:

- Financing and delivery through per capita prepayment so that the physician organization has a budget for the care it will provide and an incentive to use resources wisely
- Providers and the voluntarily enrolled population they serve, facilitating the development of health improvement programs and what the IOM calls "continuous healing relationships"
- The full spectrum of care—from primary to tertiary care, nursing home and home care—enabling the system to care for the patient in the least costly, most appropriate setting, not distorted by what an insurance company will or will not pay for
- Physicians and other clinicians in multidisciplinary health care teams that can design and execute the best care processes
- Hospitals and other facilities so that costly, complex equipment can be deployed on a regional basis where it can be used with the greatest proficiency and economy
- Information, including a complete medical record of all the health issues, treatments, and outcomes for each patient, so that each provider can quickly obtain an accurate and comprehensive picture of the patient

In addition, PGPs have numerous organizational structures that support quality. For instance, because PGPs bear financial responsibility for the continuing care of members, they must pay the cost of poor-quality care. Thanks to the physician compensation system, doctors can be assigned to quality management and improvement functions and be paid for doing so. Because the entire group of physicians and health care teams is responsible for the care of every patient, physician peer review, professional checks and balances, and mutual physician oversight are common features. And thanks to the incentives in prepayment, the overuse of medical services so common in the fee-for-service system is strongly discouraged, while early detection and treatment, prevention, and chronic disease management are strongly encouraged.

Can PGPs Satisfy Physicians?

The conventional wisdom has it that physicians prefer the solo or small single-specialty group practice style, and clearly many do. But as the flow of new medical knowledge becomes an unmanageable flood and as the pressures for cost containment intensify, that may change. Recent studies of physicians in California, in both the traditional practice setting and in prepaid group practice (specifically, Kaiser Permanente), find that "the 'California Model' of loose networks of private practice physicians organized into large managed care practice organizations ["carrier HMOs"] is unraveling. . . . [In 1997], three quarters of all office-based primary care physicians in California participated in an IPA. In 2001, fewer than two-thirds of such physicians participated in an IPA."[21]

The story was similar for specialists. On the other hand, "the organization that appears to have the most 'staying power' for California physicians is Kaiser Permanente. . . . Compared with office-based physicians, Kaiser Permanente physicians are much more likely to believe that their practice organization has advantages for shared practice responsibilities and quality of care . . .; receive financial incentives related to performance based on quality of care and patient satisfaction; rate the practice pattern information they receive from their medical group and health plan as accurate, useful, and intended to improve the quality of care; [and] disagree that they experience pressures to limit referrals to specialists or ordering of medical tests."[22]

This should not be surprising. PGP physicians deal with a *single* health plan, not many, and that plan is their partner and has a clear interest in their quality and success. This contrasts with the experience of independent, office-based physicians, who must deal with many different health insurance plans whose interests differ from their own, each with its own views of clinical policies, coverage, and formularies. Most, if not all, PGPs have an agreement that *the medical group, not the carrier,* determines clinical policies, and the physicians have the major voice in deciding which technologies and procedures will be covered. They deal with one pharmacy formulary, developed by the physicians themselves, not multiple formularies developed by outsiders, and they have freedom to override the formulary to prescribe whatever they believe is medically necessary in a particular case. Physicians' hours, workloads, and working conditions are determined by the elected, representative governance of the medical group. They have opportunities for paid time for continuing medical education and to participate fully in the development of the clinical practice guidelines they are encouraged to use.

Can PGPs Satisfy Patients?

Kenneth Chuang, Harold Luft, and Adams Dudley the authors of Chapter Three, surveyed the literature comparing PGPs with fee-for-service. They found that while PGPs provide better preventive care, and there is a pattern of evidence somewhat in their favor on processes of care and outcomes, fee-for-service definitely performs better on patient satisfaction. It may well be that the fee-for-service model focuses the attention of the physician more sharply on satisfying patients than the PGP model does. The patient who wants his or her doctor to prescribe an expensive brand-name drug that confers no incremental value compared to a cheaper generic drug is more likely to be satisfied by the fee-for-service doctor.

In the RAND Health Insurance Experiment comparing Group Health Cooperative (GHC) and traditional fee-for-service in Seattle, the only randomized controlled trial conducted to date, Joseph Newhouse reported:

> Overall, fee-for-service participants were more satisfied with their care than were those assigned to the HMO experimental group. Moreover, those who had chosen the HMO—the HMO controls—were more satisfied than those assigned to the HMO experimental status. This result is not surprising, since a substantial portion of those randomly assigned to the HMO status had had an earlier opportunity through their place of employment to choose GHC coverage and had passed it up. Although those in fee-for-service plans were more satisfied than those assigned to HMO status, there was no measurable difference in satisfaction between those in fee-for-service plans and those who had chosen the HMO.[23]

This observation points to an important finding: patient satisfaction depends a great deal on whether or not the patient became an HMO member voluntarily or involuntarily. Three studies have documented that patients are much more likely to be dissatisfied with their HMO if they were not in it by choice.[24] In thinking about consumer satisfaction, the relevant issue is whether people should have choices that include PGPs, not whether a PGP would be the most satisfactory plan for everybody.

There are aspects of PGPs that some people like and aspects that some people dislike. Among the things people like are assured access to a doctor around the clock, seven days a week; low premium and out-of-pocket costs; absence of paperwork; preventive services and disease management; and "one-stop shopping" for most, or all, of their health care needs. In addition, as discussed by Berwick and Jain in Chapter Two, PGPs have been leaders in developing processes of care that are "patient-centered" and incorporating concepts of shared patient-physician decision making, another likely satisfier. That some people like PGPs a great deal is illustrated by the fact that the average Medicare member in Kaiser Permanente of Northern California has been with the program for over fourteen years.[25]

Aspects of PGPs that people dislike include narrow provider choice in small PGPs ("I don't like either ob-gyn in that group"), fear that one will not get the best doctor for one's rare and dangerous condition, fear of being kept waiting, an impersonal and institutional style, and difficulty navigating the system. Such consumer preferences ought to be respected in the context of responsible consumer choice.

There are steps PGPs have taken to mitigate the negatives and enhance the positives. In recent years, some have built substantial bonuses into individual physician pay for achieving objective measures of patient satisfaction. Some (if not all) refer members to the best-qualified regional centers for complex problems. Kaiser Permanente has pioneered "advanced access," guaranteeing same-day access to one's doctor or health care team. Harvard Community Health Plan built a center in Cambridge, Massachusetts, in which each primary care team had its own outside entrance to its own waiting room to reproduce the ambiance of a small personal practice. Some PGPs emphasize choice of a personal primary care physician. But there is still room for improvement. PGPs could build trust through better explanation of the model, including how physicians are compensated.

The consumer-patient expectation that fits with the traditional free-choice fee-for-service model is that one can pick one's doctors à la carte when the need arises, independently of their affiliations with any group, institution, or health plan—or each other. People often identify such freedom with "quality." The choices people make are rarely based on reliable quantitative information about the outcomes different doctors can produce (or even well-founded measures of the processes of care) because such information rarely exists. Rather, choices are often based on anecdotes and the recommendations of friends. The expectation of being able to choose *any* physician one believes to be of high quality conflicts with the notion of selective provider contracting. However, much of the backlash against managed care centered on the fact that managed care organizations limit choice of providers in ways patients find arbitrary or do not understand.

One problem with the "choice equals quality" assumption is that in an era of increasingly complex and changing medical practice, people must obtain their care from "systems" or suffer from the lack of teamwork and coordination. If one suffers from a serious chronic condition, a team of health professionals is needed to provide and coordinate the care. If one is taken seriously and acutely ill, one is certain to find oneself surrounded by many unfamiliar people that one did not personally select—and it is likely to make a real difference to outcomes and safety whether those people work well together and are used to doing so. Medicine has become too complicated to be practiced by teams assembled from scratch for each episode. It takes organized systems to develop best practice guidelines and to communicate them to physicians to keep them up-to-date with the latest scientific information and to monitor their performance and to provide feedback on how well they are doing. Eventually, à la carte medicine will yield to the need for integration, and quality will be gauged by reliable measurements of outcomes and injuries associated with different systems of care.

Content of This Book

The first three chapters of this book explore both the theory and the evidence that prepaid group practices perform better than the fee-for-service system in terms of efficiency, quality, and safety. Chapter One, by Stephen Shortell and Julie Schmittdiel, places prepaid group practice within the broader context of organized delivery systems, describing the advantages inherent in several of their key organizational dimensions. These include medical groups, health care teams, defined populations, aligned financing and payment arrangements, effective partnerships between medicine and management, information management capability, and accountability. The authors explore both the early promise of organized delivery systems and their overall performance and future potential as measured against the Institute of Medicine's six criteria for evaluating health care systems.[26]

The chapter incorporates the views of the leaders of several major organized delivery systems regarding the reasons that PGPs are not more prevalent and what would need to change to make them so. The leaders also discuss the potential of PGPs to serve as models for other, less integrated health systems. Shortell and Schmittdiel conclude with their own predictions about the future organization of American health care and the role of PGPs in that system.

The second chapter, by Donald Berwick and Sachin Jain, begins with the premise that prepaid group practice has unrealized potential to deliver far better quality of care than the more prevalent disaggregated fee-for-service system. The chapter examines the quest for health care quality in the context of the modern quality movement in many industries, noting that traditional medical professional values have sometimes come into conflict with the quality movement. The authors use the Institute of Medicine's *Crossing the Quality Chasm* report (of which Berwick is an author) as a "road map" for applying modern notions of excellence to the health care system. They explore whether and how the structural characteristics of prepaid group practices may enable them to implement the IOM's "Ten Simple Rules" for care redesign in a way that is not possible in the fee-for-service world. Berwick and Jain use available evidence and examples to show how PGPs either could or do follow these rules.

Whereas Berwick and Jain describe why PGPs should, in theory, provide better, safer, and more efficient care than uncoordinated fee-for-service medicine, Chapter Three, by Kenneth Chuang, Harold Luft, and Adams Dudley, reviews the evidence on whether or not prepaid group practices actually do so. This work is based on an analysis of the literature and identification of findings in which PGPs performed better than other types of delivery models, worse than other types, or about the same.

In general, Chuang and colleagues found that PGPs perform better in the area of preventive care. There was also a weak pattern of findings in PGPs' favor on processes and outcomes, but they did not perform as well on patient satisfaction. They also found that in terms of practice patterns, clinicians in PGPs tend to use somewhat less costly and less invasive interventions. This work includes an explanation of the difficulties involved in making these comparisons using current published research. The authors conclude that "the most important task for future researchers is to separate types of HMOs according to structural characteristics so that policymakers can understand the relative performance of each."

The next five chapters describe the contributions that prepaid group practices have made (or in some cases could have made) to American health care in five specific areas: national health policy, technology assessment, pharmacy benefit management, medical workforce policy, and research.

In Chapter Four, Jon Christianson and George Avery describe the impact of prepaid group practice on U.S. health policy. They provide a historical overview of the role of PGPs in shaping major policy milestones, including the 1932 report from the Committee on the Costs of Medical Care, the Federal Employees Health Benefits Program, Medicare and Medicaid, the Federal HMO Act, the National Committee on Quality Assurance, and the Clinton administration's health care reform proposal.

The authors explain why PGPs have found it necessary to play such a prominent role in national health policy, noting the strong motivation provided by the opposition of traditional organized medicine. They find that "PGPs have been influential in the policy process . . . because they have been consistent about what they have wanted to achieve [and] they have tangible and symbolic characteristics that made them attractive to policymakers and policy entrepreneurs with a variety of agendas." The authors predict that PGPs may be challenged in the future to repeat their policy successes in an environment in which information technology allows much less structured forms of care delivery to appear "organized" and in which purchasers increasingly opt for loosely organized health plans with significant consumer cost sharing. They conclude: "If PGPs are not seen as a 'solution' endorsed by employers, their influence in the policy process is likely to be diminished."

In Chapter Five, David Eddy addresses technology assessment, an issue of growing importance to the ability of health care organizations to control costs in an environment of rapidly proliferating new medical devices and procedures. Eddy examines how technology assessment, deployment, and implementation are performed in three PGPs—Kaiser Permanente, Group Health Cooperative, and HealthPartners. Drawing on his experience as a technology assessment consultant, Eddy also discusses the strengths and weaknesses of PGPs relative to their ability to perform assessments, implement the results, and monitor outcomes. He finds that while the PGPs described have many real and potential advantages in this area, the evidence for PGPs' superior performance is mixed. The best technology assessment program in use today, says Eddy, is the Blue Cross Blue Shield Association's Technology Evaluation Center, which is now in partnership with Kaiser Permanente.

In Chapter Six, William Campbell, Richard Johnson, and Sharon Levine describe the management of prescription drug benefits in the very different contexts of prepaid group practice and carrier HMOs, which assign the task to pharmacy benefit management companies (PBMs). Drawing on theoretical perspectives and on the experiences of several PGPs, they find that a major advantage of PGPs is that the pharmacy system is integrated into the rest of the delivery system, both clinically and financially, allowing for an alignment of incentives not found in the comparatively less organized PBM world. They examine five processes necessary to integration of pharmacy benefits: administration and management, drug selection, drug prescribing, drug dispensing, and drug use and monitoring. They analyze these processes from the perspective of the known and theoretical opportunities that arise from full horizontal and vertical integration.

The authors also interviewed the leaders of pharmacy programs in several large prepaid group practices to test their theory that PGPs enjoy many potential advantages over the carrier-PBM model for delivering efficient and effective pharmacy benefits. Looking toward the future, Campbell and colleagues ask whether the lessons learned from PGPs can be translated to broad networks of physicians contracting with multiple health plans, which in turn contract with PBMs.

In Chapter Seven, Jonathan Weiner presents new, comprehensive, specialty-specific data on physician, nurse practitioner, and physicians assistant staffing patterns in each of the Kaiser Permanente regions, as well as in HealthPartners and Group Health Cooperative. A primary objective of this analysis is to identify the unique approaches that PGPs have taken to workforce deployment and to offer potential lessons for the U.S. and other health care systems. As Weiner notes, "Determining what a medical workforce should . . . look like . . . in the future is fraught with conceptual, political, and even moral challenges." Therefore, given that PGPs have expended considerable energy and expertise in workforce planning, it is natural to look to them as one source of guidance for policymakers focusing on this issue.

Although the analysis does suggest an increase in the use of specialists by an aging population, Weiner is careful to note that "although the PGP staffing levels may not translate directly into benchmarks for the nation, the findings . . . do indicate that U.S. policymakers should deliberate carefully before encouraging the costly expansion of medical training programs."

In Chapter Eight, Raymond Fink and Merwyn R. Greenlick describe the major contributions of prepaid group practice to the field of health care research, including both clinical and health services research. The authors note that prior to the 1950s, there was little information about the use of health services by noninstitutionalized populations, nor was much known about the prevalence of chronic diseases in the population. Some of the first estimates of Americans' health care use and health status were developed by researchers at Kaiser Permanente in California and at the Health Insurance Plan (HIP) in New York. This groundbreaking research was enabled by a number of attributes that were unique to PGPs at that time, among them access to both administrative and clinical data for large populations; comprehensive coverage, allowing data capture for all services used; and continuous coverage of enrollees for extended periods of time, allowing for longitudinal studies.

Highlighted research includes work on the prevalence of health conditions; the use of health services, particularly by the poor and the aged; and health screening, epidemiology, and disease management and intervention studies. The authors note that PGPs have taken a leadership role in implementing the automated medical record, a development that has enormous potential to add to the value of research conducted by PGPs.

The final four chapters collectively pose the question, If prepaid group practices are a good idea and have much to contribute to the American health care system, why have they not thrived everywhere, and what internal and external factors would need to be present to encourage their growth?

Chapter Nine looks inward at the most critical piece of prepaid group practice—the physicians themselves. Authors Francis Crosson, Allan Weiland, and

Robert Berenson explore the elements of physician leadership and "followership" that are necessary to PGP success and to bringing about changes in U.S. health care. They begin by arguing that "American health care entered the twenty-first century . . . with *no* effective leadership. . . . The contest for influence among physicians, insurers, regulators, politicians, and purchasers that ensued in the 1990s turned into a mass retreat by the end of the century, leaving the field to the de facto and somewhat reluctant leadership of the consumer (for whom retreat is not an option)." In this vacuum of leadership, the physician leaders of PGPs have an opportunity to show how accountable leadership over the direction of American health care can be reestablished through the ethic of "group responsibility," which they describe as one of the defining attributes of PGPs.

Like several of the authors in this volume, Crosson and colleagues look to the Institute of Medicine for a framework of accountability. They describe the IOM's "six challenges" for crossing the quality chasm and show how the practice principles that make up the physician culture in PGPs are uniquely designed to meet those challenges. From there they offer observations about the qualities and characteristics required to lead groups of physicians in such a way that encourages collective responsibility and dual accountability for both individual patients and populations. They conclude with observations about the relevance of PGP-based physician leadership to the broader world of American medicine.

In Chapter Ten, James Robinson sets out to explain why prepaid group practices have not been more successful outside of limited geographical areas. Robinson breaks down the concept of prepaid group practice into four elements that compose the core of the most successful examples: multispecialty physician organization, capitation payment, exclusive linkages between delivery and insurance ("vertical integration"), and a "managed competition" framework featuring multiple choice of plans, fixed employer contributions, and open enrollment. He explains why each of these elements has proved to be more difficult to implement than originally believed. Given the forces arrayed against PGPs (outside of the West Coast and parts of the Midwest), Robinson concludes that it is unrealistic to expect that PGPs will become the dominant mode of health care delivery. However, he notes that to serve as benchmarks for quality and efficiency, PGPs do not need to exist everywhere or to be available to all people. In addition, PGPs may serve as "incubators" for innovative practices that can be translated to other forms of care delivery.

In Chapter Eleven, Helen Darling draws on her own extensive experience as a corporate health care benefits manager, as well as interviews with several prominent employer purchasers, to look at employers' relationships with prepaid group practice. She describes how and why employers have either encouraged or hindered the growth of PGPs. The interviews provide both a history of employers' involvement with PGPs and a sense of what aspects of PGPs are most valued by them. For example, several large employers have used PGPs to set "benchmark" practices and prices to enhance price and quality competition among health plans. Darling also describes how large employers were instrumental in developing behavioral health performance standards for HMOs and in creating the Health Plan Employer Data and Information Set (HEDIS), both of which have allowed PGPs to showcase the strengths of their population-based approach to care delivery. She also examines why, despite their strong belief in the PGP model, employers have not been more aggressive in encouraging them.

In the last chapter, Alain Enthoven asks the question, Given what we know about the necessary elements for PGPs' success, what can private employers and public policymakers do to make market environments more hospitable to this model of care delivery? He focuses on elements that must be present to allow an efficient PGP access to the *employee* market, not just the employer market. These include a broad choice of health plans; risk adjustment to mitigate adverse selection; an employer contribution that allows employees to retain any savings resulting from an economical choice; a level regulatory playing field among HMOs, insurers, and self-insured plans; and reliable, comparable information on quality of care and consumer satisfaction.

Enthoven also argues that in addition to the right market conditions, PGPs require a certain level of start-up funding and other support from the business community. He calls for a greater commitment on the part of foundations to fund PGP start-ups, given that many health care experts believe they are the nation's best hope for improving the safety and quality of care. He also describes a less costly evolutionary path for creating PGPs not "from scratch" but from existing multi-specialty group practices that may or may not be prepaid and are not exclusively affiliated with an insurer. With appropriate market conditions, many of the roughly one thousand existing multispecialty group practices could evolve into PGPs.

Finally, a book about PGPs' contributions to, and promise for, a twenty-first-century health system would be incomplete without a discussion of clinical information systems. In the Epilogue, George Halvorson notes that prepaid groups and other large multispecialty group practices have been leaders in the implementation of what he calls "computerized caregiver support tools." This is due to a number of factors, including a culture of team-based group practice; access to capital (often through a partnership with a health plan); and in most cases, financial incentives to allocate resources to maximize the health of an entire covered population. Halvorson makes a compelling case for the vital role that clinical information systems can and must play in reducing error and inconsistency, managing chronic disease, promoting patient involvement in care, and improving system efficiency.

Notes

1. Mercer Human Resources Consulting, *National Survey of Employer-Sponsored Health Plans: 2002 Survey Report* (New York: Mercer Human Resources Consulting, 2003).

2. Hewitt Associates, "HMO Rates Continue Double Digit Trend but Are Lower Than Last Year," press release, June 23, 2003 [http://was4.hewitt.com/hewitt/resource/newsroom/pressrel/2003/06–23–03.htm].

3. R. Kronick and T. Gilmer, "Explaining the Decline in Health Insurance Coverage, 1979–1995," *Health Affairs*, 1999, *18*(2), 30–47.

4. Publications by the Institute of Medicine: *Coverage Matters* (Washington, D.C.: National Academy Press, 2001); *Care Without Coverage* (Washington, D.C.: National Academy Press, 2002); *Health Insurance Is a Family Matter* (Washington, D.C.: National Academy Press, 2002); *A Shared Destiny: Community Effects of Uninsurance* (Washington, D.C.: National Academy Press, 2003); *Hidden Costs, Value Lost: Uninsurance in America* (Washington, D.C.: National Academy Press, 2003).

5. P. Fronstin, *Sources of Health Insurance and Characteristics of the Uninsured: Analysis of the March 2002 Current Population Survey,* Issue Brief no. 252 (Washington, D.C.: Employee Benefit Research Institute, 2002).

6. Institute of Medicine, *To Err Is Human* (Washington, D.C.: National Academy Press, 1999) and *Crossing the Quality Chasm: A New Health System for the 21st Century* (Washington, D.C.: National Academy Press, 2001).

7. R. Kronick, D. C. Goodman, J. Wennberg, and E. Wagner, "The Marketplace in Health Care Reform: The Demographic Limitations of Managed Competition," *New England Journal of Medicine*, 1993, *238*, 148–152.

8. J. C. Robinson, *The Corporate Practice of Medicine: Competition and Innovation in Health Care* (Berkeley: Milbank Memorial Fund and University of California Press, 1999); J. C. Robinson, "Blended Payment Incentives in Physician Organizations Under Managed Care," *Journal of the American Medical Association*, 1999, *282*, 1258–1263.

9. United Healthcare, "United Healthcare Introduces Care Coordination," press release, Nov. 9, 1999 [http://www.unitedhealthgroup.com/news/rel1999/1109ccoord.htm].

10. See, for example, *Charles B. Shane, MD, Jeffrey Book, DO, et al., California Medical Association, Texas Medical Association, et al., plaintiffs,* vs. *Humana, Inc., Aetna, Inc., et al.,* Miami Division, Southern District of Florida, MDL No. 1334, July 2002.

11. Fronstin, *Sources of Health Insurance.*

12. J. P. Newhouse and others, "Some Interim Results from a Controlled Trial of Cost Sharing in Health Insurance," *New England Journal of Medicine*, 1981, *305*, 1501–1507.

13. Kaiser Family Foundation and Health Research and Educational Trust, *Employer Health Benefits: 2002 Annual Survey* (Menlo Park, Calif.: Kaiser Family Foundation and Health Research and Educational Trust, 2002).

14. G. C. Halvorson and G. J. Isham, *Epidemic of Care* (San Francisco: Jossey-Bass, 2003); B. Martinez, "Strong Medicine: With New Muscle, Hospitals Squeeze Insurers on Rates," *Wall Street Journal*, Apr. 12, 2002, p. A1.

15. H. S. Luft, "How Do Health Maintenance Organizations Achieve Their 'Savings'?" *New England Journal of Medicine*, 1978, *298*, 1336–1343, p. 1336.

16. W. G. Manning and others, "A Controlled Trial of the Effect of a Prepaid Group Practice on the Utilization of Medical Services," *New England Journal of Medicine*, 1984, *310*, 1505–1510.

17. Ibid, 1505.
18. J. P. Newhouse, *Free for All? Lessons from the RAND Health Insurance Experiment* (Cambridge, Mass.: Harvard University Press, 1993).
19. R. A. Dudley and others, "Selective Referral to High-Volume Hospitals, Estimating Potentially Avoidable Deaths," *Journal of the American Medical Association,* 2000, *283,* 1159–1166; T. A. Gordon, G. P. Burleyson, J. M. Tielsch, and J. L. Cameron, "The Effects of Regionalization on Cost and Outcome for One General High-Risk Surgical Procedure," *Annals of Surgery,* 1995, *221,* 43–49.
20. Institute of Medicine, *Crossing the Quality Chasm,* p. 9.
21. K. Grumbach and others, "California Physicians 2002: Practice and Perceptions," California Workforce Initiative at the UCSF Center for the Health Professions, San Francisco, Dec. 2002, p. i.
22. Ibid., p. ii.
23. Newhouse, *Free for All?* pp. 304–305.
24. K. Davis and C. Schoen, "Assuring Quality, Information, and Choice in Managed Care," *Inquiry,* Summer 1998, pp. 104–114; A. Gawande and others, "Does Dissatisfaction with Health Plans Stem from Having No Choices?" *Health Affairs* (Sept.-Oct. 1998, pp. 184–194; A. C. Enthoven, H. H. Schauffler, and S. McMenamin, "Consumer Choice and the Managed Care Backlash," *American Journal of Law and Medicine,* 2001, *27,* 1–15.
25. Kaiser Foundation Health Plan of Northern California, "Business Analysis, Strategic Market Planning," July 2003.
26. Institute of Medicine, *Crossing the Quality Chasm.* The criteria are safety, effectiveness, patient-centeredness, timeliness, efficiency, and equity.

TOWARD A 21st CENTURY HEALTH SYSTEM

CHAPTER ONE

PREPAID GROUPS AND ORGANIZED DELIVERY SYSTEMS

Promise, Performance, and Potential

Stephen M. Shortell and Julie Schmittdiel

I tell our trustees, "When you walk into [name of medical group], you are walking into the arms of an organized group practice. You walk into our competitor, you walk into the equivalent of a farmers' market where there are a bunch of people sitting there in stalls, selling their wares, and leaving at the end of the day when they are done. They don't particularly care what the farmers' market is like as long as the bathrooms are clean and the lights are on. They don't particularly care who is selling stuff next to them because they are not integrated."

PHYSICIAN LEADER OF AN ORGANIZED DELIVERY SYSTEM

The American health care system is the poster child for underachievement. As stated in the Institute of Medicine report *Crossing the Quality Chasm*, "Between the healthcare we have and the care we could have lies not just a gap, but a chasm."[1] The reasons for this are well documented.[2] The largest limiting factor is not lack of money, technology, information, or even people but rather lack of an *organizing principle* that can link money, people, technology, and ideas into a *system* that delivers more cost-effective care (in other words, more value) than current arrangements. Given the growing number of Americans with chronic illness (currently estimated at 125 million at an annual cost of $173 billion and accounting for 60 to 75 percent of personal health care expenditures),[3] the emerging application of genetic medicine, and the potential for a more health-informed and "activated" citizenry, the lack of an organizing principle for the delivery of health care in the twenty-first century has serious consequences.

The current system has been based largely on the fee-for-service or indemnity model of financing, operating within the context of highly individualistic models of care delivery. It is difficult to discern an organizing principle for such arrangements other than that of maximizing the autonomy of each of the individual parties involved. The current system might best be described as a collection of autonomous professionals providing largely self-defined expert care within organizational, payment, and regulatory environments involving conflicting incentives, goals, and objectives.

But a very different organizing principle is also available—that of prepaid group practice (PGP), which has roots going back more than sixty years. A PGP is an organized delivery system based on an accountable, multispecialty group of physicians and other health professionals who work together in teams to provide comprehensive care for a voluntarily enrolled population within a per capita, prospectively determined budget (see the Preface to this volume). This chapter examines the promise, performance, and potential of PGPs and similar organized delivery systems to address the problems of fragmentation embodied in our current health care system. In the discussion that follows, we use the term *PGP* to refer to closely related organized delivery systems as well.

Some prepaid groups, such as Group Health Cooperative and Kaiser Permanente, have an exclusive relationship between the insurance carrier and the physician organization. Such arrangements have the advantage of fully internalizing the rewards of prudent resource use. In other cases, prepaid groups may also contract with health plans other than the one owned by the system. In turn, the system-owned health plan may also contract with other physician groups. Examples of such nonexclusive arrangements include the Henry Ford Health System, Intermountain Health Care, and the Mayo Clinic. Such organized delivery systems have been defined as a "network of organizations that provides or arranges to provide a coordinated continuum of services to a defined population and is willing to be held clinically and fiscally accountable for the outcomes and health status of the population served."[4]

Table 1.1 compares the fee-for-service, indemnity, or autonomous unit model (or what Enthoven and Tollen refer to as the "carrier-HMO model" in the Preface) with the PGP model on some key parameters of health care delivery. Evidence to support the idea that organized delivery systems actually achieve the desired elements summarized in Table 1.1 is mixed (see Chapter Three).[5] The point of the table is to indicate that PGPs at least have the *potential* for achieving the desired elements, while it is clear that the fee-for-service or indemnity model that has been dominant for most of the past century cannot meet the needs of the next.

The PGP approach, however, needs to be critically examined so that its promise and potential may be realized in its actual performance. This chapter highlights the inherent promise of the PGP model as contained in its core features. Then the six aims for a quality health system identified in the Institute of

TABLE 1.1. COMPARISON OF FEE-FOR-SERVICE AND PREPAID GROUP PRACTICE OR ORGANIZED DELIVERY SYSTEM APPROACHES.

Health Care System: Ideal Elements	Fee-for-Service, Indemnity, or Autonomous Units	Prepaid Group Practice or Organized Delivery System
Focuses on meeting the population's health needs	Focuses on individual sick patient	Focuses on enrolled populations
Matches service capacity to the population's needs	Occurs by chance only	Potential for coordination and economies of scale and scope
Coordinates and integrates care across the continuum	Difficult to accomplish	Ownership and alliances provide potential for integrated care
Has information systems to link patients, providers, and payers across the continuum of care	Has neither the resources nor the elements of the system in place	Has elements in place for linkage to occur
Is able to provide information on cost, quality outcomes, and patient satisfaction to multiple stakeholders: patients, staff, payers and purchasers, community groups, and external review bodies	Insufficient volume per provider to trust the data, even if it could be produced	Infrastructure exists to provide reliable data over time
Uses financial incentives and organizational structure to align governance, management, physicians, and other caregivers in support of achieving shared objectives	Has little capacity to do this	Potential exists; some evidence that it occurs
Is able to improve continuously the care that it provides	Depends on individual motivation and skill	Potential exists given the existence of infrastructure to do it
Is willing and able to work with others to ensure that the community's health objectives are met	Highly variable, dependent on individual interest	Broad-based potential exists due to population focus

Source: Adapted from S. M. Shortell and others, *Remaking Health Care in America: The Evolution of Organized Delivery Systems,* 2nd ed. (San Francisco: Jossey-Bass, 2000), p. 21.

Medicine's *Crossing the Quality Chasm* report are used as criteria for evaluating PGP performance. Next, interview information obtained from six PGPs—Group Health Cooperative, HealthPartners, the Henry Ford Health System, Intermountain Health Care, Kaiser Permanente, and the Mayo Clinic—is used to assess the model's potential for geographical diffusion. Finally, the conclusion provides a discussion of the role of PGPs within the evolving health system of the future.

Components of Prepaid Group Practice

The key components of prepaid group practices (or organized delivery systems) are multispecialty group practices, health care teams, defined populations, and aligned financing and payment arrangements. These components combine to produce three resulting characteristics that are key to the potential success of PGPs: effective partnerships between medicine and management, enhanced information management capability, and accountability. Each of the key components and the three resulting characteristics is discussed in turn. It is the interdependence and alignment of these components and characteristics that distinguish the value of PGPs.

Multispecialty Group Practice

In 1932, the Committee on the Costs of Medical Care suggested group practice of physicians as the cornerstone for the development of an effective health care system. More than seven decades later, relatively little progress has been made in realizing this recommendation. Today, 47 percent of private physicians still work in practices of one or two doctors, and 82 percent work in practices of nine or fewer.[6] The practice of medicine, even in the twenty-first century, remains largely a cottage industry.

This is cause for concern, as the basic building block of an organized delivery system is the medical group that works together to care for a defined panel of patients. The first prepaid group practice in the United States was the Ross-Loos Clinic, founded in Los Angeles in 1929, followed by a progenitor of Kaiser Permanente in 1933. Other early group practices (although not necessarily having their origins in prepayment) include the Mayo Clinic, founded in Minnesota in 1888; the Scott White Clinic in Texas, 1897; the Geisinger Clinic in central Pennsylvania, 1915; and the Marshfield Clinic in Wisconsin, 1919 (see Appendix).

Such groups are more than collections of doctors loosely related to each other through independent practice associations. Rather, they are entities with a psychological sense of belonging and identification with the group fostered by a common vision, a shared culture, and accountable leadership. Among the advantages of such groups is the ability to consult and learn from each other, provide coverage and on-call services, coordinate specialist referrals, and achieve economies of scale and scope in staffing, facilities, supplies, and technology purchases.

Health Care Teams

The medical group is the base structure or "house" for the operation of health care teams. In organized delivery systems, teams, not individuals, deliver most health care. The importance of well-functioning teams is growing with the increased prevalence of chronic illness in the population.[7] Teams have been referred to as "microsystems," constituting the smallest replicable unit of an organization that relates to the patient.[8] Teams operating within an organized system of care are part of an *organizing principle* for health care delivery in the twenty-first century. To use a biological analogy, teams are the RNA that links the medical group structure (or protein) with the DNA of clinical information and knowledge. It is *not* information itself that integrates care but rather the team that *uses* the information, including the patient as a central member of the team. In large part, the failure of American medicine has been its resistance to the organizing principle of the team, making it difficult to link the various pieces of the system together.

Defined Populations

A third key element is that PGPs care for defined populations of potential patients and strive to "know" these people. This will vary by the extent to which the organized delivery system is an exclusive owner or contractor with a health plan (for example, Kaiser Permanente and Group Health Cooperative) or whether the organized delivery system also provides care to patients other than those of the plan owned by the system (for example, Henry Ford Health System and Intermountain Health Care). The focus on populations enables these systems to plan resources in relation to population needs. When combined with appropriate financing and payment incentives, it also results in an emphasis on disease prevention, health promotion, and appropriate longitudinal follow-up care.

Aligned Financial and Payment Incentives

The fourth key element of PGPs is the existence of financial and payment arrangements that promote cost-effective care. These include prepayments to medical groups and in turn arrangements by which a group's individual physicians have incentives to practice cost-effective care within the group's budget. Combined with the emphasis on enrolled populations, aligned financial and payment incentives provide each physician and health professional with a rationale to use resources prudently, to provide care only where evidence indicates that it would benefit the patient, and to eliminate wasteful practices that contribute to inefficient and potentially harmful care. At the same time, the prepayment or capitated payment feature can lead to the withholding of services that might benefit the patient. However, the three associated properties of organized delivery systems—medicine-management partnerships, enhanced information capability, and enhanced accountability—act as powerful countervailing forces to potential underprovision of care.

Medicine-Management Partnership

When health care teams work within the context of organized medical groups, focusing on defined populations with aligned financial and payment incentives, the ingredients for a productive interface between medicine and management are present. The technical, clinical skills of medicine and the health professions must be linked to the managerial and organizational skills of executives and managers to create a consistently outstanding experience for patients. Prepaid group practices provide the setting and incentive structure for this to occur, as everyone is focused on the same set of goals and potentially shares in the rewards of achievement. Clinical and cost performance data are shared by clinicians and managers so that priorities can be set and trade-off decisions can be made based on evidence.[9] There is a need for greater use of both evidence-based medicine and evidence-based management.[10] Prepaid group practices also provide the potential for the integration of evidence-based medicine and evidence-based management. This integration and partnership will be key to the ability of the health care industry to implement the care delivery innovations needed to meet the challenges posed by the many advances in the biomedical and informational sciences and the public's response to them.

Enhanced Information Management Capability

PGPs typically have the size and resources to invest in information technology (IT) capabilities and are in the best position to capture their benefits. Small, autonomous practices must rely on large health plans or linkages with hospitals or health systems to gain access to the capital needed for enhanced IT capability. To date, these partnerships have been largely restricted to claims processing and back-office administrative functions as opposed to enhancing clinical capabilities. In contrast, a number of organized delivery systems, such as Kaiser

Permanente, the Mayo Clinic, Intermountain Health Care, the Henry Ford Health System, and Geisinger Clinic, have made major, multibillion-dollar investments in IT over several years, some with partners such as IBM and 3M.[11] The investments are intended to lead to the development of electronic medical records that can (1) provide timely, accurate information to the health care team at the point of care; (2) provide information for continuing improvement of practice and longitudinal research; and (3) yield data for purposes of meeting the legitimate accountability demands of external groups.

Accountability

With organized groups, teams, defined populations, aligned incentives, medicine-management partnerships, and information capabilities, a basis exists for enhanced accountability to all stakeholders—governing boards, employers and purchasers, governmental and accreditation bodies, individual patients, and the community. Accountability involves taking responsibility for what one does and comparing one's performance to stated objectives or goals. It involves setting explicit standards of performance, measuring performance against the standards, communicating the results to those with legitimate interests, and following up to remedy performance deficits. Public reporting of quality and outcome data in addition to cost data is growing. The development of a national quality report card and various "pay for performance" initiatives will stimulate further demands, as will consumers who are being asked to bear more of the costs of their care. Organized delivery systems are likely to be best positioned to respond to these demands.

As we have suggested, these seven elements reinforce each other in their potential to promote value in health care delivery. Furthermore, organizational arrangements for the delivery of health care can be evaluated using these elements. The greater the extent to which each of the seven features exists, the greater the probability of providing value in health care delivery. When all seven exist to the fullest extent possible, resources and energies are focused on *care management* and *care coordination*. When various elements are missing altogether or little weight is given to them, organizational arrangements tend to maximize market power, bargaining leverage, and economies of scale but leave care management virtually untouched.

The Performance of Prepaid Group Practice

The performance, or value, created by prepaid group practice can be assessed using the six criteria for health care system quality identified in the Institute of Medicine's *Crossing the Quality Chasm* report: safety, effectiveness, efficiency, patient-centeredness, timeliness, and equity. In brief, care should be provided in such a way that patients are not injured by care that is intended to help them. Care should be provided in such a way that services are based on the best available scientific knowledge regarding effectiveness. Care should be respectful of and responsive to individual patient preferences, needs, and values, ensuring that patient preferences guide all clinical decisions. Care should also be provided in such a way that waiting time and harmful delays are reduced or eliminated to the extent possible so that waste, including waste of equipment, supplies, ideas, and energy, is kept to a minimum. Finally, care should not vary in quality because of personal characteristics such as gender, ethnicity, geographical location, or socioeconomic status. We shall use each of these criteria to provide a high-level evaluation of the performance of PGPs to date, relative to other arrangements. (More detailed assessments can be found in Chapters Two, Three, and Five.)

Safety

Since the publication of the Institute of Medicine's report *To Err Is Human* in 1999, increased attention has been given to reducing medical errors and increasing patient safety. Although a number of studies are under way, none has addressed differences in the ability of PGPs to reduce medical errors or increase patient safety in comparison with other organizational or financial arrangements. To the extent that costly electronic medical record systems, computerized drug order entry systems, and related technologies enhance patient safety, one might expect larger, better-capitalized organizations of whatever type, including PGPs, to achieve greater safety gains than independent or autonomous arrangements. This is in part because of the greater ability of the medicine-management partnership of the PGPs to focus attention, resources, leadership, and accountability on the task of reducing errors and enhancing safety. Whether or not this is true is an area for future research.

Effectiveness

Miller and Luft provide the most recent and comprehensive update on the comparative effectiveness and efficiency of health maintenance organizations (HMOs), including carrier HMOs, versus alternative arrangements.[12] Consistent with earlier research, the recent literature suggests no consistent, systematic differences in quality or outcomes of care between HMOs broadly defined and non-HMO arrangements. However, a recent national study of the management of chronic illness for patients with asthma, congestive heart failure, depression, and diabetes found that a select group of twelve large multispecialty medical groups were significantly more likely to use recommended, evidence-based care management processes (disease registries, reminder systems, guidelines, case management systems, and so on) and to report a positive financial impact from their investment in these processes than other, more loosely organized groups, including other large groups of one hundred physicians or more (see Table 1.2).

Recent evidence also suggests that groups affiliated with or owned by HMOs, hospitals, or health systems use more recommended care management processes than freestanding groups.[13] Also, recent work comparing Kaiser Permanente with the British National Health Service revealed that Kaiser Permanente patients receive more recommended treatment for diabetes and heart disease—for example, 93 percent of Kaiser Permanente heart attack patients receive beta blockers versus 42 percent in the United Kingdom.[14]

Further, for the past five years, the California Cooperative Health Care Reporting Initiative (CCHRI) has rated Kaiser Permanente among the best in the state in providing breast and cervical cancer screening, comprehensive diabetes care, cholesterol management in patients with heart disease, and follow-up care after hospitalization for mental illness. In fact, cardiovascular disease is no longer the leading cause of death among Kaiser Permanente's Northern California population, although it remains so among the population at large. The 15 percent decline in the cardiovascular death rate at Kaiser Permanente, Northern California, between 1990 and 1998 is attributed largely to a coordinated strategy of implementing guidelines.[15] In a similar example, Intermountain Health Care has increased the percentage of its post–heart attack and congestive heart failure patients on ACE inhibitors and beta blockers from 60 percent to 90 percent, saving an estimated 450 lives per year and about $3 million per year in reduced hospitalizations.[16]

Efficiency

Recent evidence suggests that HMOs continue to have lower hospital use and use less expensive technologies than other types of delivery or financing arrangements.[17] Other investigators have found that prepaid groups are associated with lower costs to patients and that groups with a strong culture of shared values among physician members had lower costs.[18] In a related study of eighty-six clinics, use of physician profiles and clinical guidelines were associated with lower costs.[19] At the level of the overall organized delivery system, it was found that more centralized systems and networks experienced significantly lower costs than more decentralized and independent systems and networks.[20] It appears that the cost savings are due to different use of resources (for example, less inpatient hospital care, more outpatient care, and possibly closer management of patients

TABLE 1.2. COMPARISON OF SELECTED PGPs TO OTHER GROUPS.

NSPO Survey Item	PGP ($N = 12$)	Groups with 100 + M.D.'s ($N = 468$)	All Other Groups ($N = 1,028$)
Percentage with financial gains in the past year	66.7%	46.7%	45.7%
Percentage whose investment in asthma had positive financial impact[a]	41.7%	32.8%	27.0%
Percentage whose investment in CHF had positive financial impact[a]	75.0%	36.8%	29.5%
Percentage whose investment in depression had positive financial impact[a]	27.3%	14.6%	13.5%
Percentage whose investment in diabetes had positive financial impact[a]	75.0%	42.0%	37.7%
Percentage with smoking cessation programs for patients	100%	42.8%	39.9%
Mean POCMI (out of 16)[b]	12.5	5.9	5.3
Mean CCMI (out of 11)[c]	9.0	4.8	4.6
Mean Clinical IT Index (out of 6)[d]	4.5	1.2	1.3
Mean External Incentives Index (out of 7)[e]	4.1	1.9	1.7

[a]For groups who treat this illness.

[b]POCMI = Physician Organization Care Management Index—use of disease registries, patient self-management, guidelines, automated reminders, performance feedback, and the like.

[c]CCMI = Chronic Care Management Index—patient self-management, linkages to community resources, delivery system redesign, decision support tools, and the like.

[d]Clinical IT = An electronic medical record for each patient—a standardized problem list, laboratory findings, medications prescribed, radiology findings, clinical guidelines and protocols, medication ordering reminders and drug interaction information—entered into an electronic medical record directly by the physician or after being dictated and transcribed and electronic reporting of the number of patients with diabetes.

[e]External Incentives = Bonuses from health plans, public recognition, better contracts with health plans, quality reporting on HEDIS data, clinical outcome data, results of quality improvement projects, patient satisfaction data.

Source: Data from *National Study of Physician Organizations and the Management of Chronic Illness* (Berkeley: School of Public Health, University of California, 2002).

with high-cost chronic illnesses) rather than economies of scale or scope.[21] This is supported by the recent Kaiser Permanente–United Kingdom study in which Kaiser Permanente averaged 270 acute bed days per 1,000 population versus 1,000 for the United Kingdom.[22]

Patient-Centeredness

A potential advantage of PGPs is that by knowing who their patient population is in advance, they can tailor treatment to meet individual patient needs and use cost-effective interventions for each patient.[23] To the extent that personalized patient care might be loosely measured by patient satisfaction with care, the bulk of the evidence suggests that patient satisfaction is lower in organized delivery system arrangements than in other arrangements.[24] The lower satisfaction appears to be true for both measures of access to care, such as difficulty in getting an appointment, and measures of patient-physician communication and quality of services received. However, these studies have included both loosely organized network-model HMOs and more highly organized group practice HMOs.

Some group practice HMO models have committed significant time and resources to improving the overall patient care experience. For example, Kaiser Permanente has established the Care Experience Council to help redesign the patient care experience throughout the Kaiser Permanente system by identifying the specific functions most strongly associated with member satisfaction and retention and then designing interventions to improve those factors. In recent years, Kaiser Permanente has received above-average marks in customer service and the ability of patients to get needed care. The California Cooperative Health Care Reporting Initiative and the California Office of the Patient Advocate gave Kaiser Permanente high marks on effective physician communication with members. Further research is needed to compare different types of HMO and PGP models in regard to patient satisfaction and personalized care.

Timeliness

The literature addresses the issue of timely care largely in the context of time to receive an appointment and waiting time in the physician's office. As previously noted, PGPs generally score lower on these aspects of the care experience. To address this issue, organizations such as Kaiser Permanente and Group Health Cooperative have implemented nurse call systems, same-day appointments, and automated reminder systems. Within Kaiser Permanente, appointments can be made online, prescription refills are available without calling or visiting a doctor, and patients referred to a specialist are seen within two weeks.

Equity

Emerging research suggests that not only are there inequities in people's access to health care services, but there are also differences by race, ethnicity, and related socioeconomic variables in the actual provision of care.[25] However, there have been no studies examining differences in care among different socioeconomic or ethnic groups within PGPs versus other care arrangements. To the extent that PGPs are more likely to use evidence-based, standardized care management processes, one might hypothesize fewer differences in quality of care by socioeconomic status within PGPs than in other arrangements subject to the greater variability in individual provider practices. Further, given the presence of prepayment, there are no differential financial incentives to use more services or treatments than the evidence and best clinical judgment suggest is necessary. Nonetheless, comparisons between PGP models and more independent or autonomous models of equity in treatment merit further study.

Summary of Prepaid Group Practice Performance

Using the Institute of Medicine's system criteria, current evidence is mixed regarding the performance of PGPs in comparison with other arrangements. It is important to note that past summaries of quality and outcomes of care have been based on HMOs broadly defined to include carrier HMOs. These reviews show no systematic differences in quality or outcomes of care between HMOs and fee-for-service arrangements. But emerging work comparing more integrated forms of PGPs suggest superior quality and outcomes of care relative to other arrangements, particularly in regard to chronic illness management.

On the efficiency front, HMOs may be somewhat less costly than other arrangements, but outpatients seem to be less satisfied with their care—at least for HMOs overall, which include network models as well as group practice models. No evidence is available regarding the provision of safe care or differences in equity of care. However, there is as much variability *within* PGPs on many of the criteria as there is between them and other arrangements.[26] In particular, research is needed that compares different types of PGPs with each other as well as with the independent, fee-for-service, and autonomous models in regard to (1) the management of chronic illness, including issues of patient safety; (2) patient satisfaction with care; (3) treatment patterns and practices by ethnicity, gender, socioeconomic status, and related variables; and (4) patterns of underuse, overuse, and misuse of services in areas where evidence-based standards exist. Research is also needed to identify the components of PGPs that can be most easily transferred to other delivery arrangements, as well as to examine the processes of transfer themselves, so that the most efficient and most effective transfer processes can be identified. In-depth comparative research on high-performing PGPs would also be useful to "unpack" the specific features of these organizations that have made them successful over time.

Next, exploratory interviews with leaders of six such organizations are used to assess their experiences to date and the future potential of the PGP model.

The Experiences of Six Selected PGPs

Twelve top executives from six of the highest performing PGPs and organized delivery systems in America were interviewed: Group Health Cooperative (Seattle, Washington), HealthPartners (Minneapolis–Saint Paul, Minnesota), Henry Ford Health System (Detroit, Michigan), Intermountain Health Care System (Salt Lake City, Utah), Kaiser Permanente (Oakland, California), and the Mayo Clinic (Rochester, Minnesota). These leaders shared their views on what they saw as the accomplishments, limitations, and future potential of this form of health care delivery.

Four themes—patient-centeredness, efficiency, effectiveness, and information technology capability—were viewed as major advantages for PGPs, while two themes—lack of a group culture and lack of financial incentives—were identified as barriers to further diffusion of the model. In regard to patient-centeredness, many of those interviewed felt that the teamwork of physicians in multispecialty group practice made the notion of a "system looking out for the patients" a reality.

Another common theme was efficiency. Many executives strongly believed their groups were started on the principle that multispecialty group practice, grafted on to the concept of prepayment, inherently provided the most efficient and cost-effective way to provide care.

Executives also cited numerous ways in which the organized delivery system enhanced patient care delivery, especially in the use of chronic care management and evidence-based medicine. As one executive stated, "The integrated model is the most advanced approach for dealing with chronic illness management and disease prevention. It is more advanced than any of the alternatives." The reasons cited for this advantage ranged from optimal alignment of interests and incentives through integration and population-based medicine; continuity of care and treatment through vertical integration of hospitals; use of a built-in network of doctors to provide a medium for diffusing best practices and innovation; and superior information technology.

Information technology was frequently cited as being a key way for health care systems to optimize efficiency. "Information technology has to become part of active health care delivery in a more effective way than it is now. We are in the dark ages compared to most other industries," said one executive. Many pointed out that PGPs have a greater ability to invest in technical infrastructure than smaller groups, and their integrated structure allows them to maximize the return on their IT investments in part because of their ability as integrated systems to offer patients online access to physicians, prescriptions, lab test results, and health care information. "We offer consumers the best available knowledge and advice to inform their health care decisions. [We put] them in the driver's seat," said an executive.

Enhanced IT capabilities offer PGPs a way to leverage their coordinated structure to lubricate the "natural friction points" between health plans, physicians, and hospitals, said many executives, who nonetheless acknowledged that managing such organizations is difficult. "I believe that there is no more complex organization on the planet than an integrated group practice," said one executive. Information technology may also prove to be a key to making such integration work for other kinds of health care organizations without necessarily integrating their structure. As one executive put it, "Information technology will be the glue for virtual groups."

Many organizations reported using their IT capabilities to implement computerized patient medical records; however, with or without paperless offices, many felt that their unified medical charts made it easier to provide continuity of care and to make that care transparent to all. "All of [the physicians] tend to have a very active peer review mechanism because of the unified chart," said one physician executive. Another pointed out that the common medical record "changes our practice style automatically because we are more prudent about what we do."

Despite the advantages, health care executives acknowledged that there were limitations to the appeal of the PGP model, including developing a culture in which physicians put the group ahead of individual entrepreneurial interests. "The group comes first," said one leader, adding, "We don't tolerate superstars here very well." Said another, "The biggest limitation is how do we take a whole group of incumbents, whether they are medical students or practicing physicians, and develop a model where they hopefully align incentives so that people can effectively sublimate their own individual ambitions and rewards to [those of] a group."

Many executives felt that the potential for PGPs to expand is held back by health care's current financial incentive system, which encourages competition among specialties and physicians rather than cooperation. They also felt that without substantial changes to the U.S. financial and regulatory systems, it would be difficult for new PGPs to develop and for many of the current ones to expand significantly beyond current markets. They specifically noted the lack of consumer motivation to demand change and the difficulty of "exporting" the group culture.

As one executive put it, "The [integrated] model is good. We see disintegration [in the health care system] because of the inability to execute it."

Nonetheless, many leaders believe that the PGP model remains a blueprint for addressing the future challenges of health care in America. As one executive noted: "Organized health care in this country is going to increase. I think it is going to increase because we are heading toward the edge of a cliff. . . . We are rapidly approaching the point where we will need some voluminous quantities of health care [provided by] fewer and fewer people. I think the only way we will be able to do that effectively is through organized delivery systems."

Conclusion: Lessons and Implications

Despite the many complaints and criticisms of the U.S. health care system, one must recognize and underscore the fact that Americans like their system, with all its faults and internal contradictions, more than the alternatives. It may not be very pretty, and at times it may look downright ugly, but it is important to remember that most of the time, most Americans do not use the health system. When they do, they are willing to put up with it because they think someone else is paying for it. Further, when Americans look around at other countries, everyone else seems to be complaining as well. All of the major stakeholders—employers and purchasers, health plans, providers, and patients—value choice and autonomy, which the system offers, and they are willing to pay for it with time, money (or at least someone else's money), and apparently, tolerance for errors and variations in treatment and outcomes. The system is not yet at the threshold or "tipping point" for fundamental change, and until it is (if that point is ever reached), the PGP model is unlikely to grow much beyond its current state. Although the fee-for-service or indemnity model is unable to meet current health care challenges, many of its core features will continue to exist because they fulfill the basic American demands for choice and autonomy. This may change as more Americans experience the mounting personal health challenges of the new century, but for now, health care is caught in a period of transition characterized by uncertainty, ambiguity, and growing anxiety. We are trapped in a maze of different delivery and financing arrangements and do not know how to get out.

In thinking about this predicament, it is useful to consider two different scenarios for the future. Each is based on the following assumptions: (1) continued growth in the number of Americans experiencing one or more chronic illnesses; (2) continued growth of new biomedical knowledge and technology and their transfer into clinical practice; (3) continued increases in costs, with consumers paying an increasing share of those costs; and (4) continued interest on the part of all parties in maintaining a pluralistic health system that features choice as one of its core values.

Evolution of the Status Quo

In the first scenario, nothing will change: the current disenchantment with managed care, the inability of PGPs (with a few exceptions) to demonstrate consistently superior performance, the aversion of most physicians to practicing in larger organizations, and the desire of most Americans for a variety of insurance products will persist, putting more pressure on consumers to pay for the cost of their care and to use the new information tools (especially the Internet) to make wise choices. Essentially, each person must make his or her own map to navigate the maze.

In this scenario, PGPs will need to compete effectively in the area of benefit design and premium rates to hold their own. PGPs are likely to continue to be major players in areas where they already enjoy a significant presence, but they are unlikely to expand beyond their current boundaries. Costs will continue to rise, and physicians and other health professionals will continue to be frustrated until enough information on system performance (cost, quality, outcomes, satisfaction, and access) is trusted by all parties to motivate a concerted search for viable alternatives. At this point, the PGP models will be looked to as possible approaches for reform, but they will be found to be too difficult to implement in most parts of the country. They will be beyond the comfort zone of most local stakeholders' tolerance for change, particularly in the absence of stronger evidence that such an approach will specifically benefit each stakeholder group—purchasers, health plans, provider organizations, and patients. However, it is possible that each party may adopt *some elements* of the PGP approach to create delivery systems that better address the challenges of the status quo. This gives rise to the second scenario.

A Coalition of Partnerships

In this second scenario, the four major stakeholder groups—purchasers, health plans, providers, and patients—join forces to create partnerships that mimic some features of the PGP model. It begins with purchasers (employers, federal and state governments) recognizing the need to obtain better value for their dollars, particularly in the areas of disease prevention and chronic illness management, and providing incentives to health plans to accomplish this. Smaller employers could come together to form "exchanges" with health plans for this purpose.[27] The plans in turn develop partnerships with their physician organizations, both large and small, to reward them on the basis of measurable quality and outcome metrics, in addition to cost considerations. Physicians and physician organizations now have financial incentives that reinforce and are congruent with professional values (in other words, paying for quality) and work to develop new models of care delivery to achieve better patient outcomes. Finally, patients, with a greater economic stake in their care and a greater knowledge base, can work in partnership with their physician organizations to maintain their health. Most important, rather than finding their providers, health plans, and employers fighting with each other, patients experience greater cooperation, exchange of information, and shared accountability.

This second scenario permits a variety of different "4P partnerships" (among purchasers, plans, providers, and patients) to exist, reflecting the diversity and pluralism of the country. Thus, while existing PGPs are not likely to "generalize" or expand to the rest of the country, they will play a leadership role in serving as incubators of better practices that can be adopted by others. This is particularly true in the area of implementing evidence-based medicine, managing chronic illness, and preventing disease. They will help set the standards by which others will be judged and will change the expectations of purchasers, plans, and patients alike. (For some idea of these new standards, see Table 1.3.)

Which of the two scenarios is likely to prevail? The "evolution of the status quo" may persist for several years as Americans search for exits from the current health care maze. But as they begin to feel the impact (again) of significant cost increases, the growing burden of chronic illness, and the growth of new technologies and biomedical advances, they will grasp (again) for some straws of a "solution" to the ever-present and latest "health care crisis."

The appeal of the "coalition of partnerships" scenario is that it allows for the possibility of multiple exits out of the maze, depending on where one is currently lost. Physicians can continue to practice in small partnerships and groups, health plans can continue to offer multiple products, purchasers can continue to engage in various cost-sharing arrangements with their employees, and patients can continue to make choices based on what they believe is best for them and their families.

So how is this different from the status quo? The answer lies in the flow of dollars attached to shared incentives driven by information technology, which makes all transactions and outcomes more transparent and accountable. Financial incentives and information technology are the primary lubricants for facilitating partnerships among purchasers, plans, providers, and patients. An early test of the feasibility and potential impact of such partnerships will come from the evaluation of demonstrations funded by The Robert Wood Johnson Foundation's Rewarding Results Program and related pay-for-performance initiatives across the country. For example, in California, employers, physician organizations, consumer advocates, and all six of the major non–Kaiser Permanente health plans have agreed to a common set of measures for purposes of providing additional payment bonuses to physician organizations for meeting selected quality targets and

TABLE 1.3. PAY-FOR-PERFORMANCE MEASUREMENT SET.

Condition	Measure Description	Weighting
Childhood immunizations	The percentage of children who turned 2 years old during the measurement year, who were continuously enrolled for twelve months immediately preceding their second birthday, who received any of the following: • Four DTaP/DT *or* • Three IPV/OPV *or* • One MMR *or* • Three H influenza type B *or* • Three hepatitis B *or* • One chickenpox vaccine	50%
Breast cancer screening	The percentage of women aged 50 through 69 years who were continuously enrolled for two years and who had a mammogram.	
Cervical cancer screening	The percentage of women aged 18 through 64 years who were continuously enrolled for three years and who received one or more Pap tests.	
Asthma	The percentage of patients with persistent asthma continuously enrolled for two years who received at least one dispensed prescription for inhaled corticosteroids. The measure should be reported for each of three age stratifications: • Ages 5–9 years • Ages 10–17 years • Ages 18–56 years	
Coronary artery disease	The percentage of patients aged 18 through 75 years as of December 31 who were discharged alive by December 31 for acute myocardial infarction (AMI), coronary artery bypass graft (CABG), or percutaneous transluminal coronary angioplasty (PTCA) and had evidence of LDL-C screening.	
Diabetes	The percentage of members with diabetes (Type 1 and Type 2) aged 18 through 75 years continuously enrolled for one year who had evidence of hemoglobin A1c (HbA1c) screening.	
Patient satisfaction	• Specialty care • Timely access to care • Doctor-patient communication • Overall ratings of care	40%
IT investment	• Integrate clinical electronic data sets at group level • Support clinical decision making at point of care	10%

Source: Courtesy of the Integrated Healthcare Association, Walnut Creek, Calif.

for purposes of public reporting (these are presented in Table 1.3). Although there are many challenges to the implementation of such arrangements, the fact that they are beginning to take place suggests that such partnerships may be a viable approach to improving the U.S. system of health care delivery.

In particular, many industry observers hope that information technology will help smaller or more loosely organized groups of physicians provide data and learn from each other. This will vary as a function of the leadership of the independent practice association or related "virtual" groups. Physicians are not likely in the short term to form larger groups, and those that do are likely to be more motivated by increasing their negotiating leverage with health plans than by improving the quality of care.[28] Thus the techniques and experiences of providing evidence-based medicine learned from the PGPs must be brought to other physicians and adapted to their needs and circumstances.

The key role of PGPs going forward will not be in replicating themselves as wholes but as parts drawn on by others. They will serve as engines of continual innovation, particularly in regard to chronic illness management, disease prevention, and the overall design of positive patient care experiences. What might be observed over the next five to ten years is a greater number of well-functioning health care teams (the organizing principle at the micro level of our health care system) operating within a coalition of partnerships among purchasers, plans, providers, and patients (the organizing principle at the macro level of the health care system).

None of this will occur, however, until Americans become more dissatisfied with the current malaise. But once this threshold is reached, the model of aligned incentive partnerships that can vary to fit local circumstances will be viewed as more achievable and less disruptive than the PGP model.

As the old Scottish proverb notes, "There is no such thing as bad weather, only inappropriate clothing." Perhaps, some day, PGPs will be the appropriate "clothing" for dealing with the maelstroms of health care in America. In the meantime, "mix and match" partnerships (facilitated, perhaps, by purchaser plan exchanges) are likely to prevail.

Notes

1. Institute of Medicine, *Crossing the Quality Chasm: A New Health System for the 21st Century* (Washington, D.C.: National Academy Press, 2001), p. 1.
2. Ibid.; Institute of Medicine, *To Err Is Human: Building a Safer Health System* (Washington, D.C.: National Academy Press, 2000); D. C. Coddington, E. A. Fischer, and K. D. Moore, *Strategies for the New Health Care Marketplace: Managing the Convergence of Consumerism and Technology* (San Francisco: Jossey-Bass, 2001); J. D. Kleinke, *Bleeding Edge: The Business of Health Care*

in the New Century (Gaithersburg, Mo.: Aspen, 1998); D. Lawrence, *From Chaos to Care* (Cambridge, Mass.: Perseus, 2002); I. Morrison, *Health Care in the New Millennium* (San Francisco: Jossey-Bass, 2000); J. C. Robinson, *The Corporate Practice of Medicine: Competition and Innovation in Health Care* (Berkeley: University of California Press, 1999); S. M. Shortell and others, *Remaking Health Care in America: The Evolution of Organized Delivery Systems*, 2nd ed. (San Francisco: Jossey-Bass, 2000).

3. C. Hoffman, D. Rice, and H. Y. Sung, "Persons with Chronic Conditions: Their Prevalence and Costs," *Journal of the American Medical Association*, 1996, *276*, 1473–1479.

4. S. M. Shortell and others, *Remaking Health Care in America: The Evolution of Organized Delivery Systems* (San Francisco: Jossey-Bass, 1996), p. 7.

5. See also J. B. Christianson, R. A. Taylor, and D. J. Knutson, *Restructuring Chronic Illness Management* (San Francisco: Jossey-Bass, 1998); T. S. Snail and J. C. Robinson, "Organizational Diversification in the American Hospital," *Annual Review of Public Health*, 1998, *19*, 417–453; Robinson, *The Corporate Practice of Medicine;* Shortell and others, *Remaking Health Care in America*, 2nd ed.; R. H. Miller and H. S. Luft, "HMO Plan Performance Update: An Analysis of the Literature, 1997–2001," *Health Affairs*, 2002, *21*(4), 63–86.

6. L. P. Casalino and others, "Benefits of and Barriers to Large Medical Group Practice in the United States," *Archives of Internal Medicine*, 2003, *163*(16), 1958–1964; P. I. Havlicek, *Medical Groups in the U.S., 1999.* Chicago: American Medical Association, 1999.

7. Lawrence, *From Chaos to Care.*

8. J. B. Quinn, *Intelligent Enterprise* (New York: Free Press, 1992).

9. R.G.A. Feachem, N. D. Sekhri, and K. L. White, "Getting More for Their Dollar: A Comparison of the NHS with California's Kaiser Permanente," *British Medical Journal*, 2002, *324*, 135–141.

10. J. M. Eisenberg, *Doctors' Decisions and the Cost of Medical Care* (Ann Arbor, Mich.: Health Administration Press Perspectives, 1986); A. R. Kovner, J. J. Elton, and J. Billings, "Evidence-Based Management," *Frontiers of Health Services Management*, 2000, *16*(4), 3–46; K. Walshe and T. G. Rundall, "Evidence-Based Management: From Theory to Practice in Health Care," *Milbank Quarterly*, 2001, *79*, 429–457.

11. Coddington, Fischer, and Moore, *Strategies for the New Health Care Marketplace.*

12. Miller and Luft, "HMO Plan Performance Update."

13. Casalino and others, "Benefits of and Barriers to Large Medical Group Practice."

14. Feachem, Sekhri, and White, "Getting More for Their Dollar."

15. E. Levin and others, "Innovative Approach to Guidelines Implementation Is Associated with Declining Cardiovascular Mortality in a Population of Three Million" (abstract.) Presented at the American Heart Association's Scientific Sessions 2001, Anaheim, Calif., Nov. 12, 2001.

16. C. Sorensen, Chief Operating Officer, Intermountain Health Care, personal communication, Dec. 2002.

17. Miller and Luft, "HMO Plan Performance Update."

18. J. E. Kralewski, T. Wingert, D. Knutson, and C. Johnson, "The Effects of Medical Group Practice Organizational Factors on Physicians' Use of Resources," *Journal of Healthcare Management*, 1999, *44*, 167–182.

19. J. E. Krawleski and others, "The Effects of Medical Group Practice and Physician Payment Methods or Costs of Care," *Health Services Research*, 2000, *35*, 591–613.

20. G. J. Bazzoli, B. Chan, S. M. Shortell, and T. D'Aunno, "The Financial Performance of Hospitals Belonging to Health Networks and Systems," *Inquiry*, 2000, *37*, 234–252.

21. M. V. Pauly, "Will Medicare Reforms Increase Managed Care Enrollment?" *Health Affairs,* 1996, *15,* 182–191.

22. Feachem, Sekhri, and White, "Getting More for Their Dollar."

23. M. R. Greenlick, "The Impact of Prepaid Group Practice on American Medical Care: A Critical Evaluation," *Annals of the American Academy of Political and Social Science,* 1972, *399,* 100–113.

24. Miller and Luft, "HMO Plan Performance Update."

25. B. D. Smedley, A. Y. Stith, and A. R. Nelson, eds., *Unequal Treatment: Confronting Ethnic and Racial Disparities in Health Care* (Washington, D.C.: National Academy Press, 2002).

26. Miller and Luft, "HMO Plan Performance Update."

27. A. C. Enthoven, "Where Are Health Care's 'Hondas'?" *Wall Street Journal,* Oct. 24, 2002, p. A16.

28. Casalino and others, "Benefits of and Barriers to Large Medical Group Practice."

CHAPTER TWO

SYSTEMS AND RESULTS

The Basis for Quality Care in Prepaid Group Practice

Donald M. Berwick and Sachin H. Jain

Prepaid group practices (PGPs) have the potential to deliver greater health care quality than is provided in the more prevalent, disaggregated, fee-for-service care system.

It would be hard to find an assertion in American health care policy discourse that invites more controversy and doubt than this statement. Yet in the face not only of evidence but also of logic, enormous segments of both the public and the professional communities persist in suspecting that organized, prepaid systems of care often behave in bureaucratic, stingy, and impersonal ways to the great disadvantage of both patients and their well-meaning clinical staffs. "Managed care" has become a bogeyman.

One problem is in the words. When words lose consistent meaning, rational discourse suffers, and that is exactly where the public debate about managed care and quality has run aground. In the public imagination, managed care (a category into which PGPs are often lumped) largely represents a Rube Goldberg machine designed to limit access to necessary services. Stabilizing the terms so that "prepaid group practice" and "quality of care" both mean something specific should help reilluminate the relationship between the two.

This chapter will examine recent efforts to promote quality improvement from the most general level down to the specific prescriptions for improved quality health care as articulated by the Institute of Medicine (IOM). It will specifically examine how PGPs have lived up to their potential for realizing quality improvements in the four levels of health care outlined in the IOM report *Crossing the Quality Chasm*, citing specific examples wherever possible.[1] We will then consider seven institutional and cultural barriers that may be holding PGPs back from realizing their full potential for quality improvement, and we will conclude with some suggestions for how a select group of PGPs could provide a leadership vanguard to promote quality improvements across the entire American health care system.

Definitions: "PGPs" and "Quality"

Alain Enthoven and Laura Tollen provide a comprehensive definition of "prepaid group practice" in the Preface to this book. To restate it in different terms that illuminate ideas relevant to this chapter, a "prepaid group practice" is an organized group of primary care clinicians and specialists, including but not limited to physicians, who are paid under a common corporate mechanism for the ongoing care of a defined population of enrolled patients. The group knows its budget for that care in advance of giving that care and has the ability to form extended relationships with hospitals, home health care agencies, skilled nursing facilities, and numerous other types of organizations that together can meet the health care needs of the client population. A "prepaid group practice" is guided and assisted by a management system that has the "whole" in mind—both the whole of the financing and the whole of the care. The management system can also engage in strategic activities, such as capital development, human resource development, and new program plans.

"Quality of care" is a bit more difficult to define and requires an excursion into recent history. Health care is not the only sector concerned about quality. In fact, it is a latecomer into a vast social movement occupying a good portion of the twentieth century. That social movement has had numerous aliases, including total quality management, continuous quality improvement, reengineering, and Six Sigma, but these monikers belie the underlying unity of the modern view of excellence in complex, human production systems. Across schools, consultants, labels, and theories, one finds remarkable consistency about the elements necessary for success in making products and services better and better, including the following:

- A *focus on customers* (the parties who depend on the product or service) as the ultimate source of direction—"meeting and exceeding" their needs, both manifest and latent.

- A belief that *many improvements to quality also reduce costs,* especially in terms of reducing waste (defined as activities and products that do not meet customers' needs).
- A strong *investment in innovations,* some of which reduce costs to customers and others of which raise costs but add sufficient value to be worth it. (These latter improvements are sometimes called "features"; cruise control in an automobile is an example.)
- *Systems thinking* deeply embedded in management and strategy; that is, a strong understanding that performance is a property of the design and management of processes, much as the top speed of a car is a property of that car. Systems thinking leads to the inevitable conclusion that better performance requires changes in processes and design.
- *Specific views of the workforce* that generally involve trust in intrinsic motivation (such as pride, joy, and the motivation to learn) and the value of total participation in the improvement of services and products.
- *Investments in continuous learning and change* in the day-to-day activities of the organization: for example, fostering widespread, real-time experiments by workers at all levels, all the time—the so-called "plan-do-study-act" cycle in day-to-day work—and the closer linkage of research and development, on the one hand, with production and the "shop floor," on the other hand, such that research, development, redesign, and production are parallel and simultaneous.
- An *emphasis on leadership* as coaching and support, rather than strictly as control and problem solving. This includes a focus by leaders on change and improvement as strategies, tightly linked to the pursuit of organizational sustainability.

Health care in recent years has become much more familiar with principles like these, but many clinicians and organizations have had a tough time acting on them. In some cases, the modern theories of quality run headlong into contradictory beliefs in traditional medical care. For example, true "customer focus" is not easily compatible with the idea that "the doctor knows best," "systems thinking" and its consequent emphasis on teamwork can run upstream against medical hierarchies and the prerogatives that the profession of medicine has accrued, and "leadership" in health care organizations is sometimes unhelpfully divided among, say, physician-leaders, nurse-leaders, and executives, who experience tension, not teamwork, among themselves.

Even when beliefs are not a barrier, other real-world conditions can be. For example, to a remarkable extent, health care financing systems pay quite well for defects in care. A computer company whose equipment fails will find itself with high warranty costs and departing market share. A hospital with high complication rates may, in contrast, get paid more as its patients migrate to higher-paying diagnosis-related groups (DRGs) or collect new fees as it repeats laboratory tests to replace lost ones.

To help it emerge from such ambiguity about the meaning of "quality," American health care received a major support in the form of two Institute of Medicine reports as the century turned. *To Err Is Human*, released in November 1999, and *Crossing the Quality Chasm*, published in March 2001, were book-length statements by the IOM's Committee on Quality of Health Care in America on what the nation should do to move its care toward markedly improved quality.[2] The former focused on changes to achieve higher levels of patient safety; the latter was a more comprehensive prescription for improvement in many dimensions of performance, including but not limited to safety.

Both reports sent deep roots into the modern quality movement. Both called for much greater customer focus, systems thinking, and workforce involvement, for example, but they carefully connected their agendas to the health care research literature and to the special needs and contexts of health care as a system.

Briefly, the IOM reports, especially *Crossing the Quality Chasm*, called for changes at four levels of the American health care system:

1. Changes in *aims*, offering a bold array of six objectives for improvement in patient safety, effectiveness of care (that is, reducing overuse of unnecessary care and underuse of effective care), patient-centeredness (with a rather radical call for patients' greater individual control over their own care), timeliness, efficiency (reducing waste and thereby reducing costs), and equity (especially closing racial and socioeconomic gaps in health status).
2. Changes in the *"microsystems"* of care, such as office practices, surgical teams, and chronic disease care programs, guided by a set of new "simple rules" for redesign.
3. Changes in the *organizations* that house and support the actual care microsystems, involving information technology, human resource development and training, teamwork, cooperation with other organizations, and measurement and reporting systems.
4. Changes in the *environment* of care, such as in payment, regulation, accreditation, professional training and licensure, and legal liability systems.

The *Chasm* report was a remarkably sweeping proposal, suggesting an integrated vision of new approaches at all levels of system aggregation, all focused on the single, unifying purpose of providing better care to individuals and communities. In its proposed aims for improvement, linked to ideas about the redesign of care, organizations, policy, and finance, it offers the health care industry as a whole a sophisticated definition of quality itself.

Prepaid Group Practice and the IOM's Prescription for Change

The *Chasm* report also offers a chance at a rational formulation of the question about the quality of prepaid group practice. The formulation is this: "Why might PGPs be better able to turn the vision of the *Chasm* report into reality? Or why not?"

A simple comparison of properties of prepaid group practice with a disaggregated, fee-for-service care system shows some of the advantages immediately apparent in the former (see Table 1.1 in Chapter One).

Comparing these systems with reference to the modern, general principles of quality management, prepaid group practices seem, in theory at least, to be better positioned to learn and improve continuously and to focus those efforts especially on the needs of the chronically ill, which account for the large majority of health care expenditures and among whom the defects in care cited by the *Chasm* report may today be most egregious and costly.

A more detailed look at the *Chasm's* four-level vision for change may be helpful.

Changes in Aims

With respect to aims, prepaid group practices have the capacity to set such aims self-consciously, to assign responsibility to someone for their pursuit, to measure progress, and at an emotional level to link the aims with a sense of duty or commitment to population-based care. An individual physician-practitioner or a free-standing hospital with no links to an integrated delivery system could "adopt" a subset of the *Chasm* aims, of course. A physician could seek to use pedigreed scientific care protocols in his or her own practice (thus improving "effectiveness") or to introduce shared decision-making technologies for patients (thus improving "patient-centeredness"), but it is hard to imagine how the physician would then proceed to monitor progress meaningfully or address alone the needed information technologies, business case issues, or the more difficult aim of "equity." A hospital could make its care of diabetic ketoacidosis more scientifically effective, but it would have difficulty investing in the continual improvement of diabetic control in its geographical region. Broad aims—system-level aims—require a system to see and to manage, a vision and an opportunity beyond the conventional horizon of solo-practice doctors and freestanding hospitals. Aims in the disaggregated system therefore tend to be more local and more timid than the *Chasm* report proposes.

Changes in Microsystems: Care Redesign

With respect to care redesign, the PGP is in a far stronger position than a fragmented system is. Following are the Institute of Medicine's "Ten Simple Rules" for care redesign and some ideas and evidence from the world of prepaid group practice regarding action on those rules. Most of these examples will be drawn from three of the oldest and best-established PGPs: Kaiser Permanente, Group Health Cooperative (formerly "of Puget Sound"), and HealthPartners.

Care as Relationship, Not Just Visits. The *Chasm* report asserts that the needs of chronically ill people render the current system's emphasis on encounters and episodes as the primary product dysfunctional. The main population need today is for continuing relationships over time and place, integrating care with a memory. Prepaid groups have been leaders in exploring nonvisit alternatives to care, such as e-mail use between patients and physicians, group visits, phone consultations, and outreach to homes. In addition, several of the most successful planned care models for specific chronic illnesses have emerged in prepaid groups.

In one example of PGP innovation in going beyond visits, Kaiser Permanente in Northern California demonstrated improved outcomes in care for depression patients by placing supportive phone calls to patients between office visits.[3] During calls, they inquired about reactions to antidepressants and side effects and provided emotional support when necessary. Patients had markedly higher satisfaction ratings and lowered depression scores on standard scales. Kaiser Permanente's Care Management Institute is aimed at improving care in several key chronic disease areas: diabetes, asthma, heart failure, coronary artery disease, and depression, among similar systemic care designs.

Such results are not limited to Kaiser Permanente. Ed Wagner and his colleagues at Group Health Cooperative have a long history of innovation in chronic care by integrating the use of regular office visits, group visits, and directed self-care.[4] The results are reflected in improved clinical outcomes and decreased utilization of health services. Though this integrated model of care is being introduced nationally in a variety of practice settings, its development was clearly favored by the PGP model of care, in which physicians from diverse specialties are best positioned to coordinate care.

Customization to Patient Needs. The *Chasm* report severely calls into question the widespread variation in practice that characterizes American health care and strongly suggests much more standardization and reliability for delivery of care of proven effectiveness while avoiding care of no known effectiveness. It does, however, call for an *increase* in one form of variability, namely, variation in response to different patients' needs, values, cultures, and circumstances. In calling for "customization," the Institute of Medicine asks that the system of the future listen more closely to patients and value diversity in its work to match diversity among the people it is trying to help.

Indeed, PGPs have actively taken on this challenge of introducing valued diversity into care. Kaiser Permanente, for example, has established the Institute for Culturally Competent Care and developed highly customized systems for people of different languages, income groups, national backgrounds, and sexual orientations. The institute and its expert staff support and facilitate Permanente physicians interested in researching the needs of specific populations and developing responsive programs to address them.[5] The institute has fueled six centers of excellence that have grown to respond to the group practice's changing demographics: African American populations (West Los Angeles), Latino populations (Colorado), linguistic services (San Francisco), women's health, members with disabilities, and Eastern European populations.

Besides considering cultural and social factors that might alter patients' care experience, Permanente physicians have actively sought to design care programs to respond to individual patient needs.[6] In a trial introduction of the cluster visit model, Kaiser Permanente surveyed patients to identify the topics about which they needed education. A series of presentations, ranging from podiatric health to sexual dysfunction to exercise, were organized according to the requests of each individual patient cluster. Several months following the completion of the program, patients who had participated in the cluster visits had higher levels of adherence to a self-care routine and had demonstrably lower glycosylated hemoglobin levels.

The "shared decision-making technologies" of John Wennberg and his colleagues were first developed, and remain most actively used, in prepaid group settings.[7] Prepaid groups were the first to help develop and test the most widely used patient satisfaction and feedback systems. Furthermore, prepaid systems have often been the primary sites for workforce innovations that have given patients new types of relationships as options, such as the increased use of nurse practitioners and other allied health professionals as caregivers.

Patient as the Source of Control. The *Chasm* report contains a surprisingly radical—some might say subversive—call for a redistribution of power and control over health care: more to patients and communities and somewhat less to hegemonic professions and corporate executives. It was prepaid group practices such as Group Health Cooperative and HealthPartners in Minneapolis that were among the first and most effective in building systems to reflect patients' voices in the governance of their organizations at the level of the board of directors.

Thirteen of HealthPartners' fifteen board members are patients elected by other patients.[8] At Group Health Cooperative, all consumers age eighteen and older can register to become voting members at no cost; voting members elect the eleven-member board of trustees and vote on the bylaws that guide the organization. Furthermore, all members can attend board meetings, speak at open-microphone sessions, and join an advisory council.[9]

The opportunity for recipients of health care services to govern their delivery seems to have subtle but important effects on member experience. Both Group Health Cooperative and HealthPartners members have a well-enumerated set of rights and robust systems through which to report concerns to management.

Free Flow of Information. The *Chasm* report emphasizes both the crucial role of information exchange, with and about patients, as a form of care ("information is care") and the importance of modernizing information systems to support that exchange. Prepaid groups, partly because they can manage capital and make plans and partly because they can organize around population-based needs, have been at the forefront of development of useful computerized medical record systems, as well as in developing computer-based decision support systems for clinicians and patients. They have also experimented widely with information systems to support outreach and prevention for their enrolled patients.

Robert Thompson and his colleagues at Group Health Cooperative have been national leaders in researching and designing interventions to improve preventive care. This wide-ranging work addressing HIV,[10] domestic violence,[11] and immunizations,[12] among other areas, has typically involved collecting specific information from patients to better predict and understand their care needs. In example upon example, Group Health Cooperative has demonstrated ways in which improving flow of information between patients and care providers can prevent health risks, decrease care utilization, and lead to better outcomes. The drive for this important research is certainly grounded in the PGP's strong incentive to limit preventable illness wherever possible.

Evidence-Based Care. In its prominent call for more "effective" care, the Institute of Medicine is suggesting much tighter links between scientific evidence and actual practice. Much actual practice today departs from the clinical science base, either through overuse (giving patients tests, treatments, and medicines that scientifically cannot help them) or underuse (failing to make reliable use of interventions of known benefit, even inexpensive ones). To accomplish this requires support systems that can (1) find the science, (2) embed the science in sound standards of practice, (3) make the relevant knowledge available to clinicians and patients at the point of care and at the time of care, and (4) track performance and improve it continually. In the development of these systems, prepaid group practices have been at the forefront. The Institute for Clinical Systems Integration (ICSI) in Minneapolis, for example, is a national treasure in its approach to the formulation and spread of scientifically grounded care protocols. Though it now assists physicians and organizations well beyond "managed care," its roots and support lie deeply in the PGPs of that region—particularly Bloomington-based HealthPartners. Diabetes care programs, prevention protocols, and asthma care systems have all been developed to the highest state in the nation within prepaid groups.

Safety as a System Property. The sister report to the *Chasm, To Err Is Human,* is an extended call for a safer care system. It describes a large family of needed changes that fall roughly into two categories: technical changes and cultural changes. Prepaid groups have not been alone in the seriousness with which they have taken on the challenge of reducing patient injuries, but several have done so with vigor. The prepaid group practice model is particularly conducive to improving safety and reducing the misuse, underuse, and overuse of care because the practice itself (and not the insurers or patients) must pay the costs of poor quality. Kaiser Permanente has publicly set bold aims for improved safety, has conducted some of the most active internal cultural assessments in all of health care, has instituted a vast organizationwide training initiative to improve its "culture of safety" and teamwork, and has fostered valuable research on the topic.

Interestingly, the Veterans Health Administration (VHA) has become one of the most active of all systems in pursuit of safety, and it is no coincidence that its core structure—a salaried clinical system with a central budget, a client population, and an integrated view of care across boundaries—is essentially that of an extremely large prepaid group practice, with associated inpatient facilities as owned entities. The VHA has created the National Center for Patient Safety, which aims to "foster a culture of safety . . . by developing and providing patient safety programs and delivering standardized tools, methods, and initiatives." The center advocates a "non-punitive approach to patient safety activities that emphasizes systems-based learning, the active seeking out of close calls, which are viewed as opportunities for learning and investigation, and the use of interdisciplinary teams to investigate close calls and adverse events through a root cause analysis process."[13] In its short existence, the center has helped develop the infrastructure for computerized medical records, order entry, laboratory imaging results, and encounter notes; furthermore, it has enabled VHA hospitals to bar-code all medications. The centralized structure of the organization has allowed well-conceived safety ideas to be rapidly disseminated and implemented for the benefit of patients.

Transparency. The *Chasm* report asserts that health care ought to measure and report on its performance, partly to motivate change, partly to allow consumers more choice, and partly to speed the identification of best practices in support of an agenda for learning. Of course, many prepaid groups have joined others in health care in their concern and fear about open measurement and reporting. On the whole, however, if any sector of care has begun to drive toward greater transparency, it has been the prepaid group sector. It was the staff and group model health maintenance organizations (HMOs) that initially sparked the health care measurement and reporting system that has become known as HEDIS (Healthplan Employer Data and Information Set), now administered by the National Committee for Quality Assurance. In a dramatic show of investment in the value of openness, HealthPartners publicly announced its intention to improve appointment access times dramatically *before* it actually achieved its new targets. Many large prepaid group practices have for decades supported strong research units, publishing their findings and evaluations openly in peer-reviewed journals.

HealthPartners offers members and prospective members unprecedented access to patient satisfaction data and clinical quality information. The company's Web site (www.healthpartners.com) features easy access to clinic satisfaction data (collected by an independent market research firm) to help inform patients' decisions about providers and group clinic sites. Patients can gauge whether members are satisfied with their "overall care," "availability of medical advice by phone," "ability to schedule appointments," "waiting room times," and "ease of seeing the doctor of your choice," among other aspects of care. Clinical quality information, providing measures of clinic sites' outcomes and compliance with standard clinical practices, is also available. A diabetic patient might learn of the "percentage of members with diabetes 18 through 75 years of age who have optimally managed risk factors including glycosylated hemoglobin levels, LDL, aspirin use, blood pressure, and tobacco." Likewise, a cardiac patient can learn about the "percentage of members with a diagnosis of coronary artery disease 18 through 75 years of age who have optimally managed risk factors including LDL, lipid-lowering medication, aspirin use, blood pressure, and tobacco."

The clinical data presented on the Web site are not risk-adjusted and hence are not fully illustrative of the disparities that might exist between clinic sites. To be fair, many of these clinical measures might be difficult for patients to interpret. Still, the availability of any kind of information to help inform decisions, particularly satisfaction and access information, represents an important leap in transparency.

At the very least, the availability of such data informs important internal discussions about differences in clinical outcomes that can drive change.

Anticipation, Not Reaction. The *Chasm* report calls for much more sophisticated use of modern scheduling, planning, and modeling capacities, such as queuing theory, industrial engineering, and dynamic modeling, to better design patient flow, access systems, and resource use. Many of the successes that build confidence in such analytical approaches come from prepaid group practice, such as "open access" and "advanced access" scheduling at HealthPartners and resource planning in Kaiser Permanente. These groups, perhaps as a result of their early reputations for long waits, have made early, aggressive efforts to revamp their scheduling practices to reduce waiting times in clinics and physicians' offices. HealthPartners, for instance, was able to decrease average waiting times from twenty minutes to less than twelve minutes at several clinic sites by scheduling more complex patients at the ends of sessions, communicating on-time status to care team members, and using exam room waiting time for preventive services, among other changes.[14]

Kaiser Permanente's size and resources have allowed it to shift and allocate resources as necessary to reduce wait times. For instance, in 2001 and 2002, Kaiser Permanente Colorado recognized that increasing demand for radiology services was beginning to translate into longer delays in receiving necessary tests. Accordingly, it invested $7 million to purchase faster machines and add capacity.[15] The size and associated capacity of PGPs means that the practice can often respond to larger infrastructure needs that might go unmet in other types of practice settings.

Focus on Reducing Waste. The *Chasm* report shows moderate confidence that waste levels in health care are very high and that better management of inventory, the supply chain, job allocations, and protocols to reduce overuse of unhelpful care could lead to enormous savings. Of course, prepaid groups were pioneers in reducing unnecessary hospital days in decades past, but by now most of the rest of American health care has taken instruction from them and caught up. New frontiers of waste reduction lie in finding superior substitutes for encounters and visits, in helping both patients and clinicians identify and reduce overuse in the ambulatory care system and, through anticipation, outreach, and care planning, reduce complications, mishaps, and errors with costly downstream consequences. Recent progress, for example, in reducing hospital admissions for people with congestive heart failure suggests that such savings are within reach for an integrated care system, though possibly out of reach for a less organized system.

Given the costliness of diagnostic procedures, some PGPs have worked to systematically study the efficacy of different disease detection procedures.[16] The provider attention paid to issues such as cost effectiveness in PGP drives the production of care that is delivered with a rational consideration of the cost of its delivery.

Cooperation. The premier idea and cultural value espoused by the *Chasm* report as a guideline for redesign of care is cooperation. All patients depend on it, but the chronically ill depend on it most of all. Yet the Institute of Medicine has documented pervasive failures of cooperation among disciplines, organizations, and social sectors, with patients' paying the bulk of the resulting toll. The nature of a well-run, values-oriented prepaid group practice offers high potential for giving cooperation the pedestal it deserves. The group culture of the Mayo Clinic, though not a PGP, has been famously oriented around teams and teamwork, with the patient at the center. Care management systems within PGPs have succeeded perhaps most of all because of the clinical teamwork they tend to put into their genetic code and processes.

This issue is well addressed in Chapter Nine of this book. However, an outstanding example of integration and cooperation across disciplines is the way in which Kaiser Permanente manages the care of diabetes patients. Care teams include endocrinologists, primary care physicians, nurses, pharmacists, and psychologists. The inclusion of such a diverse set of professionals is intended to address patient care issues from a multidisciplinary perspective. Imprinted in the care system's design is the notion that appropriate disease management is not restricted to the domain of a single specialty but requires the coordinated input of a diverse set of care providers.

Physician and Staff Satisfaction. An important element that is not included in the Institute of Medicine's "Ten Simple Rules" but remains a key topic in the *Chasm* report is provider satisfaction and providers' own perceptions of the care they provide. Most discussions of health care quality appropriately have patients at their center. But consideration of provider satisfaction is also especially relevant, given the strong link between a satisfied workforce and quality care. Two additional factors are also relevant: (1) controversy surrounding managed care organizations' use of financial incentives and capitation to limit utilization and (2) widespread reports of declining physician career satisfaction.

Fortunately for this analysis, providers' satisfaction and their perceptions of quality of care provided are two of the few areas in which prepaid groups have been studied separately from other types of managed care organizations. Strong empirical evidence suggests that physicians in prepaid groups have higher job satisfaction rates and feel less compromised than colleagues in other practice types by the constraints imposed by systems of payment. A 1998 study by Kevin Grumbach and his colleagues advised that "compared to solo practitioners, physicians in staff-model or group-model HMOs felt less pressure to limit referral in a way that they felt compromised care or to limit what they told patients about treatment options in a way that compromised care, but they also felt greater pressure to see more patients."[17] This study, based on a large survey of California physicians, found that prepaid group physicians (primarily from Kaiser Permanente) were more likely than solo practitioners to experience payment incentives linked to quality of care and patient satisfaction.

Another California-based study by Eric Chehab and his colleagues examined physician job satisfaction and perceptions of managed care for PGP and office-based practitioners. In a multifactorial analysis, similarly situated PGP physicians were found to be "significantly more satisfied with quality of practice and patient care than physicians in [office-based practice]."[18] This satisfaction runs deep and is linked strongly to the extent to which the different practice settings were seen as making work more difficult. Some 39 percent of survey respondents in office-based independent practice reported that managed care treatment guidelines made work relatively harder for office-based independent practice physicians; only 4 percent reported that it makes work easier. Among PGP physicians, 56 percent reported that treatment guidelines made work easier; only 12 percent reported that it made it harder. The differences are more profound in a consideration of drug formularies. A healthy 42 percent of PGP physicians found that formularies make their practice easier, whereas only 1 percent of office-based physicians could make the same statement.

In the aggregate, the two groups of physicians differed significantly in their perceptions of how managed care affected the quality of patient care. Compared with office-based practitioners, PGP physicians were significantly more satisfied with the quality of care, "had more positive viewpoints on the effects of treatment guidelines and drug formularies on the quality of patient care, and had more favorable perceptions of the impact of managed care on patient care."[19] The sources of these strong differences seem intimately tied to the nature of the practice environment.

The data suggest that physicians who provide care to patients covered by a number of different insurance plans may be overwhelmed. A formulary or treatment plan might be regarded as helpful to the practitioner or beneficial to the patient when it is uncomplicated, but it is understandable how a physician forced to operate under multiple systems of compensation might become frustrated and confused. Furthermore, in large group practices such as Kaiser Permanente, an administrative staff might handle many of the administrative responsibilities that frustrate providers in single-physician office-based practices. The economies of scale and the simplicity of the prepaid group practice model—a single payer and a single set of accompanying administrative guidelines—might make practice more rewarding.

There are a few important caveats to reading too deeply into the results described. The most important of these is the difference in the types of providers and patients who are attracted to the PGP model of practice. It is quite possible that PGP physicians have chosen that particular style of practice because of personal preferences and that dissatisfied solo practitioners would not necessarily be any happier working in a staff-model HMO than they are in their solo practice. Furthermore, although many practice parameters were roughly equivalent across practice types in Chehab's study, it is possible that the different case mix across practice types may have altered the study's results.

Still, the theoretical basis for the claim that providers are more satisfied in prepaid group practice is strong. Physicians operate under a single system of compensation and administrative guidelines and have a well-aggregated set of resources and colleagues to which they may refer patients. These attributes—coupled with the fact that physicians are usually active participants in developing these administrative guidelines—contribute to legitimately high levels of satisfaction and perceptions of quality care.

Changes in Organizations: Investments in Quality

The nature of prepaid groups favors more than other settings the development of practices and behaviors in accord with the Institute of Medicine's "Ten Simple Rules." These practices and behaviors cannot, however, emerge of their own accord, since they depend on organizational supports and supplies. It is at the organizational level, in fact, that the advantage of PGPs is greatest, since by their nature they can move resources around and make plans to support changes in care. At a lower level of aggregation, such as the individual, freestanding office practice, the flexibility to do so is largely absent; resources are bottled up too tightly in small jars.

Four organizational investments are most critical to improving quality the way the *Chasm* report defines it.

Human Resource Strategies. The pursuit of the vision of the *Chasm* report requires both new skills in the workforce (consider, for example, the skill to use e-mail or shared decision-making technologies with patients or the skill to use an evidence-based care protocol or an electronic medical record) and, even more challenging, new jobs and roles. Prepaid groups have been stronger at the former than the latter—they, like all care systems, have some very strong beliefs about who can do what in giving care—but they have great potential for making progress in both areas through investments and innovative trials. On the reverse side, PGPs are also better able to address concerns associated with impaired and nonproficient providers. Because providers are employed by the practice, the practice can recognize problems and direct staff to counseling, training, and appropriate resources when necessary.

Information Technologies. In the area of information technology (IT), prepaid groups are not at all alone, since most hospitals are equally compelled to enter the modern era in information. Some PGPs have been pioneers in using electronic medical records, and many have developed helpful patient support and education systems. Group Health Cooperative has long relied on IT systems to support its world-class preventive care and outreach programs. Prepaid groups have in common with hospitals the problem of raising capital for initial IT investments, but for obvious reasons, they are more likely to be able to do so than disaggregated, smaller organizations. Kaiser Permanente, for its part, announced in 2002 a $2 billion dollar investment in a new IT infrastructure that will allow for immediate access to medical records and test results, with clinical decision support, in addition to online scheduling, medication refill, and referral requests.[20]

Financial Planning and Budgeting Capabilities. In developing innovative care, it is crucial to be able to track financial flows clearly and accurately. With a population perspective, integrated group practices can think as few others can about the total flow of funds to serve a population and thus can plan integrated services as a whole.

Leadership Systems. Since improvement always requires changes, and large improvements such as those proposed in the *Chasm* report require large changes, the burden on leaders for promoting improvement is great. They must provide much of the will, ideas, resources, optimism, measurement, and consequences that large human systems need to get unstuck and make progress. Prepaid group practices, especially large ones, can appropriately tackle the related leadership development needs strategically and directly, through training, review, supervision, and career development planning, in ways that leaders, particularly physicians, are not prepared to do. Kaiser Permanente has created a special executive position to manage leadership development. The physician who has assumed this role has made developing a curriculum for core leadership skills a top priority and has established an intensive leadership institute in North Carolina, where physician-leaders can gain management and administration skills. The formal nature of this program and the range of skills emphasized suggest that strong leadership systems are a cornerstone of Kaiser Permanente's strategic vision (see Chapter Nine).

Changes in the Environment of Care

The fourth and final level of change contemplated in the *Chasm* report is in the environment of care, a catchall category comprising many factors, some troublesome, that affect the opportunities and will of organizations, professionals, and the workforce as a whole to try to make changes that are improvements.

Managing and changing the environment of care is extremely difficult, and no single formula for success is apparent. Nonetheless, prepaid groups have a better shot than most of the rest of the care system at changing, or at least blunting or mitigating, toxic features of the environment.

The primary environmental hazards are probably financial. Historically, payment for care was built around the concept that care is episodic, that visits are crucial, that treatment occurs in specific places, and that patients get sick and either die or get well rather quickly—over days or weeks, for example. When a child breaks an arm or a well adult gets a case of pneumonia, that paradigm may apply. But it does not meet the needs for most care in America today, which does not involve episodes of transient illness but rather long-term chronic illnesses that do not go away. The needs are for relationships, not just visits, across boundaries of location, and with temporal perspectives that last years or even lifetimes. Relevant resources lie well outside classical health care boundaries, and the best experts are often not the caregivers but the patients and families themselves.

It is possible to devise payment schemes that can help integrate care—in fact, they exist in the Indian Health Service, the Veterans Health Administration, and the National Health Service in the United Kingdom. Such payment schemes have become one of the babies in the bathwater of managed care, now so reviled. However, the fact is that most American care payment today is "dis-integrative."

Prepaid groups can help mitigate that problem primarily through creative deals with payers who do feel responsible for populations. Unlike disaggregated care systems, PGPs stand a chance of proposing successfully to such aggregate payers that they be given the flexibility to move resources around, to reconfigure care according to actual needs, especially for the chronically ill. A wise payer would be unlikely to agree to that on faith but may do so in return for some guarantees about performance and total cost. This trade—flexibility in return for performance—is plausible for PGPs as for almost no other form of care organization. In addition, given their scale, PGPs may also be in a good position to make and execute plans for quality-enhancing capital formation (for example, information technology development) that is prohibitively costly for other types of practice.

Clinicians often cite another environmental barrier to change: the tort system. Improvement of care requires transparency, learning from defects, and "plan-do-study-act" trials of change,[21] all of which become more difficult in a climate of vicious litigation. At the time of this writing, prepaid groups are not on a strong footing to change malpractice laws, but as managed entities, they do have an opportunity to insulate their own clinical staffs to some small degree from the fear and consequences of threatened lawsuits by providing them with legal counseling and representation and by indemnifying them under the proper circumstances against the most harmful and unfair effects of misguided lawsuits.

As for the regulatory and accreditation system, prepaid group practices have already had a favorable effect through their support and development of the National Committee for Quality Assurance and its quality measurement processes. Many have also begun to innovate in the professional education pipeline through creative medical school and residency projects and by forming relationships with local academic medical centers.

Barriers to Improvement in Prepaid Group Practice

As the foregoing has suggested, research and logic argue strongly that prepaid groups have often led in the pursuit of quality of care and that they have even more potential than they have yet realized. But all is not rosy. Prepaid groups are participants in the greater health care system, with all of its warts, and many of the defects in that system have affected them as well. At least seven institutional and cultural barriers have retarded change.

Professional Autonomy

The primary confounder of cooperation, which is the central asset for change, remains professional isolation and autonomy. Many prepaid groups have made good progress with regard to teamwork, but still too often professionals, and most commonly physicians, exercise their prerogatives to the disadvantage of patients and the system of care. Even the best of PGPs have met opposition from physicians who fear evidence-based care protocols as handcuffs or for whom transparency and sharing is uncomfortable. At Kaiser Permanente, this concern has become deeply embedded in a nearly unassailable cultural norm that the tension between the Permanente Medical Groups and the Kaiser Foundation Health Plan is somehow healthy. To an outsider, it is quite clearly unhealthy. It diverts enormous energy to internal battles of no consequence to care or patients other than to drain energy from their care. "Tension" is a euphemism for wasted effort, yet this tension is so deeply habitual at Kaiser Permanente that to question its value is to be automatically marginalized.

Old Habits

Habits continue in prepaid groups that directly block the redesigns contemplated in the *Chasm* report. The three largest obstacles are opposition to transparency, customization, and authentic patient control over care.

To be transparent and open about results, PGPs would have to overcome their own fears of public disclosure, embarrassment, and "bad press" about less than ideal care. They would do so only if they became convinced, as most are not yet, that the bright side of transparency is "learning."

To customize care would require a much deeper respect for the variability in legitimate patient needs than many American care systems now evince. Instead of asking patients how they want their care to go, American health care organizations are generally more comfortable informing patients of the standard rules and procedures to which patients must conform.

To give patients firm control over their own care requires a level of trust and risk taking that the health care system has trouble accepting. The first step toward this, as specifically articulated in the *Chasm* report, would be to offer patients "unfettered access" to their own medical records. Yet very few organizations of any type do this. They may say they do, but the fetters are all too evident.

Waste

Like much of American health care, prepaid groups still seem not to believe that the levels of waste in their own care are as high as the *Chasm* report implies they are. Perhaps they simply do not see the waste. Perhaps they regard the payoff of waste reduction as too small or remote in time. Perhaps it is politically or managerially inconvenient for their leaders to suggest that the waste exists. Or maybe they do not have strong ideas about how, through redesign and "lean production" methods, they could remove the waste without damaging their own providers and patients.

Culture of Blame

When they experience or identify defects in care, prepaid group practices are as likely as any other health care organizations to cast blame on their own patients—their customers. Some continue to attribute high costs, overuse, or waste to unrealistic patient expectations or high demands. Some build high fences around all patients because they can imagine problems with some patients ("We cannot give patients their medical records because some patients would become very worried and have no way to handle their concerns. . . ."). The most creative PGPs recognize that the patients' expectations are largely of the group's own making and that systematic efforts can change expectations just as surely as unsystematic miscommunication created them in the first place.

Information Technology Issues

Prepaid groups are encountering major hurdles in developing information systems. They, like all others, lack confidence that standards will be stable for coding and interfacing. They must deal with multiple, cacophonous vendors of software and hardware, making investments risky and incompatibility a constant threat. And the nonprofit groups especially may lack sufficient access to capital.

"Managed Care" Backlash

The alleged failure of "managed care" continues, by reputation, to plague the most ambitious of the prepaid group practice quality agendas, which proceed from the understanding that "managing care" is the only way to give patients and families what they truly need. Yet PGPs' every move is suspect, including efforts to standardize according to science, to try to reduce wasteful and risky overuse, to help patients and their loved ones become more self-sufficient and skilled in self-care, to keep people from unnecessary hospital days that put them at risk and drain their energies, to rationalize pharmaceutical testing and diagnostic imaging, to insist on evidence before promoting invasive care, to innovate in the workforce so that the best people do the best jobs, and to improve safety by supporting disclosure. Each of these steps and more toward rational, customized, dignified, safe, responsive, transparent care can be interpreted, wrongly but convincingly, as withholding, controlling, stingy, unprofessional, or otherwise wrong. Sadly, many and skilled are the forces who want nothing more than to convince America's patients and families that the last thing they should want is change.

Leadership Void

Finally, prepaid group practices are experiencing a leadership gap. Leading these changes in health care in small or large organizations is a daunting job, and health care has underinvested substantially in helping leaders build their skills and experience in mastering organizational change. Until recently, management and leadership roles in PGPs have often been sidebar assignments or assumed to be within the skill base of clinicians automatically, even if they had had no training in executive leadership and management. That is changing fast, but the gap is still large, and therefore the pool of skilled managers—clinical and nonclinical—remains too small for our needs.

The Future: Meeting the Leadership Challenge

Far from a disappointment, the sector of "managed care" represented by progressive prepaid group practice provides one of the brightest hopes for the leadership of needed changes in American health care, such as those described in the

Chasm report. To maximize delivery on that promise, PGPs that seek to lead will have to assure their continuing investment in innovation. They will do this best in a spirit of openness, not just because transparency is the right rule but also because it gives them the best chance of learning from one another.

Not all prepaid group practices will be up to the challenge, but leadership of change does not require them all. It requires only that a sufficient minority of prepaid groups self-consciously become a vanguard, a movement for change, not unlike the initial wave of bold, exciting changes that the original, classical PGP HMOs—the Kaiser Permanentes, Group Health Cooperatives, and Harvard Community Health Plans—brought into health care in the middle of the twentieth century. Their appearance brought discomfort for the medical mainstream, but it meant enduring and still-persistent benefit for millions of patients.

That vanguard will have to pursue its agenda in daylight, to build trust and to speed learning. It would do best to treat improvement knowledge as a public good, relying on reputation and success, not intellectual property rights, to yield local advantage.

Changing the policy environment is not absolutely essential to this leadership role, but it certainly would help. Perhaps somewhere there is a state (or maybe the Centers for Medicare and Medicaid Services would like to try) where optimism about integrated health care is great enough that the following circumstances could emerge, at least for a while, to give the forces of productive change a shot in the arm:

- Expanding opportunities to consolidate budgets for the care of populations rather than continuing to pay for events. The larger the boundary around that consolidated budget, the greater the potential for improving care.
- Introducing a no-fault compensation system for injuries to patients, with enterprise liability, on a temporary basis, with rules of immediate disclosure to patients, apology, compensation, and learning.
- Supporting changes in curricula for medical students and residents, centered on the new care design and with training experiences in the prepaid group practices.
- System-level performance measures, openly shared and actively used to stimulate learning.
- A well-supported program for leadership development.
- An investment in a computerized medical record system, offered at no cost in the public domain and suitable for a small office as well as for a large prepaid group practice.
- At the national level, decisions on a small but necessary set of information technology standards for coding and interfacing.

The most important change that would improve the adoption of prepaid group practice lies in a cultural transformation in which health care consumers begin to think of health care quality as more than just provider choice. Over the course of the past decade, much of the managed care backlash has centered on the fact that managed care organizations often limit choice of providers.[22] Accordingly, there has been a logical (yet misguided) public tendency to equate health care quality with choice. This is well illustrated in the discussion surrounding the patient's bill of rights, where choice was defined as the foremost quality issue.

This relatively shallow approach to defining quality has hindered a more complex and useful approach to defining quality that includes the benefits of integrated and coordinated care delivery systems. Often these benefits are most easily obtained when choice is restricted. For prepaid group practices to achieve greater acceptance, there must be a simultaneous transformation in how the public defines quality; the current definition seems to oppose the PGP, not support it. Advocates for prepaid group practice must be able to convincingly align the PGP mode of operation with the more expansive notion of quality described in the *Chasm* report.

Since the public has expectations of unfettered choice based on the fee-for-service insurance model's long history, a change in public opinion will be gradual. A more plausible, short-term approach will be not to rely on a change in public attitudes but for PGPs to employ a strategy of attraction.

In response to patient expectations of choice, PGPs should allow patients to opt out of the group for their care, as in a preferred provider organization, while simultaneously educating patients about the high quality of care that remaining in the integrated system affords. In this way, the PGP can preserve the patient's expectation that he has the right to choose his doctor, all the while pursuing the fundamental change in attitudes that needs to take place.

Conclusion

Health care has been called the nation's most complicated industry. This characterization has historically been attributed to the complexity of the associated bioscience and the truism that "no two patients are ever alike." More recently, we have been attributing this to the extraordinary web of regulation, paperwork, and administration with which most health care providers grapple. The complexity of multiple insurance companies, multiple plans, different formularies, and even more methods of compensation creates a difficult environment in which to function, for patients and doctors alike.

The prepaid group practice has tremendous potential to simplify the work of everyone involved. The economies of scale associated with practicing in a multi-specialty group practice have meant that many patient care and administrative functions that might be shared by all members of the staff of less integrated health care organizations can be specialized. Patients interact with a common administrative body with common regulations and a well-developed infrastructure through which providers can communicate about their care. A large practice group has more opportunities to consolidate costs and greater freedom to pursue integration across practice styles. It is this consolidation and associated coordination that ensures care that is high in value and quality.

Notes

1. Institute of Medicine, *Crossing the Quality Chasm: A New Health System for the 21st Century* (Washington; D.C.: National Academy Press, 2001).
2. Institute of Medicine, *To Err Is Human: Building a Safer Health System* (Washington, D.C.: National Academy Press, 2000); ibid.
3. E. Hunkeler and others, "Efficacy of Nurse Telehealthcare and Peer Support in Augmenting Treatment of Depression in Primary Care," *Archives of Family Medicine*, 2000, *9*, 700–708.
4. T. Bodenheimer, E. H. Wagner, and K. Grumbach, "Improving Primary Care for Patients with Chronic Illness," *Journal of the American Medical Association*, 2002, *288*, 1775–1779.
5. A. J. Karter, "Self-Monitoring of Blood Glucose: Language and Financial Barriers in a Managed Care Population with Diabetes," *Diabetes Care*, 2000, *23*, 477–483.
6. C. Sadur and others, "Diabetes Management in a Health Maintenance Organization: Efficacy of Care Management Using Cluster Visits," *Diabetes Care*, 1999, *22*, 2011–2017.
7. D. L. Frosch, R. M. Kaplan, and V. Felitti, "The Evaluation of Two Methods to Facilitate Shared Decision Making for Men Considering the Prostate Specific Antigen Test," *Journal of General Internal Medicine*, 2001, *16*, 391–398; P. H. Barrett, "Treatment Decisions About Lumbar Herniated Disk in a Shared Decision-Making Program," *Joint Commission Journal of Quality Improvement*, 2002, *28*, 211–219.
8. HealthPartners, "Learn About Board Elections," 2003 [http://www.healthpartners.com].
9. Group Health Cooperative, "Leadership," 2003 [http://www.ghc.org/about_gh/leadership/index.jhtml].
10. W. T. Dodge and others, "Enhancing Primary Care HIV Prevention: A Comprehensive Clinical Intervention," *American Journal of Preventive Medicine*, 2001, *20*, 177–183; J. Bluespruce and others, "HIV Prevention in Primary Care: Impact of a Clinical Intervention," *AIDS Patient Care and STDs*, 2001, *15*, 243–253.
11. Y. C. Ulrich and others, "Medical Care Utilization Patterns in Women with Diagnosed Domestic Violence," *American Journal of Preventive Medicine*, 2003, *24*, 9–15.
12. R. L. Davis and others, "Impact of the Change in Polio Vaccination Schedule on Immunization Coverage Rates: A Study in Two Large Health Maintenance Organizations," *Pediatrics*, 2001, *107*, 671–676.
13. J. R. Heget, J. P. Bagian, C. Z. Lee, and J. W. Gosbee, "John M. Eisenberg Patient Safety Awards: System Innovation: Veterans Health Administration National Center for Patient

Safety," *Joint Commission Journal of Quality Improvement,* 2002, *28*(12), accessed online, Nov. 19, 2003 [http://www.jcrinc.com/subscribers/journal.asp?durki=3629&site=14& return=1535].

14. T. W. Nolan, M. W. Schall, D. M. Berwick, and J. Roessner, *Reducing Delays and Waiting Times Throughout the Health Care System* (Boston: Institute for Healthcare Improvement, 1996).

15. S. Krizman, "Kaiser Permanente Shows Growth, Financial Stability in 2001," Feb. 28, 2002 [http://www.kp.org/locations/colorado/newsroom/releases/co022802.html].

16. A. M. Garber and N. A. Solomon, "Cost-Effectiveness of Alternative Test Strategies for the Diagnosis of Coronary Artery Disease," *Annals of Internal Medicine,* 1999, *130,* 719–728.

17. K. Grumbach and others, "Primary Care Physicians' Experience of Financial Incentives in Managed-Care Systems," *New England Journal of Medicine,* 1998, *339*(21), 1519.

18. E. L. Chehab and others, "The Impact of Practice Setting on Physician Perceptions of the Quality of Practice and Patient Care in the Managed Care Era," *Archives of Internal Medicine,* 2001, *161*(2), 202.

19. Ibid., p. 205.

20. B. Hayon, "Marriage Between Nation's Largest Health Care Group and Most Advanced Technology to Revolutionize Health Care," press release, Kaiser Permanente, Feb. 4, 2003 [http://www.kaiserpermanente.org/newsroom/releases/020403.html].

21. G. J. Langley and others, *The Improvement Guide: A Practical Approach to Enhancing Organizational Performance* (San Francisco: Jossey-Bass, 1996).

22. D. Stone, "Managed Care and the Second Great Transformation," *Journal of Health Politics, Policy and Law,* 1999, *24,* 1213–1219.

CHAPTER THREE

THE CLINICAL AND ECONOMIC PERFORMANCE OF PREPAID GROUP PRACTICE

Kenneth H. Chuang, Harold S. Luft, and R. Adams Dudley

The first two chapters in this volume documented deficiencies endemic in the United States health care system. A telltale sign of these deficiencies is the tremendous variation in quality of care from one provider organization to the next. These variations are substantial enough to be observed even across large geographical regions of the country.[1]

There are also potentially important variations in the structure and organization of care in the United States. Organized forms of care have become the norm in some parts of the nation but not others,[2] and the forms that exist vary from small group practices with no hospital affiliation or rural hospitals without official connections to any providers to large integrated delivery systems that include physicians in almost every specialty and other types of practitioners, hospitals, and home health organizations.

Some investigators have asked whether the structure and organization of care influence quality and whether dissemination of such structural changes could improve quality. Increasingly, policymakers want to know what they can do to improve care.[3] The Institute of Medicine (IOM) has argued that greater integration of care is needed.[4] This chapter reviews the evidence that prepaid group practices (PGPs) provide better care than indemnity insurance with no attempt

Kenneth Chuang's work on this chapter was supported by the Veterans Affairs Quality Scholars program.

to organize care, also known as fee-for-service, or than other forms of managed care (nongroup managed care organizations, or "carrier HMOs").

An important finding is that relatively little is known about the performance of PGPs, primarily because most prior research does not distinguish between PGPs and other types of HMOs. However, based on the available data, PGPs do seem to deliver preventive services more often and have lower utilization and costs than other plans but also have lower patient satisfaction.

Conceptual Model: Prepaid Group Practice Versus Other Types of Care Delivery

Prepaid group practices differ not only from the fee-for-service (FFS) model of care delivery but also from other forms of "managed care."

Prepaid Group Practice Versus Fee-for-Service

Several characteristics that distinguish PGPs from fee-for-service might be expected to improve care (see Exhibit 3.1). The first of these is the prepayment mechanism itself. Prepaid group practices have more information about the upcoming year's budget than do organizations that receive payments based on care provided. This

EXHIBIT 3.1. CHARACTERISTICS OF PREPAID GROUP PRACTICE THAT MAY CONTRIBUTE TO IMPROVED QUALITY RELATIVE TO FEE-FOR-SERVICE.

Prepayment for a defined population creates budgetary certainty at the start of each planning period and:

- May facilitate investments needed to reorganize care
- Creates a financial incentive to optimize care
- Encourages a population focus and responsibility that could justify outreach from plan to enrollees

Group practice integrates care across multiple specialties and settings and:

- Can spread the cost of improvement over a larger population of providers and patients
- Can consider novel arrangements for professional teams
- Allows benefits from shared governance
- Allows access to clinical data across care sites and providers
- Can adjust the supply of providers to match expected demand

Cultural insulation allows a more internal focus on processes to demonstrate improved overall quality and effectiveness, rather than a focus on performance of individual clinical specialties and expectations.

knowledge may facilitate the planning of investments needed to improve care or provide the opportunity to reorganize care for maximum efficiency and quality. The fixed budget also gives the PGP, relative to FFS providers, a financial incentive to provide optimal initial treatment of a medical problem (for example, education for asthmatics as outpatients to avoid future unnecessary hospitalizations). Similarly, in established patients, investments in primary or preventive care may pay off as reduced health care needs in the future (a penalty in FFS). In addition, the population focus created by prepayment could lead to more of the outreach from plan to enrollees that the IOM says is necessary (for example, bringing enrollees in for screening or early treatment).[5]

One might argue that large fee-for-service multispecialty clinics or faculty practice plans could roughly estimate their revenues and expenses for the next year in much the same way as a PGP can. However, the fact that revenues in such settings are tied to services rendered by specific specialties and departments places an enormous hurdle in the way of resource allocation. Thus it may not be that physicians in the PGP are more effective at making the case for prevention than clinicians in a FFS setting but rather that they do not have to contend with the internal politics of wresting revenue from the "profitable units" to support less profitable services, such as preventive visits.

The structure of group practice may also create opportunities to improve care through integrated decision making and to offer services that usually are not feasible in fee-for-service. Scale alone could be an important issue. Investments in process change could benefit larger populations of providers and patients than is possible in FFS. This is particularly true because some PGPs have integrated medical groups with hospitals and home care providers. This integration allows for novel arrangements of care, both between physicians and allied health providers and among groups of physicians. In PGPs, for instance, a pulmonologist might teach primary care physicians how to take better care of asthma patients so that unnecessary specialist visits are avoided. In contrast, under an FFS arrangement, the pulmonologist would have no incentive to reduce the number of referrals from primary care physicians (whether necessary or not) because more referrals result in more revenues.

The group practice form also incorporates shared governance across specialties so that decision making can be brought to a higher level than isolated departments focusing on their own expertise and budgets. This may increase the probability that the larger investment pool will encourage decisions that lead to novel or efficient arrangements. Finally, integration across providers and sites of care means that the group can share clinical data about a patient across sites without having to deal with legal concerns about sharing data with an outside organization.

Prepaid group practice may also benefit from cultural insulation. That is, to the extent that a PGP is large enough to provide its clinicians with an internal peer support group, it may be easier to institute cultural or process change within the organization. For instance, a PGP may more readily implement a new clinical practice guideline than an academic institution or a fee-for-service private practice because the PGP physicians benefit from shared governance and are motivated by a population focus rather than an individual patient focus. Even if a small FFS group decided to implement a practice style that encouraged prevention and discouraged high-tech interventions, its clinicians would always have to "explain themselves" and be on the defensive when meeting their professional colleagues. The history of PGPs being attacked by organized medicine for allegedly providing poor quality of care may have led to a sense among PGPs that they are outsiders and must prove themselves and the quality of their care. This attitude may engender greater willingness to accept the changes needed to excel. The central management mechanism of the PGP allows it to limit the influence of other parties whose goals it does not share. For example, a PGP may be able to force all direct pharmaceutical marketing efforts to be funneled through a pharmacy and therapeutics committee (see Chapter Six).

Prepaid Group Practice Versus Other Forms of Managed Care

Several characteristics distinguish prepaid group practice from other forms of managed care, specifically carrier HMOs (see Exhibit 3.2). Prepaid group practice usually involves significant clinical integration across the spectrum of physician care. In contrast, carrier HMOs cannot plan for the allocation of resources across types of care and therefore have limited opportunities for innovation. For example, carrier HMOs typically have physicians who are still actively engaged

---

EXHIBIT 3.2. CHARACTERISTICS OF PREPAID GROUP PRACTICE THAT MAY CONTRIBUTE TO IMPROVED QUALITY RELATIVE TO CARRIER HMOS.

- **Greater integration** across specialties and sites of care, allowing flexibility about reorganization
- **More complete "capture" of providers,** allowing greater goal congruence and consistency of incentives and potentially decreasing conflict among clinical protocols
- **Larger scale**
- **Stable enrollee population**

---

in both capitated and FFS practice and thus encounter multiple and perhaps conflicting incentive arrangements. Even when the incentives between plan and
provider are aligned, the providers often see patients from many different HMOs,
which may all have different protocols. In practice, PGPs have typically had very
tight affiliations with hospitals. This gives PGPs both the flexibility to reorganize
care across the full spectrum of providers and clinical sites and to spread investments across a large number of providers. Such close relationships with hospitals
are not often found in carrier HMOs.

Because prepaid group practice, by its nature as a closed network, requires
patients to change physicians to enroll (and again if they disenroll), after the first
one to two years, continuing enrollees are far more likely to stay members than is
the case for other HMOs.[6] Thus PGPs generally retain members longer than
carrier HMOs do, giving providers more reason to believe that long-term investments might pay off. For example, Kaiser Permanente has actively pursued screening for colorectal cancer by sigmoidoscopy among its members even though its
own cost-benefit analyses showed that the technology only begins to reduce
expenditures after ten years of enrollment.

Factors Mitigating Actual and Measured Prepaid Group Practice Performance

While there are theoretical reasons to believe prepaid group practice may be able
to outperform fee-for-service medicine and carrier HMOs, there are also practical realities that may reduce the impact of the structural characteristics that favor
PGPs (see Exhibit 3.3). These include factors that may affect both the actual
performance of PGPs, as well as their measured performance (in other words,
their ability to demonstrate superior performance given measurement tools and
methods available).

Actual PGP Performance

Although there is less turnover in PGPs than in other types of plans, enrollee
turnover still exists and can reduce the return on any investment. Turnover may
influence PGPs' willingness to make the long-term commitments one would otherwise hope for but could also result in patterns that decrease apparent (but not
necessarily actual) quality. For example, if new PGP enrollees with hypertension
have worse blood pressure control than longtime members, a cross-sectional
analysis of blood pressure might underestimate the impact of PGP efforts to improve quality.

EXHIBIT 3.3. POTENTIAL FACTORS MITIGATING REALIZATION OF PREPAID GROUP PRACTICE PERFORMANCE POTENTIAL.

- **More complete "capture" of providers:**
  Potential tension around clinician autonomy versus shared governance and central decision making

- **Measurement of performance:**
  No incentive for performance documentation

  Selected population effect of plan choice on satisfaction

  Spillover of PGP performance into local system

- **Larger scale:**
  Economies of scale still may not be enough to overcome costs of implementation of new technologies

  One standard of care for all patients can lead to diseconomies of scale

- **Relatively stable enrollee population**

- **Spread of PGP from original site**

In addition, the extent to which the benefits of administrative and financial integration in a PGP actually translate into better performance may depend on the degree to which the medical group feels it is working in concert with its partner health plan (for example, the extent to which the Permanente Medical Group physicians believe they can trust Kaiser Foundation Health Plan to work for the patients' best interests). If there is distrust of centralized decision making (a common finding in U.S. political systems), clinicians may be unwilling to give up their individual autonomy to achieve group goals.

The greater scale of most PGPs (relative to provider organizations under FFS arrangements and carrier HMOs) may still be insufficient to reduce the per-member costs of some investments to low enough levels to allow PGPs to pursue change. For instance, although the potential to use electronic medical records to eliminate duplication of tests and improve communication has been obvious for years, the costs were such that even the largest PGP, Kaiser Permanente, did not develop an electronic information system until the mid-1990s. Many other PGPs are further behind.

Conversely, the scale of some PGPs may be so large as to create managerial diseconomies. Very large organizations may find it especially difficult to respond to the rapid technological changes occurring in medicine. When an organization feels that it needs to offer comparable care to everyone, decisions about making practice changes may be time-consuming due to the scale on which the changes must be implemented. Furthermore, the organizational separation between health plans and medical groups required by some states results in a dual governance structure, which, again, may slow decision making.

Measured PGP Performance

In addition to the possibility that PGPs may not live up to theorists' expectations for their performance, inadequate measurement may reduce their ability to demonstrate superior performance. For example, in the assessment of influenza vaccination rates, fee-for-service providers are paid only if they can prove they have given the vaccine. As a result, they have reason to ensure that vaccine administration is documented in clinical and, especially, administrative data. Prepaid providers have no such incentive to document procedures. Despite having provided the vaccine, prepaid providers may not take the time to write it down because it does not affect their finances, leading to a reporting bias. Thus documentation alone may lead to imprecise quality measurement in some cases.

Finally, studies have shown that trends in HMO care can influence local standards of practice, even outside the HMO. For instance, Laurence Baker showed that increased HMO market share can lead to decreased Medicare expenditures and overall plan costs.[7] Paul Heidenreich and his colleagues showed that areas with greater HMO penetration had better delivery of beta-blockers and aspirin following a heart attack and had slightly lower rates of utilization of angiography and reperfusion surgery than areas with lower HMO penetration.[8] Most assessments of HMO versus fee-for-service care come from geographically defined databases (for example, state hospital discharge databases), so it may be that spillover effects reduce the measured impact of HMOs on quality or efficiency of care. That is, if HMOs improved quality and these new practice patterns disseminated rapidly, comparisons between HMOs and FFS could consistently show no difference.

Other Confounding Issues

Several additional factors may confound analyses of prepaid group practice performance relative to other types of plans, although the direction of the resulting bias is not clear. For instance, patients who enroll in PGPs know that they are accepting some limitation on their choice of providers relative to other types of plans. Is it possible, then, that there are inherent differences in the personality traits of PGP enrollees relative to other plans? There is some evidence to support such a difference. One study found that enrollees who are "somewhat dissatisfied" or "very dissatisfied" with care are less likely to leave a PGP than enrollees who are similarly unhappy but are members of a FFS or carrier-model plan.[9] This may reflect the fact that disenrollment from a PGP almost always means changing providers, whereas FFS and carrier HMO members can often change plans without changing providers. This phenomenon may also be a function of the type of patient who chooses a PGP. If there are differences in enrolled populations, how will that influence apparent quality?

In addition, historically, PGPs have grown from a founding site, illustrated, for example, in Kaiser Permanente's expansion from its West Coast birthplace. However, much of the research comparing PGPs to other models of care delivery focuses on the care provided in the original PGP sites. Continuing with the Kaiser Permanente example, most of the comparative research comes from the Northern California and Northwest regions. Much less is known about the care provided when Kaiser Permanente expanded to the East Coast and Hawaii. It is possible that care differs in these locations and that the measured performance of PGPs is biased or incomplete if it includes only the original sites.

Comparing the Performance of PGPs, Carrier HMOs, and Fee-for-Service: Methods and Results

Several studies synthesize the literature comparing HMOs (in general) to fee-for-service.[10] Rather than repeat those studies, we used them as primary sources for the general HMO-to-FFS comparison.

To identify literature comparing PGPs specifically to other plans (both FFS and managed care plans), we performed a search of the English-language literature, limiting the search to studies of U.S. health plans. Since such articles are often poorly indexed, we conducted a broader Medline search, using a number of keywords.[11]

We also searched by hand *Health Affairs, Health Services Research, Inquiry,* the *Journal of the American Medical Association,* and *Medical Care.* As a last step, we reviewed the references of all articles pulled.

Unfortunately, there is little literature comparing prepaid group practice specifically to other types of plans. Many more studies compare HMOs or managed care in general to fee-for-service, but few of these disaggregate HMOs by type.

HMOs and Fee-for-Service

The general comparisons of HMOs to fee-for-service show little difference in actual clinical performance.[12] In general, HMOs have slightly lower patient satisfaction, although these studies were not corrected for patients' freedom of choice across plans.[13] The only other differences are in *clinical performance*—HMOs provide better preventive care and FFS plans more home care.[14] HMOs do, however, appear to reduce utilization without reducing quality.[15]

Prepaid Group Practice and Other Types of Plans: Clinical Practice and Patient Satisfaction

The initial Medline search yielded 1,146 abstracts, which were reviewed for likely relevance. Of these, 208 were identified for full text review. Only 22 studies compared clinical performance in prepaid group practice specifically to fee-for-service. Each study could have more than one dependent variable measured, and therefore we made 108 comparisons of PGPs to FFS from these 22 studies. Only one study compared PGP to carrier HMO performance, and it included three comparisons.

Prepaid Group Practice and Fee-for-Service. The available literature shows a spread of results for patient satisfaction, processes of care (for example, prescription of antihypertensive medications to patients with elevated blood pressure), intermediate outcomes (for example, blood pressure control), and outcomes (for example, stroke or mortality from hypertension). Table 3.1 shows the distribution of the findings in these domains in five categories:[16]

- PGP performs statistically significantly better than FFS ($p < .05$).
- PGP performs more than 5 percent better than FFS, but the difference is not statistically significant.
- PGP and FFS performance results are not significantly different (and the absolute value of the difference is within 5 percent).
- PGP performs more than 5 percent worse than FFS, but the difference is not statistically significant.
- PGP performs statistically significantly worse than FFS ($p < .05$).

As the table shows, there is no unequivocally consistent pattern except that PGPs provide better preventive care. There may be a slight tendency for PGPs to have better processes of care and FFS plans to have better patient satisfaction.

Prepaid Group Practice and Carrier HMOs. Only one paper specifically compared PGPs to carrier HMOs.[17] Nancy Miller found one process and one outcome measure in which PGP performance was better (statistically significant)

TABLE 3.1. PERFORMANCE OF PREPAID GROUP PRACTICE VERSUS FEE-FOR-SERVICE HEALTH PLANS.

Domain	Measure	PGP Better (statistically significant)	PGP Better (not statistically significant)	No Difference Between PGP and FFS	FFS Better (not statistically significant)	FFS Better (statistically significant)
Processes of care	Number of comparisons	6	5	5	1	2
	Number of studies	5	2	3	1	2
Preventive care	Number of comparisons	15	3	4	0	0
	Number of studies	4	2	2	0	0
Patient satisfaction	Number of comparisons	3	5	5	15	13
	Number of studies	2	1	1	4	5
Clinical outcomes	Number of comparisons	1	10	11	4	1
	Number of studies	1	4	7	2	1
Summary[a]	**Number of comparisons**	**25**	**23**	**25**	**20**	**16**
	Number of studies	**12**	**7**	**12**	**7**	**8**

[a] Summary number of studies may not equal sum of individual categories due to multiple outcomes (preventive and satisfaction) within a study.

than carrier HMOs and one outcome for which PGPs were worse (not statistically significant).

Prepaid Group Practice and Other Types of Plans: Costs of Care

No papers compared actual costs within a PGP to costs within another plan type. Three papers compared an imputed cost to the health system based on utilization of resources (defined as hospitalizations or number of ambulatory visits). Costs were imputed based on the average cost of a visit or hospitalization within a particular geographical area and thus may not be equal to the actual savings realized within the system. Given those caveats, all three studies showed that costs were about 25 percent lower in PGPs than in other types of plans. However, other studies have shown that hospital utilization in large multispecialty group practices such as the Mayo Clinic and the Palo Alto Medical Clinic is similar to that in PGPs. Thus the lower utilization and imputed costs may reflect integration of the delivery system more than a specific physician payment mechanism.[18]

Conclusions

The clearest thing that can be said is that relatively little is known about the performance of prepaid group practices. PGPs seem to deliver preventive services more often and have lower patient satisfaction but also lower costs and utilization than their counterparts. However, the literature does not demonstrate that they add significantly to the quality of processes of care or to patient outcomes. On the other hand, there is no evidence that they are the major threats to quality that their early detractors claimed.

To a substantial extent, the lack of evidence in either direction is due to the fact that there is not a large literature that addresses this question. In part, this may reflect the reliance on data sources that do not disaggregate prepaid group practice from other types of HMOs. Since there is a theoretical rationale to believe that HMOs that are more integrated can achieve better performance, further research aimed at distinguishing the relative performance of different forms of HMOs versus each other and versus fee-for-service may show that PGPs do outperform other types of plans.

There may also be more that can be learned from the unpublished literature, which could be unpublished for a variety of reasons. For example, most PGPs are not academically oriented and may not have the resources or incentives to pursue publication. In fact, at the meetings during which this book was developed, several participants mentioned findings that suggest better results have recently been documented for PGPs but not published. These include suggestions that PGPs have better HEDIS scores than the National Committee for Quality Assurance average and can be more successful at reducing smoking rates. These findings suggest the need for ongoing evaluation of PGP performance versus other types of plans.

Another possibility is that PGPs' theoretical advantages will take some time to manifest themselves in superior performance such that research in the future will show more quality benefit than has research to date. This could be the case for several reasons, the most important of which are the slow development of consensus about quality indicators and the fact that PGPs are not isolated from other forms of care and must compete with them. With respect to quality indicators, only recently has agreement about how to measure quality reached the point where the Joint Commission on the Accreditation of Healthcare Organizations and the National Committee for Quality Assurance have added a significant number of clinical measures to their standards. Therefore, until recently, it may have been difficult for PGP managers to know where to focus their resources and attention to achieve the benefits of integration. As the clinical community comes to more agreement about the definition and measurement of quality, PGPs may now be more able to leverage their organizational advantages to achieve superior performance.

There may also be an issue of what aspects of clinical performance are chosen for study. Historically, quality measures have been selected for development and study based primarily on issues of feasibility, with a focus on indicators that can be derived from administrative data (such as vaccinations) or tied in a simple way to a clinical event (such as aspirin use after myocardial infarction, or MI). It may be that more sophisticated or more complicated quality measures that capture aspects of integration are needed to understand the relative contribution of PGPs to quality. For example, most assessments of health plan performance focus on the outpatient arena, whereas few evaluations of hospital care have included type of plan as a predictor variable. Perhaps close connections between primary care physicians and those who manage most inpatient care lead to superior inpatient processes, but this has not been examined. Similarly, one might expect integration to lead to higher levels of appropriateness for surgery or other procedures. Measures that assess follow-up of patients after events usually managed by specialists (for example, MI or gastrointestinal bleeding) also might reflect benefits of integration if primary care physicians in PGPs are more aware of and able to carry out postevent management guidelines. For instance, one might assess long-term management of patients after MI (what proportion are on anticholesterol therapy or in a smoking cessation program six months post-MI?)

or cirrhotics who have a variceal bleed (what proportion are on beta-blockers six months after their hemorrhage?). Finally, as the population ages, it will be important to be able to assess how plans handle patients with multiple chronic conditions. Prepaid group practice may have a special advantage in this area because of its capacity to create links among specialists and between primary care physicians and specialists.

In terms of competing with other forms of care, most prepaid group practices are still working to establish and justify their place in the system. In the absence of research showing superior performance of PGPs, both providers and patients may have resisted the restriction of choice that participating in a PGP usually implies. Having to address and overcome these hurdles may also have taken some PGP management attention away from maximizing the benefits of integration. For example, if a PGP is competing for providers with systems or clinical practices that offer more autonomy, this may make PGP managers more reluctant to use the central decision-making mechanisms that would allow them to integrate care. As PGPs become more accepted—a change that may accelerate now that other plans are raising the costs of choice by raising patient copayments—PGPs may find it easier to integrate and reorganize care to optimize quality.

Without clear outcome measures, PGPs may be hesitant to alter the processes of care in ways that are contrary to the conventional clinical wisdom, especially if it might appear that such changes are designed to save money rather than to improve quality. For example, if a PGP were to reduce its use of revascularization immediately after heart attack, this might appear to be an effort to control costs at the expense of quality, even if a protocol of stabilization and then readmission might yield better outcomes.

In general, without appropriate risk adjustment of premiums, HMOs have little incentive to become visibly better if doing so will attract sicker enrollees. Instead, HMOs may focus much of their attention on improving the quality of their service and on increasing patient satisfaction, rather than on clinical quality. Thus even though the potential for improved quality may be present, there may be disincentives to actively pursuing those opportunities.

In summary, there is ample theoretical reason to believe that prepaid group practice can achieve better clinical performance than other types of health plans. However, the evidence available to date neither confirms nor refutes this hypothesis, primarily because there is so little of it. The most important task for future researchers is to separate types of HMOs according to structural characteristics so that policymakers can understand the relative performance of each. There may also be work for PGPs themselves to do to maximize the potential benefits of their organizational forms.

Notes

1. S. F. Jencks and others, "Quality of Medical Care Delivered to Medicare Beneficiaries: A Profile at State and National Levels," *Journal of the American Medical Association,* 2000, *284,* 1670–1676; S. F. Jencks, E. D. Huff, and T. Cuerdon, "Change in the Quality of Care Delivered to Medicare Beneficiaries, 1998–1999 to 2000–2001," *Journal of the American Medical Association,* 2003, *289,* 305–312.

2. R. A. Dudley and H. S. Luft, "Managed Care in Transition," *New England Journal of Medicine,* 2001, *344,* 1087–1092.

3. M. N. Marshall, P. G. Shekelle, S. Leatherman, and R. H. Brook, "Public Disclosure of Performance Data: Learning from the U.S. Experience," *Quality Health Care,* 2000, *9,* 53–57; A. Mehrotra, T. Bodenheimer, and R. A. Dudley, "Employers' Efforts to Measure and Improve Hospital Quality: Determinants of Success," *Health Affairs,* 2003, *22,* 60–71.

4. Institute of Medicine, *Crossing the Quality Chasm: A New Health System for the 21st Century* (Washington, D.C.: National Academy Press, 2001).

5. Ibid.

6. M. Schlesinger, B. G. Druss, and T. Thomas, "No Exit? The Effect of Health Status on Dissatisfaction and Disenrollment from Health Plans," *Health Services Research,* 1999, *34,* 547–576; R. N. Forthofer, J. H. Glasser, and N. Light, "Life Table Analysis of Membership in an HMO Retention," *Journal of Community Health,* 1979, *5,* 46–53.

7. L. C. Baker, "Association of Managed Care Market Share and Health Expenditures for Fee-for-Service Medicare Patients," *Journal of the American Medical Association,* 1999, *281,* 432–437.

8. P. A. Heidenreich, M. McClellan, C. Frances, and L. C. Baker, "The Relation Between Managed Care Market Share and the Treatment of Elderly Fee-for-Service Patients with Myocardial Infarction," *American Journal of Medicine,* 2002, *112,* 176–182.

9. Schlesinger, Druss, and Thomas, "No Exit?"

10. R. H. Miller and H. S. Luft, "Managed Care Plan Performance Since 1980: A Literature Analysis," *Journal of the American Medical Association,* 1994, *271,* 1512–1519; R. H. Miller and H. S. Luft, "HMO Plan Performance Update: An Analysis of the Literature, 1997–2001," *Health Affairs,* 2002, *21,* 63–86; R. A. Dudley, R. H. Miller, T. Y. Korenbrot, and H. S. Luft, "The Impact of Financial Incentives on Quality of Health Care," *Milbank Quarterly,* 1998, *76,* 649–686.

11. Keywords included (managed care) or HMO or (health maintenance organization) or prepaid or (prepaid group practice) or (organized delivery system) AND indemnity or (preferred provider organization) or PPO or PPOs or fee-for-service or (traditional insurance) or (non-HMO) or (regular Medicare) OR (HMO market share) OR (HMO market penetration) OR (managed care market penetration).

12. See note 10.

13. Miller and Luft, "HMO Plan Performance Update."

14. Dudley, Miller, Korenbrot, and Luft, "The Impact of Financial Incentives."

15. Miller and Luft, "Managed Care Plan Performance"; Miller and Luft, "HMO Plan Performance Update."

16. The following studies were used:

    Carey, T. S., and others. "The Outcomes and Costs of Care for Acute Low Back Pain Among Patients Seen by Primary Care Practitioners, Chiropractors, and Orthopedic

Surgeons: The North Carolina Back Pain Project." *New England Journal of Medicine,* 1995, *333,* 913–917.

Cummings, S. R., and others. "Smoking Counseling and Preventive Medicine. A Survey of Internists in Private Practices and a Health Maintenance Organization." *Archives of Internal Medicine,* 1989, *149,* 345–349.

Druss, B. G., Schlesinger, M., Thomas, T., and Allen, H. "Chronic Illness and Plan Satisfaction Under Managed Care." *Health Affairs,* 2000, *19,* 203–209.

Every, N. R., and others. "Resource Utilization in Treatment of Acute Myocardial Infarction: Staff-Model Health Maintenance Organization Versus Fee-for-Service Hospitals: The MITI Investigators. Myocardial Infarction Triage and Intervention." *Journal of the American College of Cardiologists,* 1995, *26,* 401–406.

Gordon, N. P., Rundall, T. G., and Parker, L. "Type of Health Care Coverage and the Likelihood of Being Screened for Cancer." *Medical Care,* 1998, *36,* 636–645.

Hsia, J., and others. "The Importance of Health Insurance as a Determinant of Cancer Screening: Evidence from the Women's Health Initiative." *Preventive Medicine,* 2000, *31,* 261–270.

Lee-Feldstein, A., Feldstein, P. J., Buchmueller, T., and Katterhagen, G. "The Relationship of HMOs, Health Insurance, and Delivery Systems to Breast Cancer Outcomes." *Medical Care,* 2000, *38,* 705–718.

Lubeck, D. P., Brown, B. W., and Holman, H. R. "Chronic Disease and Health System Performance. Care of Osteoarthritis Across Three Health Services." *Medical Care,* 1985, *23,* 266–277.

Manton, K. G., and others. "Social/Health Maintenance Organization and Fee-for-Service Health Outcomes over Time." *Health Care Financial Review,* 1993, *15,* 173–202.

Merrill, R. M., and others. "Survival and Treatment for Colorectal Cancer Medicare Patients in Two Group/Staff Health Maintenance Organizations and the Fee-for-Service Setting." *Medical Care Research Review,* 1999, *56,* 177–196.

Miller, N. A. "An Evaluation of Substance Misuse Treatment Providers Used by an Employee Assistance Program." *International Journal of Addiction,* 1992, *27,* 533–559.

Potosky, A. L., and others. "Prostate Cancer Treatment and Ten-Year Survival Among Group/Staff HMO and Fee-for-Service Medicare Patients." *Health Services Research,* 1999, *34,* 525–546.

Reschovsky, J. D., Kemper, P., and Tu, H. "Does Type of Health Insurance Affect Health Care Use and Assessments of Care Among the Privately Insured?" *Health Services Research,* 2000, *35,* 219–237.

Retchin, S. M., and Brown, B. "The Quality of Ambulatory Care in Medicare Health Maintenance Organizations." *American Journal of Public Health,* 1990, *80,* 411–415.

Rubin, H. R., and others. "Patients' Ratings of Outpatient Visits in Different Practice Settings: Results from the Medical Outcomes Study." *Journal of the American Medical Association,* 1993, *270,* 835–840.

Safran, D. G., Tarlov, A. R., and Rogers, W. H. "Primary Care Performance in Fee-for-Service and Prepaid Health Care Systems: Results from the Medical Outcomes Study." *Journal of the American Medical Association,* 1994, *271,* 1579–1586.

Safran, D. G., and others. "Organizational and Financial Characteristics of Health Plans: Are They Related to Primary Care Performance?" *Archives of Internal Medicine,* 2000, *160,* 69–76.

Schlesinger, M., Druss, B. G., and Thomas, T. "No Exit? The Effect of Health Status on Dissatisfaction and Disenrollment from Health Plans." *Health Services Research,* 1999, *34,* 547–576.

Spetz, J., Smith, M. W., and Ennis, S. F. "Physician Incentives and the Timing of Cesarean Sections: Evidence from California." *Medical Care,* 2001, *39,* 536–550.

Starr, A., and others. "Is Referral Source a Risk Factor for Coronary Surgery? Health Maintenance Organization Versus Fee-for-Service System." *Journal of Thoracic and Cardiovascular Surgery,* 1996, *111,* 708–716; discussion 716–727.

Wells, K. B., and others. "Detection of Depressive Disorder for Patients Receiving Prepaid or Fee-for-Service Care: Results from the Medical Outcomes Study." *Journal of the American Medical Association,* 1989, *262,* 3298–3302.

Yelin, E. H., Criswell, L. A., and Feigenbaum, P. G. "Health Care Utilization and Outcomes Among Persons with Rheumatoid Arthritis in Fee-for-Service and Prepaid Group Practice Settings." *Journal of the American Medical Association,* 1996, *276,* 1048–1053.

17. N. A. Miller, "An Evaluation of Substance Misuse Treatment Providers Used by an Employee Assistance Program," *International Journal of Addiction,* 1992, *27,* 533–559.
18. F. T. Nobrega and others, "Hospital Use in a Fee-for-Service System," *Journal of the American Medical Association,* 1982, *247,* 806–810; A. A. Scitovsky and N. McCall, "Use of Hospital Services Under Two Prepaid Plans," *Medical Care,* 1980, *18,* 30–43.

CHAPTER FOUR

PREPAID GROUP PRACTICE AND HEALTH CARE POLICY

Jon B. Christianson and George Avery

This chapter describes the impact of prepaid group practice (PGP) on health care policy in the United States. Its scope is broad, addressing how the PGP concept has shaped policy and the perspectives of policy entrepreneurs, as well as how it has been used by advocates of particular policy initiatives to further their objectives. For expositional convenience, the discussion is organized around three familiar health policy themes: financial access to medical care, cost containment, and quality. Although these issues overlap in the evolution of U.S. health policy, they represent three distinct policy "regimes" in which PGP has played important but somewhat different roles.[1]

For each of the three themes, we describe the role that PGPs played in promoting or defining policy alternatives, as well as the actions taken by individuals with influence over policymaking who either sought to advance the political interests of PGPs or saw PGPs as central to furthering other political purposes. Because this discussion spans a period from the Great Depression to the present,

Most of the material used in developing this chapter was drawn from published sources. In addition, interview data were collected from participants knowledgeable about various issues discussed in the chapter. We thank our interview respondents for sharing their insights with us. We also thank Robert Crane, Laura Tollen, and Alain Enthoven for their counsel, as well as for their assistance in scheduling some of the interviews, and Robert Berenson for his helpful comments on an earlier draft. Finally, we thank our families for their support.

it necessarily sacrifices depth for breadth of scope. Greater detail is provided where it is essential in understanding the role of PGPs in key policy "regime shifts," but the intent is to paint a broad picture of PGP interest and involvement in U.S. health policy over time.

Overall, we find that the relationship between PGP and public policy has been quite complex—sometimes direct and easily observable, but often indirect and more speculative in nature. We conclude that PGP has played a substantial but generally underappreciated role in the development of U.S. health policy, particularly during periods of changing policy emphasis.

The Health Policy Process: A Conceptual Overview

There is a well-developed literature on the public policy process in general, with health policy frequently offered as an example or a case study.[2] In addition, numerous analyses of specific health policy initiatives have been published.[3] Together, their perspectives on public policymaking are useful in framing the ways in which PGPs and the PGP concept have intersected with the health policy process.

We begin with Anderson's definition of a public policy as a "course of action followed by [governmental bodies and officials] in dealing with a problem or matter of concern."[4] This definition underscores two important points: a policy is different from a discrete "decision," and a policy may consist of doing nothing—maintaining the status quo—in response to a particular demand. The general literature on public policy typically portrays the policy process (or the "policy cycle") as consisting of different stages, with each stage having its own body of research. Rushefsky and Patel, for instance, describe four stages in the cycle: agenda setting, policy formulation and adoption, policy implementation, and policy evaluation.[5] The first stage encompasses how policy issues emerge as part of the political agenda.[6] Intellectuals and other "policy entrepreneurs" can play a key role in this first stage by attracting media attention and establishing credibility for the policy issue.[7] Roberts and King state that the policy entrepreneur is someone who does his or her work without holding a formal position in government,[8] but this is not always a useful distinction in practice because policy entrepreneurs can move into and out of government service with relative ease. A more common role for the policy entrepreneur emerges in the second stage—policy formulation and adoption. When an issue finds a place on the policy agenda, an opportunity is created for policy entrepreneurs to propose "solutions." However, this "policy window" may not stay open long and can close if the policy entrepreneur is not prepared with an alternative that seemingly addresses the issue.[9]

Financial Access to Medical Care

Health policy analysts often point out that the United States is the only industri-alized country without some form of comprehensive, centralized, governmentally financed health insurance. Many argue that this leaves "holes" in America's health insurance system, creating problems of financial access to health care for subsets of the population. The continuing search for a policy "solution" to this problem has taken a variety of turns, with PGPs frequently playing a central role.

PGPs Enter the Health Policy Debate

In 1926, a group of leaders in medicine, public health, and the social sciences met in Washington to discuss perceived problems with the organization and delivery of health services in the United States. Out of this meeting grew the Committee on the Costs of Medical Care, a private sector organization that embarked on a five-year program of research and debate. Although the committee presumed that its primary focus would be on costs, the onset of the Great Depression shifted its attention to financial access to care. The committee concluded that overall expenditures for medical services were probably adequate but that medical care resources were not being allocated effectively.

Among other initiatives, these early health care policy entrepreneurs recom-mended the formation of multispecialty group practices, with associated hospi-tals, for the delivery of health services. These groups would provide complete medical, dental, preventive, and other services for patients in their communities and would be governed by community boards. The patient's primary contact with the group would be through a general practitioner, who would maintain an ongoing relationship with the patient. The committee urged that the groups be organized on a nonprofit basis and in fact argued against for-profit organizational forms. The groups were to receive their revenues through payments made by insurers (with insurance provided by employers or individuals), taxes, or some com-bination of the two. The committee's preference was that individual contributions toward the costs of insurance be set at levels that working families could afford, with government (primarily at the local level) paying the rest, in order to distrib-ute the costs of care across the population.[10] The credibility of this model relied heavily on studies of alternatives to the solo-practice, fee-for-service delivery sys-tem then dominant in the United States. These alternatives included the mili-tary health care system at Fort Benning, Georgia; industrial health care delivery systems established by Endicott-Johnson; and the Ross-Loos medical group practice in Southern California.

A compulsory health insurance program, influenced by the committee's work,[11] was proposed by the Roosevelt administration but withdrawn in the face of heavy opposition from organized medicine. Although it did not result in the immediate enactment of legislation, the committee's work was crucially important for PGPs, for three reasons. First, it argued forcefully for the legitimacy of the PGP model of health care delivery. The quest for legitimacy was to be a major goal of PGPs for several decades, but the committee's "endorsement" provided credibility for PGPs early in that quest. Second, the committee's report linked PGPs to major health care reform in the United States for the first time, establishing a precedent that was to reemerge many times in the half-century that followed. Third, the PGP example, as underscored by the committee, spurred private sector innovation in the financing of American health care.[12]

Henry Kaiser as Policy Entrepreneur

During the Second World War, the PGP concept grew in significance on the national health policy stage. This was largely due to the efforts of an unlikely health policy entrepreneur, the industrialist Henry Kaiser. Kaiser financed a PGP plan created by the physician Sidney Garfield during the late 1930s to provide health care for workers on Kaiser's Grand Coulee Dam project. (The story of the formation of Kaiser Permanente is well known and will not be repeated here.) When Kaiser turned to shipbuilding at the beginning of World War II, he was faced with the problem of how to provide health care to tens of thousands of workers who threatened to overwhelm the capabilities of local health care systems. Garfield responded by establishing a health care arrangement, patterned after the successful Grand Coulee Dam effort, that served workers in Kaiser shipyards on the West Coast.

Kaiser used his considerable influence in Washington, garnered through his key role in the industrial war effort, to overcome local opposition by organized medicine to these arrangements.[13] At the national level, he participated in contentious U.S. Senate hearings in 1942 that pitted the editor of the *Journal of the American Medical Association*, Morris Fishbein, against Garfield and congressional allies over the scope and legitimacy of Kaiser's health care initiative.

Inevitably, Kaiser was drawn into the national health insurance debate during this time and was asked to provide public support for compulsory national health insurance. He rejected this approach, proposing in its place his own national health insurance alternative: "a vast system of prepayment through the place of employment to medical-care organizations operated in conjunction with a physician's group. . . . These organizations would operate in facilities financed by a Federal Health and Housing Agency. . . . The national program would serve

100 million people and cost each member only fifty-eight cents per week. . . . It would employ another 1.8 million health care workers and professionals. To Henry Kaiser, his National Health Plan made such absolute economic and moral sense that he viewed meaningful opposition as impossible."[14]

From a political standpoint, the Kaiser plan did make sense. Positioned between the liberals and the conservatives in the health insurance debate, it appeared to have potential as a "compromise" plan. However, other forces overtook Kaiser's efforts. Support for Kaiser's proposal suffered during the post–World War II period as a result of rising concerns about the power of organized labor and the possible infiltration of labor unions by communists. Organized labor had become a strong supporter of Kaiser Permanente, which may have diminished the appeal of the Kaiser plan to some legislators.

Although Kaiser's plan was not passed, it did have a tangible and immediate impact on health care legislation. Its provisions regarding federal financing for facility construction helped shape the Hill-Burton Act, which funded hospital construction throughout the United States.[15] More important, Kaiser's efforts as a health policy entrepreneur set the stage for much of the policy effort involving PGPs for decades to come. First, it positioned the PGP concept as a "compromise" in the health policy landscape, ground that it was to occupy often in the future.[16] Second, it articulated a vision for health care reform on which many future policy entrepreneurs built their efforts. Third, the visibility and favorable publicity that Kaiser's efforts generated for PGPs helped establish their legitimacy as alternatives to traditional medicine. This was critically important in the judicial battles that PGPs fought with organized medicine over the next forty years. Finally, Kaiser's public policy advocacy provided a platform that was used by PGPs to insert themselves into future health policy discussions, especially discussions around the redesign of the federal employees health care system.

Redefining the Scope of the Financial Access Debate

National health insurance remained on the political agenda with a relatively low profile until 1958, when Social Security amendments were introduced to provide hospital coverage to the elderly.[17] Although the proposal failed, medical care for the elderly became an important issue in the 1960 presidential campaign, and immediately after John F. Kennedy was elected president, work began on drafting a health insurance proposal. At an initial strategy meeting that included Scott Fleming of Kaiser Permanente, sympathy was expressed for a model incorporating PGPs. However, the Department of Health, Education and Welfare (HEW) argued against this approach out of concern for the still formidable opposition of organized medicine to the PGP concept.[18]

Legislation for what later became Medicare failed to pass Congress until after the 1964 election, when it was enacted as a three-part package consisting of Medicare Part A, Part B, and Medicaid. Initial versions of the proposed legislation posed problems for PGPs because PGP members would not be able to file claims under Part B, where payment was based on encounters. Wilbur Cohen, at the time secretary of HEW, was a member of the Group Health Association of Washington, D.C., and a longtime friend of the PGP model. He was sympathetic to this issue but was reluctant to advocate for capitated payments for fear that this would generate opposition from organized medicine to the carefully negotiated legislation. The problem was resolved when Henry Kaiser discussed it with President Johnson at a social event. The president intervened to include a payment option under Part B that preserved, at least in theory, a "place at the table" for PGP under Medicare.[19] However, this option was cumbersome to implement in practice and provided little in the way of incentives for PGPs to participate.

The Battle with Organized Medicine

Even though PGPs had become active participants in the legislative process by the mid-1960s, they continued to battle with organized medicine for survival. The primary weapon used by organized medicine was denial of county medical association membership to PGP physicians, which made it virtually impossible for them to become board certified in some specialties or to gain admitting privileges at some hospitals,[20] thus discouraging physicians from joining or forming PGPs. During the McCarthy era, organized medicine also accused PGPs of being under communist influence and later used control of local health planning bodies to deny PGPs permits to construct facilities.[21] PGPs turned to the courts for relief.

A series of judicial decisions in favor of PGP positions, based on application of existing antitrust law, weakened the ability of organized medicine to impede PGP growth. In 1959, the American Medical Association ended its formal opposition to the PGP concept with the publication of the Larson Report, a document authored by a North Dakota physician sympathetic to the consumer cooperative movement.[22] Nevertheless, some local medical societies continued to oppose PGPs until in 1981 the Supreme Court affirmed a Federal Trade Commission finding that medical society ethical restrictions on advertising and contract practice violated antitrust laws. Although the legal battles waged with organized medicine were crucial to PGPs' survival, the results of these battles had much more far-reaching implications for national health policy.[23] By removing many of the legal protections that organized medicine had enjoyed as a profession, they arguably, and ironically, paved the way for the "corporatization" of medicine.

Controlling Medical Care Costs

Although financial access to medical care has remained an important part of the health policy agenda to the present, the passage of Medicare and Medicaid shifted the focus of the policy debate to the need to control rising medical care costs. Arguments in favor of national health insurance increasingly emphasized the need to control costs as well as ensure financial access. The growing importance of cost control on the policy agenda has been attributed to the fact that Medicare and Medicaid spending competed with other public spending priorities and had implications for tax policy as well.[24] We shall describe how the stressor of increasing costs created an opportunity for a policy proposal that featured PGPs as its cornerstone, furthering the legitimacy of the PGP concept, as well as the concept of choice between PGPs and traditional delivery systems. The foundation for these efforts, however, was established prior to the creation of Medicare and Medicaid in the design of the Federal Employees Health Benefits Plan.

The Federal Employees Health Benefits Plan: A PGP Success

In 1959, the Eisenhower administration proposed a uniform health insurance program for federal employees modeled after the General Electric Association Major Medical Program and managed by a private insurer. This concerned PGPs, as it would have excluded them from participation in the largest national employer group. Also, Kaiser Permanente would have lost about fifty thousand existing members from this group under the administration's proposal. Representatives from Kaiser Permanente (Arthur Weissman and Avram Yedidia) met with Senator Richard Neuberger, chairman of an important Senate subcommittee and a former member of a Kaiser Permanente dual-choice group in Oregon, to present their case.[25] Subsequently, Weissman and Yedidia testified before the senator's committee, arguing for the importance of offering federal employees a choice of plans rather than having a single uniform system.

Kaiser Permanente sent Gibson Kingren, its lobbyist in California, to Washington to head its advocacy effort on this issue. Kingren secured support for a "multiple option plan" among key legislators in the House of Representatives. Scott Fleming, Kaiser's general counsel, provided technical expertise in the drafting of the legislation. In his own words, "I personally drafted the choice-of-plan features of this legislation, and despite numerous proposed amendments, they survived the legislative process virtually intact."[26]

The legislation creating the Federal Employees Health Benefit Plan (FEHBP) was a watershed event for PGPs in the health policy process, for four reasons. First, in the words of Kaiser Permanente's Yedidia, "It was the first time Congress had acted to legitimize the existence of health service programs such as Kaiser's and other prepaid group practice medical programs."[27] Second, the inclusion of "multiple choice" in the program ratified a central tenet of the PGP philosophy, particularly as espoused by Kaiser. Third, the plan provided a "working model" for subsequent proposals that would place prepaid groups squarely in the middle of the debate over cost control for decades. Fourth, participation in the legislative process around passage of the FEHBP provided valuable experience and visibility for Kaiser health plan leaders that they would later use to their advantage.

The FEHBP legislative process also highlighted, for other PGPs, the need for more effective group representation in policy development. Consequently, in 1959, the American Labor Health Association, representing union-sponsored plans, and the Cooperative Health Federation, representing consumer cooperative model PGPs, merged to form the Group Health Association of America. The new organization had no influence on the FEHBP legislation, but from that point forward, it would serve as a vehicle for coordinating PGP participation in the policy process.

PGPs and the Nixon Administration

The late 1960s marked the beginning of an era, extending to the present, in which restraining the rise of health care costs became a major concern, if not the principal concern, of health care policy in the United States. At that time, it was widely accepted that the passage of Medicare and Medicaid had led to "demand pull" inflation for medical care. However, some analysts believed that these programs had simply added to an existing problem. In their view, the fundamental flaws in the system were that providers were paid on a fee-for-service or "cost-plus" basis in an environment of increasingly comprehensive private sector insurance coverage supported by tax incentives.[28]

During the early months of the Nixon administration, growing health care costs were elevated to "crisis" status. A report by the Department of Health, Education and Welfare cited "a crippling inflation in medical costs causing vast increases in government health expenditures for little return, raising private health insurance premiums and reducing the purchasing power of the health dollar of our citizens."[29] In July 1969, President Nixon put cost control at the top of the policy agenda when he stated, "We face a massive crisis in this area, and unless action is taken both administratively and legislatively to meet that crisis within the next two to three years, we will have a breakdown in our medical care system which could have consequences affecting millions of people throughout this country."[30] Even though the Nixon administration was quick to identify rising health care costs as a crisis, it had no policy solution to put forward.[31] Thus a "policy window" was open; there was an "opportunity for advocates of proposals to push their pet solutions."[32]

A policy entrepreneur, Paul Ellwood, who had the beginnings of a solution to the Nixon administration's problem, quickly sought out Kaiser Permanente officials who had worked on the passage of the FEHBP legislation. Fleming's visibility in the FEHBP legislative process had led to an appointment in 1968 to an HEW committee charged with addressing rising health care costs. He was distressed by the committee's conclusions, which emphasized the need to put more "teeth" in the health planning process, and he drafted a strongly worded minority dissent. This dissent came to the attention of Ellwood, a physician from Minneapolis who had personal connections to high-ranking HEW officials that provided him the opportunity to put forward a proposal to solve the health care cost "crisis." As Fleming characterized the meeting with Ellwood, it was "the beginning of the HMO [Health Maintenance Organization] Act. After two or three hours' discussion, we dictated a conceptual outline that was the starting point of the HMO legislation and gave it to Ellwood to use as he wished."[33]

The story of the federal HMO Act of 1974 has been well documented by several authors.[34] In Fleming's opinion, the act turned out to be a decidedly "mixed blessing" for prepaid groups. For example, it established the legitimacy of "foundation" independent practice association (IPA) type plans, lumping them with PGPs under the label "health maintenance organizations." These plans were cheaper to establish than PGPs (construction subsidies for PGP start-ups had been deleted from the legislation) and ultimately grew to dominate the market. However, Kaiser Permanente executives hoped that inclusion of IPAs would increase acceptance of the PGP model, and some PGP representatives expected that over time, the IPAs would evolve toward PGPs in their structure.[35]

Almost from the time of the HMO Act's passage, PGPs began to work to change its provisions. The Group Health Association of America collaborated with the Health Insurance Association of America (which represented indemnity insurers) in support of certain amendments to the act, which were passed in 1975. As part of this process, an amendment to the FEHBP was also passed, requiring the program to offer employees any available federally qualified plan, thereby increasing the access of PGPs to the federal employees group.

In retrospect, the HMO Act virtually ended the debate over the legitimacy of PGPs. In the words of Frank Seubold, director of the federal Office of HMOs in the early 1980s, "When the history books look back on this experience, I suspect that the lasting contribution that they may identify from the government's efforts is the stamp of legitimacy that it placed on prepaid group practice."[36] The act also provided firm support for the principle of multiple choice, long viewed by

PGPs as essential in establishing a level playing field with fee-for-service medicine. However, it also marked the beginning of a two-decade period during which IPA-type plans grew to dominate the managed care market in numbers of providers, enrollment, and arguably, influence in the political process.

Cost Control Meets Financial Access

The HMO Act, still in its early implementation stages, had not cured the problem of rising health care costs at the time the Carter administration assumed office in 1977. Thus the window for policy entrepreneurs remained open. Most new proposals put forward by these entrepreneurs featured federal financing of health insurance coverage in combination with some type of price-setting or budget-setting process. An exception was a proposal developed by Alain Enthoven, a professor at Stanford University and a former colleague at the Department of Defense of Joseph Califano, the HEW secretary during the early years of the Carter administration. As a consultant to HEW, Enthoven developed a national health insurance proposal known as the Consumer-Choice Health Plan (CCHP), which required federal financing but relied on a restructured, competitive health care system to control costs.[37] It was based on four principles: multiple choice among health plans for consumers, a fixed government subsidy toward whatever plan was chosen by the consumer, uniform rules applying to all health plans, and the organization of physicians into "competing economic units."

Enthoven's proposal was clearly in the lineage of Kaiser's National Health Plan, the Federal Employees Health Benefits Plan, and Ellwood's Health Maintenance Strategy.[38] In fact, Enthoven frequently referred to the federal employees plan as a real-world example illustrating the feasibility of the multiple-choice, fixed-contribution provisions of his own plan. However, the role envisioned for PGPs was reduced under Enthoven's plan. In contrast, under Kaiser's plan, the entire American health care system would be restructured into PGPs serving designated areas. Under Ellwood's plan, PGPs would be the cornerstones in a restructured deliver system (financing reform was secondary in Ellwood's proposal). Enthoven positioned his proposal differently.

In advocating for his plan, Enthoven characterized the policy choice as "competition versus regulation," with the CCHP relying on private sector competition to control costs.[39] For this to be effective and for the plan to be implemented on a widespread basis in a timely manner, it would be necessary to quickly establish clusters of competing provider groups. PGPs were expected to be successful participants in the plan, but Enthoven realized that a large number of alternative organizational forms were also needed for his plan to succeed. Nevertheless, Enthoven's proposal was attractive to PGPs because it incorporated two of the critical policy goals that they had pursued since World War II: multiple choice (including PGPs and other plans) and a "fair playing field" for PGPs.

In Enthoven's words, "The Carter administration was internally divided on the competition strategy. . . . President Carter incorporated some of the principles in his proposed National Health Plan. [But] . . . the Carter administration had committed itself early to a regulatory approach as exemplified by the twice-defeated Hospital Cost Containment bill. By the time the CCHP was developed in late 1977, the administration's course had already been set."[40] When Ronald Reagan defeated President Carter, it appeared that Enthoven's plan might have new life. Enthoven has noted that the Report of the Chairman of the Health Policy Advisory Group to President-Elect Ronald Reagan recommended that priority be given to pro-competitive health care legislation.[41] This group also recommended a phased-in Medicare reform patterned after the federal employee plan, a proposal that was strongly supported by PGPs.

Medicare and PGPs

As already noted, PGPs were allowed to participate in the Medicare program, but under a payment approach that provided weak incentives for participation. Actual participation was minimal, and PGPs continued their advocacy for payment reforms. As Iglehart noted in 1982, "The Nixon, Carter, and Reagan administrations have all expressed support for proposals that would encourage HMOs through incentives to enroll more Medicare beneficiaries and for the elderly to seek out such plans, but these efforts have been thwarted by congressional opposition or indifference, by the failure of the DHHS [Department of Health and Human Services] to focus sufficient energies on this policy objective, and by the technical problems that need resolution before sound legislation can be designed."[42]

The Reagan administration proposed a voucher system for Medicare that was patterned very closely after Enthoven's plan. While the voucher system was being debated in Congress, "competition demonstration" programs were launched by the Health Care Financing Administration (HCFA, now the Centers for Medicare and Medicaid Services). These demonstrations offered beneficiaries in a small number of locations a choice of plans, with the plans paid on a prospective, or "risk," basis. Prepaid group plans participated in these programs, including Kaiser Permanente-Northwest, Fallon Community Health Plan in Massachusetts, and Group Health in Minnesota. By 1985, with Republicans in control of the Senate, the main design features of the Medicare "competition demonstration" had been incorporated into a continuing program, providing PGPs with an attractive, risk-based payment option under Medicare for the first time.

For the next dozen years, participation by HMOs (including PGPs) in the Medicare program was highly variable. HMOs expressed a great deal of dissatisfaction with the payment approach, seeking more stable payments with less year-to-year fluctuation.[43] Others, however, suggested that payment reform was needed to address windfall profits allegedly being earned by HMOs in some communities. A major overhaul of the conditions under which HMOs participated in Medicare occurred in 1997 with the passage of Medicare+Choice. Counter to its objectives, Medicare+Choice resulted in a massive exit of HMOs from Medicare.[44]

There have been various efforts to address the perceived shortcomings of Medicare+Choice. For example, health plan representatives, including individuals from Kaiser Permanente, HealthPartners, and Group Health Cooperative, worked with HCFA to redesign the risk adjustment feature of the payment model. On a broader scale, the National Bipartisan Commission on the Future of Medicare (chaired by Senator John Breaux, D.-La., and Congressman Bill Thomas, R.-Calif.) considered several options for reform that would use different components of the federal employee plan and Enthoven's Consumer-Choice Health Plan, including offering a choice of plans and providing beneficiaries with an incentive to choose a lower-cost plan.[45]

These ideas were embodied in legislation proposed in 1995 by Senator Breaux and Senator William Frist (R.-Tenn.), a cardiac surgeon who would be elevated to the position of Senate majority leader in 2003. Under their proposal, beneficiaries would choose from private sector plans and a fee-for-service plan sponsored by the government, with a defined government contribution of 89 percent of costs for the government-sponsored plan and 85 percent for the private plan.[46] The 1995 proposal did not pass, but a modified version emerged in President George W. Bush's 2003 proposals to restructure Medicare, underscoring the enduring relevance of the federal employee plan as a model for Medicare reform. It is interesting to note that in 1980, the incoming Reagan administration's Health Policy Advisory Group recommended "a phased Medicare reform modeled on the Federal Employees Health Benefits Program."[47]

Extension of the Federal Employees Model

During the 1980s and early 1990s, Medicare was only one of several government agencies and programs that turned to a variant of the Federal Employees Health Benefits Plan in hopes of containing costs. For instance, by 1994, forty-four state governments had implemented FEHBP-type programs to insure their employees. These programs featured a choice from among multiple plans for employees and, in twenty-two states, employed fixed contributions.[48]

The military also found that the federal employees plan and Enthoven's Consumer-Choice Health Plan provided a useful framework for restructuring the delivery of medical services to active personnel, retirees, and civilian dependents. Faced with rising costs in the late 1980s, the Department of Defense initiated a five-year demonstration project in California and Hawaii. The project led to a new "managed care" program called TRICARE that had over 5 million enrollees by 2000.[49] The program offers three options: an HMO, a PPO, and a fee-for-service plan, with active personnel required to enroll in the HMO. For retirees and dependents, there is choice among plans, as in the federal employees plan and as proposed in Enthoven's Consumer-Choice Health Plan.[50] It has been argued that the structure of TRICARE's financing creates competition between military hospitals and health plans.[51] Prepaid groups have also been used as standards for evaluating staffing within the military system.[52]

Perhaps the greatest impact of the FEHBP, in combination with Enthoven's managed competition concept, has been in the restructuring of state Medicaid programs. Arizona created a Medicaid program in 1982 based entirely on prepaid health plans, with the principle of offering beneficiaries a choice wherever possible.[53] At the same time, plans in other states were participating in the Medicaid competition demonstration. The transition to managed care was gradual in most states, but enrollment in prepaid plans increased from 2.5 million in 1991 to over 13 million in 1996.[54] A dramatic conversion to managed care occurred in 1994 in Tennessee, where 700,000 beneficiaries were enrolled in prepaid plans during two months.[55]

Although the concept of multiple choice, as found in the FEHBP and advocated by Enthoven, is a key feature of most Medicaid managed care programs, administration of these programs has proved to be a challenge. Most states now employ a management approach using many of the proposed components of Enthoven's Consumer-Choice model, including a highly structured selection process coupled with substantial effort devoted to quality assurance and the monitoring of plan performance. At present, PGPs are not major contractors under Medicaid managed care; none are included among the twenty-five largest Medicaid contractors nationwide.[56]

The federal employees plan has also been viewed by some policymakers as a vehicle by which the government can expand its support of health care for low-income people beyond Medicaid. Senator Bill Bradley, in his 2000 presidential bid, suggested that low-income adults be given vouchers that could be used to purchase coverage through an existing employer plan or the FEHBP.[57]

In an ambitious but ultimately unsuccessful attempt at health care reform, the Clinton administration developed an approach that clearly drew from the experience of the FEHBP and the principles of Enthoven's Consumer-Choice Health

Plan.[58] It included a choice of health plans, with information to be provided to consumers to assist them in selecting a plan. However, PGPs were not directly involved in developing the Clinton proposal and had little representation on the administration's working task forces. Instead, they served in a consulting role, providing information to the task forces as requested.

Concerns About Quality

As enrollment in managed care organizations grew during the 1980s and early 1990s, so did employer and consumer concerns about quality of care. Until the late 1980s, it was typical for employers to offer managed care organizations to their employees along with traditional insurance plans (the multiple-choice approach advocated by PGPs). In this situation, consumers could select other alternatives if they were concerned about the quality of care they would receive from managed care plans. Furthermore, enrollees in managed care plans could switch to other options if they were unhappy with their managed care experience. When managed care plans essentially replaced traditional insurance in employer health benefits offerings during the early 1990s, a well-publicized managed care "backlash" ensued. Media stories about managed care enrollees who allegedly received inappropriate treatment because of health plan care management policies and physician payment incentives were frequent and compelling, creating the appearance of a quality "crisis" and undermining public confidence in managed care plans. The first attempts to both anticipate and address quality-of-care concerns originated in the private sector, where they were supported, and in some instances led, by PGPs. These efforts soon had an impact on public sector programs as well.

Addressing the Quality Issue

Addressing concerns about quality of care was not a new challenge for PGPs, which, from their inception, had been attacked by organized medicine for the quality of care they provided.[59] Typically, they responded by pointing to the superior coordination of care that could be achieved by group practices, the solid credentials of group practice physicians, and the opportunities that an enrolled population provided for health promotion and prevention activities. Some of the largest PGPs, including Kaiser Permanente-Northwest, Group Health Cooperative of Puget Sound, Kaiser Permanente-Northern California, and Group Health of Minnesota, formed internal research groups that published studies in peer-reviewed journals addressing their care processes and patient outcomes, using enrollee data (see Chapter Eight). These research groups have become a major source of evidence concerning the effectiveness of different models for the management of chronic illnesses, for instance.[60] Ultimately, these studies helped establish PGPs as "benchmarks" against which outcomes in other health plans, as well as in traditional insurance plans, could be compared. By the late 1990s, PGPs were being cited as the best model for the management of the patient concerns that gave rise to the managed care backlash.[61]

At the same time that this was occurring, concern was mounting in many quarters regarding the perceived ineffectiveness of competition among health plans in improving quality of care. Paul Ellwood gave voice to this concern and, in his highly publicized Shattuck Lecture on "outcomes management," called for the development of better ways to assess the "value" of the medical care delivered through health plans, urging the development of a standardized system for measuring and tracking patient outcomes.[62]

Prepaid group practices were hearing a similar message from large employers. In the words of Henry Berman, former chief executive of Group Health-Northwest:

> At a meeting of the Board of Directors of the HMO Group (now the Alliance of Community Health Plans) in 1989, we board members were complaining, as usual, about the demands from employers for claims data to justify our rate increases. The member plans had two problems with the requests: We could not provide them with cost data (as prepaid group practices, we did not create encounter forms for each visit), and we knew that these data would not tell purchasers what they most wanted to know: Were they getting their money's worth? George Halvorson, President and Chief Executive Officer of Group Health, Inc., proposed that we work with some of the more sophisticated employers to develop a set of measures that could demonstrate that their money was well spent. The HMO Group and Kaiser Permanente put together a task force that included several influential employers who were active in the Washington Business Group on Health, and Towers Perrin, to develop this set of measures.[63]

These meetings resulted in the Healthplan Employer Data and Information Set (HEDIS). The first version of HEDIS, published in 1991, included measures of quality, access, satisfaction, utilization, and financial performance.[64] The clinical measures dealt primarily with prevention, which, according to Berman, was "an area that was noncontroversial, relatively easily measured, and a historic strength of HMOs."[65] To continue the development of HEDIS, the group turned to the National Committee for Quality Assurance (NCQA), a private, not-for-profit organization that accredited managed care plans.

Just as PGPs played a catalyst role in the development of HEDIS, they were also crucial to the establishment of NCQA, which was created in 1979 under the sponsorship of the American Managed Care and Review Association and the Group Health Association of America.[66] In 1990, the founding organizations decided that, to be credible, NCQA needed to be independent. Financed in part by funding from the HMOs and The Robert Wood Johnson Foundation,[67] NCQA transitioned to an independent body capable of assuming responsibility for the further development of HEDIS and its incorporation into the health plan accreditation process.

The Washington Business Group on Health (now known as the National Business Group on Health) transferred HEDIS stewardship to NCQA with an agreement on the part of the PGPs to support development of the next version of HEDIS (2.0). From 1993 to 1994, participating HMOs collected and independently published data on their HEDIS performance, and Kaiser Permanente produced the first report card using HEDIS 2.0. Dr. Don Nielson of Kaiser Permanente chaired the performance measurement committee for HEDIS and along with Dr. Mike Ralston, also of Kaiser Permanente, was involved in the development of HEDIS 3.0.

Although HEDIS development was undertaken in response to the demands of private purchasers, it soon expanded to incorporate measures that addressed specific issues in the Medicaid and Medicare programs. An integrated set of Medicaid measures was released in 1997 as part of HEDIS 3.0. At that time, Arnold Epstein reported that the "majority of states with managed care programs now plan to require participating health plans to produce HEDIS data on samples of their Medicaid enrollees."[68] Also beginning in 1997, HMOs with Medicare risk contracts were required to submit HEDIS data to the Health Care Financing Administration, which planned to use the data to monitor the performance of health plans serving Medicare enrollees.[69]

HEDIS measures have widely acknowledged limitations as a method for determining the relative quality of care and service provided by health plans.[70] However, they helped shape a national debate about how to define and measure quality of care for populations, as opposed to individuals. HEDIS measures, and the process by which they continue to evolve, have brought public and private purchasers together as participants in this debate. Berman notes, "One veteran physician HMO executive close to HEDIS has described it as 'the closest thing we have to a national health policy.'"[71]

The Institute of Medicine Reports: A Shift in Emphasis

In 1999, public concerns about quality of care, along with the concerns of policymakers and health policy analysts, were redirected from the health plan to the provider level in a dramatic way with the release of the Institute of Medicine's report on patient safety, *To Err Is Human: Building a Safer Health System,* followed two years later by *Crossing the Quality Chasm: A New Health System for the 21st Century.*[72] These documents clearly elevated quality as a health policy issue, concluding that "quality problems are everywhere, affecting many patients. Between the health care we have and the care we could have lies not just a gap, but a chasm."[73]

In effect, the Institute of Medicine reports created a new health care "crisis," redirecting attention from health plan to health system quality. Although PGPs did not play as direct a role in shaping the development of the reports as they played in the HEDIS movement, they were nonetheless active participants on the committees that produced the reports (including, for example, George Isham of HealthPartners and David Lawrence of Kaiser Permanente). One of the committee chairs was Dr. Donald Berwick, formerly affiliated with Harvard Community Health Plan, a PGP at that time. The reports contain numerous examples of organizations that have taken steps to implement care processes with demonstrated effectiveness in improving quality, such as the work of Ed Wagner and colleagues at Group Health Cooperative with respect to the treatment of chronic illness (see Chapter Two).

Conclusions

This chapter has provided an overview of both the involvement and the influence of prepaid group practice on American health care policy over a seventy-year period. That overview suggests some of the reasons why PGPs have been so consistently involved in major health policy debates and why that involvement has influenced policy in so many different ways. For one thing, the need to establish the legitimacy of prepaid group practice in the face of opposition from organized medicine was crucial in providing the motivation for the early involvement of PGPs in the policy process. Challenges from organized medicine occurred over decades at all levels of government (local, state, and federal) and across a variety of public policy initiatives and programs (for example, national health insurance, provision of services to workers and dependents in defense plants, regional health planning, Medicare, and Medicaid). For PGPs, participation in the policy process was essential, even as recently as the 1980s, to achieve legitimacy and secure and maintain a place in the U.S. health care system.

With respect to the effectiveness of PGPs in the policy process, the explanation rests with the interplay of three factors: the clear policy objectives developed by PGPs and their tenacity in adhering to those objectives over time, the characteristics of PGPs and the appeal of those characteristics to policymakers, and the ability of PGPs to form alliances with policy entrepreneurs during policy regime changes that protected or furthered PGP interests.

Clarity of Purpose

One key to the influence that PGPs have exerted on health policy is their focus on a relatively limited but crucial set of objectives and their single-minded pursuit of those objectives. The first objective was to establish and protect the legitimacy of the PGP model. In their early years, when the threat from organized medicine was the strongest, PGPs worked hard to serve the needs of policymakers, when possible, in order to secure political allies in the battle with organized medicine. The second objective was to gain access to potential enrollees or, stated differently, to avoid being closed off from access to large groups of potential enrollees. PGPs consistently promoted public policies that enhanced access, typically in the name of "choice," and supported policy entrepreneurs with proposals that did this. Once access was attained, however, the next concern of PGPs was that they not be disadvantaged in the competition for enrollees. Consequently, PGPs supported rules, regulations, and concepts that encourage a "level playing field" in this competition. Finally, and more recently, PGPs entered the policy process to oppose legislation or regulation that would, in their opinion, unfairly penalize them (for example, so-called managed care backlash regulation).

Attractiveness of PGP Features

A second factor explaining the influence of PGPs in the policy process is that they had something important to offer, in both a tangible and a symbolic sense, to health care policymakers and policy entrepreneurs. Prepaid group proponents mobilized data and research findings to argue that PGPs provided care of comparable, and in some cases better, quality using fewer resources than other organizational structures.[74] In the policy process, proponents were able to assert, with some credibility, that PGPs represented a better way to organize and deliver medical care.

The fact that care delivered by PGPs is "organized," "managed," and "measured" is also important because, in combination with performance data, it positions PGPs symbolically as a technocratic solution to the health care system's problems. The literature on the role of "scientific illusion" in public policy is complex but suggestive in this regard. For instance, Gary Belkin asserts that there is an "important connection between being convincingly scientific and being successfully powerful in health policy. . . . Otherwise difficult, if not impossible, power shifts can instead be understood as shifts to 'better' knowledge [and] more scientific and rational practice, but where the very credibility of knowledge or practice as in fact scientific and better is shaped by its social need, use, and source."[75] In an argument that could easily be applied more specifically to PGPs, Belkin concludes that "managed care's value and success are significantly tied to the degree that it offers an objectivity that is specifically needed to resolve current political and economic tensions around health care."[76] Thus positioned, PGPs have been attractive to health policy entrepreneurs of various persuasions.

For the Committee on the Costs of Medical Care, the PGP concept offered the possibility of stretching the limited health care resources in the Great Depression through better organization of care delivery, with the goal of freeing up resources to provide more Americans with access to care. Henry Kaiser similarly argued for PGPs as a "technological imperative" for American health care. In the late 1960s, when the cost side of the cost-quality-access triangle was preeminent, the perceived efficiency and rationality of PGPs once again secured them a prominent place in the discussion. These qualities were crucial in attracting conservative support for a major federal government health care initiative, the HMO Act. In the "competition versus regulation" debate of the late 1970s and 1980s, the perceived ability of PGPs to deliver quality care at a (relatively) low price made them a key part of the competitive model. They were expected to provide the market discipline under managed competition that would hold down the prices of competitors and drive out alleged waste and inefficiency from the fee-for-service sector.

When quality of care issues rose to prominence in the 1990s, PGPs were used as examples of how the health of populations could be improved through better application of information technology and evidence-based medicine. They served as laboratories for testing process improvement models and provided benchmarks against which the performance of plans in the Medicaid and Medicare programs could be assessed, again introducing a "scientific basis" for health policy decisions.

Strategic Alliances

While these qualities made PGPs attractive to policy entrepreneurs in crafting their "solutions" to health care crises, PGPs themselves were able to form alliances at critical times that served their objectives. In some instances, their very survival in the face of opposition from organized medicine depended on being skillful in developing these alliances. Although PGP advocates rarely assumed the mantle of policy entrepreneur (Henry Kaiser provides an example to the contrary), they frequently sought common cause with others when their own objectives could be furthered through an (active or passive) alliance. These alliances entailed some risk if the proposals advocated by policy entrepreneurs were broader than the limited policy objectives being pursued by PGPs. One risk was that unanticipated consequences from implementation of the entrepreneur's policy solution could adversely affect PGPs. A second was that the political response to the proposed policy or the policy entrepreneur could be negative, and PGPs could be "tarred with the same brush," thereby diminishing their future effectiveness in the health policy process. For the most part, however, PGPs skillfully avoided these pitfalls in forming alliances that furthered their objectives.

Future Prospects

The success of PGPs in the health policy process can be attributed to strong motivation, coupled with a carefully considered, multifaceted strategy that has evolved over time to take advantage of the changing health care landscape. PGPs have been influential in the policy process over a long period of time because they have been consistent about what they have wanted to achieve, they have tangible and symbolic characteristics that made them attractive to policymakers and policy entrepreneurs with a variety of agendas, and they have been able to structure selective alliances with policy entrepreneurs or interest groups that in most cases have benefited them. But will PGPs continue to be active, successful participants in the policy process in the future? This will depend in large part on how the greater health care finance and delivery system evolves.

The perils in attempting to predict the future direction of American health care are well known. However, even in the absence of a clear crystal ball, it seems reasonable to suggest that PGPs will be challenged to repeat their past successes. First, they will need to find a new motivation that replaces their need to establish legitimacy. Their past success has led to their acceptance as legitimate components of the health care system. Second, the aura of the technocratic solution that has benefited PGPs may be weakening. New developments in information technology now allow much less structured forms of care delivery to argue that they also are "organized, managed, and measured." Third, at least at present, many purchasers do not view PGP as a potential solution to their health care purchasing problems. Instead, large purchasers are relying heavily on relatively loosely organized health plans with overlapping provider networks (that may or may not contain PGPs) and consumer cost sharing in designing their health benefits plans. Some employers likely associate PGPs with a previous strategy to contain health benefits costs that relied on competing provider groups, a strategy that, in their opinion, failed. If PGPs are not seen as a solution endorsed by employers, their influence in the policy process is likely to be diminished. Of course, this could change if medical care costs continue to increase at double-digit rates, but for the present, PGPs are challenged to find new allies in the health policy process.

Notes

1. C. Wilson, "Policy Regimes and Policy Change," *Journal of Public Policy*, 2000, *20*, 247–274.
2. See, for example, J. W. Kingdon, *Agendas, Alternatives, and Public Policies* (New York: HarperCollins, 1984).
3. Seminal pieces in this literature include T. R. Marmor, *The Politics of Medicare* (Hawthorne, N.Y.: Aldine de Gruyter, 1973), on Medicare; E. Redman, *The Dance of Legislation* (New York: Simon & Schuster, 1973), on the National Health Service Corps; L. D. Brown, *Politics and Health Care Organization: HMO as Federal Policy* (Washington, D.C.: Brookings Institution, 1983), J. D. Faulkson, *HMOs and the Politics of Health System Reform* (Chicago: American Hospital Association, 1980), and P. Starr, "The Undelivered Health System," *Public Interest*, Winter 1976, pp. 66–85, on the federal HMO Act; and J. S. Hacker, *The Road to Nowhere: The Genesis of President Clinton's Plan for Health Security* (Princeton, N.J.: Princeton University Press, 1997), and H. Johnson and D. S. Broder, *The System: The American Way of Politics at the Breaking Point* (New York: Little, Brown, 1996), on the Clinton health care reform initiative.
4. J. E. Anderson, *Public Policymaking: An Introduction*, 2nd ed. (Boston: Houghton Mifflin, 1984), p. 5.
5. M. E. Rushefsky and K. Patel, *Politics, Power and Policy Making: The Case of Health Care Reform in the 1990s* (Armonk, N.Y.: Sharpe, 1998).
6. Kingdon, *Agendas, Alternatives, and Public Policies*.
7. Wilson, "Policy Regimes and Policy Change."
8. N. C. Roberts and P. J. King, *Transforming Public Policy: Dynamics of Policy Entrepreneurship and Innovation* (San Francisco: Jossey-Bass, 1996).
9. Kingdon, *Agendas, Alternatives, and Public Policies*.
10. Committee on the Costs of Medical Care, *Medical Costs for the American People: The Final Report of the Committee on the Costs of Medical Care* (Chicago: University of Chicago Press, 1932).
11. C. Evans, "The Medical Guild Plan," in B. Aly, ed., *Socialized Medicine* (Columbia, Mo.: Lucas Brothers, 1935); V. Tereshtenko, *The Problem of Cooperative Medicine* (New York: Edward A. Fillene Goodwill Fund and Federal Works Agency, Works Project Administration, 1942); J. P. Warbasse and others, *The Vital Importance and Functions of Cooperative Health Associations* (New York: Bureau of Cooperative Medicine, Cooperative League of America, 1937); D. S. Hirshfield, *The Lost Reform: The Campaign for Compulsory Health Insurance in the United States from 1932 to 1943* (Cambridge, Mass.: Harvard University Press, 1970).
12. L. E. Weeks and H. J. Berman, eds., *Shapers of American Health Care Policy: An Oral History* (Ann Arbor, Mich.: Health Administration Press, 1985).
13. R. L. Hendricks, "Liberal Default, Labor Support, and Conservative Neutrality: The Kaiser Permanente Program After World War II," *Journal of Policy History*, 1989, *1*, 156–180; R. L. Hendricks, *A Model for National Health Care: The History of Kaiser Permanente* (New Brunswick, N.J.: Rutgers University Press, 1993).
14. Hendricks, "Liberal Default," p. 174.
15. Hendricks, "Liberal Default."

16. S. Steinmo and J. Watts, "It's the Institutions, Stupid! Why Comprehensive National Health Insurance Always Fails in America," *Journal of Health Politics, Policy, and Law,* 1995, *20,* 329–372.

17. P. Starr, *The Social Transformation of American Medicine* (New York: Basic Books, 1982).

18. S. Fleming, "History of the Kaiser Permanente Medical Program: Interviews Conducted by Sarah Smith Hughes," Kaiser Permanente Oral History Project, Bancroft Library, University of California, Berkeley, 1990.

19. A. Yedidia, "History of the Kaiser Permanente Medical Program: Interviews Conducted by Ora Huth," Kaiser Permanente Oral History Project, Bancroft Library, University of California, Berkeley, 1985.

20. Starr, *Social Transformation of American Medicine.*

21. Hendricks, *Model for National Health Care.*

22. "Report of the Commission on Medical Care Plans: Findings, Conclusions and Recommendations, Part 1," *Journal of the American Medical Association,* 1959, special edition, 34–42, 63.

23. C. Ameringer, "Organized Medicine on Trial: The Federal Trade Commission vs. the American Medical Association," *Journal of Policy History,* 2000, *12,* 445–472; W. Brandon and E. Lee, "Evaluating Health Planning: Empirical Evidence of HSA Regulation of Prepaid Group Practices," *Journal of Health Politics, Policy, and Law,* 1984, *9,* 103–124.

24. E. W. Saward and M. R. Greenlick, "Health Policy and the HMO," *Milbank Memorial Fund Quarterly,* 1972, *1,* 147–176.

25. Yedidia, "History."

26. Fleming, "History."

27. Yedidia, "History."

28. Faulkson, *HMOs and the Politics of Health System Reform;* Brown, *Politics and Health Care Organization.*

29. R. Finch and R. Egeberg, *A Report on the Health of the Nation's Health Care Systems* (Washington, D.C.: Office of the Secretary of Health, Education and Welfare, 1969).

30. Quoted in Faulkson, *HMOs and the Politics of Health System Reform,* p. 6.

31. T. R. Mayer and G. G. Mayer, "HMOs: Origins and Development," *New England Journal of Medicine,* 1985, *312,* 590–594.

32. Kingdon, *Agendas, Alternatives, and Public Policies,* p. 173.

33. Fleming, "History."

34. See, for instance, Brown, *Politics and Health Care Organization;* Faulkson, *HMOs and the Politics of Health System Reform;* Starr, "The Undelivered Health System"; and Kingdon, *Agendas, Alternatives, and Public Policies.*

35. S. J. Tillinghast, "Competition Through Physician-Managed Care: The Case for Capitated Multispecialty Group Practices," *International Journal for Quality in Health Care,* 1998, *10,* 427–434.

36. J. K. Iglehart, "The Future of HMOs," *New England Journal of Medicine,* 1982, *307,* 456.

37. A. C. Enthoven, "Sounding Boards: The Competition Strategy: Status and Prospects," *New England Journal of Medicine,* 1981, *304,* 109–112.

38. P. M. Ellwood and others, "Health Maintenance Strategy," *Medical Care,* 1971, *9,* 291–298.

39. A. C. Enthoven, "Consumer-Choice Health Plan (First of Two Parts)," *New England Journal of Medicine,* 1978, *298,* 650–658; A. C. Enthoven, "Health Care Costs: Why Regulation Fails, Why Competition Works, How to Get There from Here," *National Journal,* 1979, *11,* 885–889.

40. Enthoven, "Sounding Boards," p. 111. See also J. Hacker and T. Skocpol, "The New Politics of U.S. Health Policy," *Journal of Health Politics, Policy, and Law,* 1997, *22,* 315–338.

41. Enthoven, "Sounding Boards."

42. Iglehart, "The Future of HMOs," p. 454.

43. B. Dowd and others, "Issues Regarding Health Plan Payments Under Medicare and Recommendations for Reform," *Milbank Quarterly,* 1992, *70,* 423–453; R. J. Jackson, statement before the Select Committee on Aging, House of Representatives, June 11, 1987.

44. J. Oberlander, "Managed Care and Medicare Reform," *Journal of Health Politics, Policy, and Law,* 1997, *22,* 595–631; S. Makhorn, *How Not to Reform Medicare: Lessons from the Medicare+Choice Experiment* (Washington, D.C.: Heritage Foundation, 1999); General Accounting Office, *Medicare+Choice Plan Withdrawals Indicate Difficulty of Providing Choice While Achieving Savings* (Washington, D.C.: General Accounting Office, 2000); M. Casey, A. Knott, and I. Moscovice, "Medicaid Minus Choice: The Impact of HMO Withdrawals on Rural Medicare Beneficiaries," *Health Affairs,* 2002, *21,* 192–199.

45. R. Feldman, K. E. Thorpe, and B. Gray, "Policy Watch: The Federal Employees Health Benefits Plan," *Journal of Economic Perspectives,* 2002, *16,* 207–217.

46. W. Frist, "The Future of Medicare," *Health Affairs,* 1995, *14,* 82–88.

47. Enthoven, "Sounding Boards," p. 112.

48. M. L. Maciejewski, B. Dowd, and R. Feldman, "How Do States Buy Health Insurance for Their Own Employees?" *Managed Care Quarterly,* 1997, *5,* 11–19.

49. S. Johnson, "TRICARE: The Military's Version of Managed Care," *Medical Interface,* 1996, *9,* 86–89; J. Zwanziger and others, "Providing Managed Care Options for a Large Population: Evaluating the CHAMPUS Reform Initiative," *Military Medicine,* 2000, *165,* 403–410.

50. TRICARE, "TRICARE Management Activity Fact Sheet," Apr. 23, 2000 [http://www.tricare.com].

51. J. Gardner, "The TRICARE Debate: Restructured Financing of New Military Managed-Care Contracts Raises Questions," *Modern Healthcare,* 1997, *27,* 49.

52. G. Johnson, "Primary Care Enrollment Levels in Staff- and Group-Model Health Maintenance Organizations: A Standard to Compare Military Enrollment with Civilian Organizations," *Military Medicine,* 2002, *167,* 370–373.

53. J. Christianson and D. Hillman, *Health Care for the Indigent and Competitive Contracts: The Arizona Experience* (Ann Arbor, Mich.: Health Administrative Press Perspectives, 1986).

54. A. M. Epstein, "Medicaid Managed Care and High Quality: Can We Have Both?" *Journal of the American Medical Association,* 1997, *278,* 1617–1621.

55. R. Hurley and S. Somers, "Medicaid Managed Care," in P. Kongstvedt, ed., *Essentials of Managed Health Care* (Gaithersburg, Md.: Aspen, 2001).

56. InterStudy, *Competitive Edge 12.2, Part II: HMO Industry Report* (St. Paul, Minn.: Inter-Study, 2002).

57. Feldman, Thorpe, and Gray, "Policy Watch."

58. Johnson and Broder, *The System.*

59. Starr, *Social Transformation of American Medicine.*

60. J. Christianson and others, *Managed Care and the Treatment of Chronic Illness* (Thousand Oaks, Calif.: Sage, 2001).

61. T. Bodenheimer, "The HMO Backlash: Righteous or Reactionary?" *New England Journal of Medicine,* 1996, *335,* 1601–1604; P. R. Alper, "The Doctor-Patient Breakdown: Trouble at the Core of the Medical Economy," *Policy Review,* 2002, *12,* 53–71.

62. P. M. Ellwood, "Shattuck Lecture: Outcomes Management: A Technology of Patient Experience," *New England Journal of Medicine*, 1988, *318*, 1549–1556.

63. H. S. Berman, "Performance Measures: The Destination or the Journey?" *Effective Clinical Practice*, 1999, *2*, 284.

64. A. G. Mainous III and J. Talbert, "Assessing Quality of Care via HEDIS 3.0: Is There a Better Way?" *Archives of Family Medicine*, 1998, *7*, 410–413.

65. Berman, "Performance Measures," p. 284.

66. J. K. Iglehart, "The National Committee for Quality Assurance," *New England Journal of Medicine*, 1996, *335*, 995–999.

67. Ibid.

68. Epstein, "Medicaid Managed Care and High Quality," p. 1618.

69. P. Grimaldi, "HMOs Must Submit Medicare HEDIS," *Nursing Management*, 1997, *28*, 54–55.

70. See, for instance, D. O. Farley, E. A. McGlynn, and D. Klein, "Assessing Quality in Managed Care: Health Plan Reporting of HEDIS Performance Measures," Commonwealth Fund, Sept. 1998 [http://www.cmwf.org/programs/quality/farley_assessingquality_pb_298.asp]; Berman, "Performance Measures"; and Mainous and Talbert, "Assessing Quality of Care via HEDIS 3.0."

71. Berman, "Performance Measures," p. 286.

72. Institute of Medicine, *To Err Is Human: Building a Safer Health System* (Washington, D.C.: National Academy Press, 2000); Institute of Medicine, *Crossing the Quality Chasm: A New Health System for the 21st Century* (Washington, D.C.: National Academy Press, 2001).

73. Institute of Medicine, *Crossing the Quality Chasm*, p. 1.

74. For early examples of this research, see G. Williams, "Kaiser: What Is It? How Does It Work? Why Does It Work?" *Modern Hospital*, 1971, *116*, 67–69, and Saward and M. R. Greenlick, "Health Policy and the HMO."

75. G. S. Belkin, "The Technocratic Wish: Making Sense and Finding Power in the 'Managed' Medical Marketplace," *Journal of Health Politics, Policy, and Law*, 1997, *22*, 510–511; see also J. Morone and G. S. Belkin, "The Science Illusion and the Triumph of Medical Capitalism," paper presented at the annual meeting of the American Political Science Association, Chicago. Sept. 2, 1995.

76. Belkin, "The Technocratic Wish," p. 512.

CHAPTER FIVE

TECHNOLOGY ASSESSMENT, DEPLOYMENT, AND IMPLEMENTATION IN PREPAID GROUP PRACTICE

David M. Eddy

New medical technologies are appearing at a rapid and steadily accelerating pace. Unfortunately, many of them are introduced and aggressively promoted before there is good evidence that they are effective and beneficial. For instance, of the last fifty-six new technologies recently assessed by the Blue Cross Blue Shield Association's Technology Evaluation Center, thirty-nine, or nearly three-fourths, failed to meet minimum standards for evidence of effectiveness.[1]

Any organization that has contracted to provide high-quality health care to a group of people within a budget has a responsibility to ensure three things: (1) members should have access to new technologies that are known to be effective and safe, (2) members should not be exposed to technologies whose effects are unknown or known to be ineffective or harmful, and (3) members' money should be spent in the most efficient way to improve their health. The programs that organizations use to achieve these objectives are called "technology assessment," "technology deployment," and "technology implementation." This chapter describes these programs generically and in the context of three prepaid group practices (PGPs). The chapter also analyzes the theoretical reasons why PGPs might be expected to excel at technology assessment, deployment, and implementation and then examines the evidence on whether or not they do in

The author wishes to thank Robin Cisneros for her valuable assistance.

fact excel. (Note that although pharmaceuticals are considered "technology" and may be included in the technology strategies described here, this chapter focuses only on nonpharmaceutical technologies. Pharmaceutical technology in prepaid group practice and elsewhere is discussed in Chapter Six.)

The Formal Approach to New Technologies

An organization can respond to the appearance of a new technology in primarily two ways, which can with some simplification be called "formal" and "informal." The informal approach allows new technologies to drift into practice and counts on physicians to sort everything out as they incorporate the technologies into their practice. Although some organizations may take this approach, organizations that are committed to quality and efficiency do not. The reason is that this approach cannot be relied on to assess the effects of a technology accurately. This is not the fault of clinicians. It is caused by several factors, including the probabilistic nature of health outcomes, the relatively small effects of treatments (the "signal") compared to the effects of other nontreatment factors (the "noise"), the difficulty of assigning patients to different treatments in a way that evens out the nontreatment factors, the difficulty of following patients for long periods of time, and the difficulty of measuring patient outcomes.

Taken together, these factors make it virtually impossible for clinicians to accurately see the outcomes of a technology. The problem is well documented by numerous examples of failures to spot ineffective or even harmful technologies, in many cases despite decades of use in hundreds of thousands of patients. To cite just two of many examples, radical mastectomy, despite almost a century of "time-honored" use, has now been shown to be no more effective than breast-conserving surgery, and long-term hormone replacement therapy, despite the conventional wisdom and results of halfway research, is now known to actually increase the risk of coronary artery disease.

Given the shortcomings of the informal approach, most organizations that are committed to quality and efficiency use a formal approach.

Technology Assessment

There are five main steps in a formal technology assessment. The first is to formulate the assessment problem: precisely define the technology that is to be assessed, the patient population to whom it will be applied, the alternative technologies against which it will be compared (including no treatment or doing nothing), the providers who will use it, the setting in which it will be used, and the health outcomes that it will affect. The second is to identify all the evidence that addresses the assessment as formulated. The third is to analyze and summarize the evidence. The fourth is to make judgments about whether, given the available evidence, the technology meets agreed-on criteria of effectiveness and benefit. The fifth step is to write an explicit rationale for the conclusions reached.

The crux of the assessment is the application of the criteria in the fourth step. An example of such criteria is the list developed by the Blue Cross Blue Shield Association's Technology Evaluation Center. In paraphrased form, and with comments in parentheses, they are as follows:[2]

1. The technology must have final approval from the appropriate government regulatory bodies, if applicable.
2. The scientific evidence must (be of sufficiently good quality to) permit conclusions concerning the effects of the technology on health outcomes. (Health outcomes are the outcomes that patients experience and care about, such as heart attacks, strokes, and hip fractures.)
3. The technology must improve the net health outcome. (That is, the expected benefits must be judged to outweigh any side effects or risks.)
4. The technology must be as beneficial as any established alternatives.
5. The improvement must be attainable outside the investigational setting.

The details of these steps can vary from organization to organization, but the hallmarks are that the conclusions are based on evidence from well-designed studies, not just expert opinions, a professional consensus, or the prevailing practice in a community; the analysis of the evidence is comprehensive and open-minded; the evidence and rationale are written down so that everyone can review them; and the entire process is orderly, open, and accountable.

Assessments that follow these steps are called "evidence-based assessments." For some assessments, there will be an additional step, which is to estimate quantitatively the expected effects of the guideline on the health outcomes of the patients to whom the guideline is to be applied. Assessments that provide this type of quantitative information are called "outcomes-based." Some assessments also include a formal analysis of costs. Two examples of evidence-based assessments are presented in the appendix to this chapter.

To have a technology assessment program that has these qualities, an organization must address the following issues:

1. Centralization of the assessment process to avoid duplication of effort and inconsistencies in conclusions
2. The use of a team that includes not only physician experts but also individuals trained in research and other analytical methods

3. A commitment by team members to set their personal biases aside and let the evidence drive the conclusions
4. A commitment by the organization to provide the necessary resources (a formal technology assessment is far more expensive than simply convening a group of experts and asking their opinions)
5. An institutional commitment to withstand the social pressure that comes with unpopular decisions

This last requirement arises because patients, their families, the press, the courts, legislators, and even professional societies can exert enormous pressure to provide a treatment before its effects have been documented. An organization that wants to provide high-quality care efficiently has to be able to withstand that pressure. The reasons include protecting patients from technologies whose benefits are unknown but whose harms might be great; conserving people's money so that it can be applied to technologies that are known to be effective; preventing an unproven technology from creeping into widespread use, after which it can be very difficult to withdraw; not fostering an impression that a technology's effectiveness is known when it is not; and not stifling the additional research that will need to be done to determine its effectiveness. The tangible justification for this stance is the long list of instances where patients, families, courts, the press, and physicians have jumped the gun and been wrong, with disastrous long-term consequences for patients.

Technology Deployment

If the assessment of a technology shows that it meets the agreed-upon criteria for effectiveness and benefit (and possibly cost effectiveness), the next step is to determine how it should be deployed. This step is especially important if the technology involves expensive supplies, equipment, or capital expenditures, or if proper use of the technology requires people with specialized skills or coordination across disciplines. The issues to be addressed include such questions as which brand to use; how many units to obtain; where to place them; whether to buy, lease, or contract out; and how to get the best deal.

To address these types of issues, an organization must have at least three capabilities. The first relates to the decision-making structure: the organization must have sufficient vertical integration to control these decisions, and it must place the decision in a committee that is sufficiently high in the organization to have an overview of and responsibility for the entire group of members, the authority to make the decisions, and the authority to negotiate with vendors. In general, the higher in the organization these decisions are made, the greater the opportunities to achieve efficiency. In contrast, if these decisions are left to local units—individual medical centers, clinics, or physicians—there are higher risks of inefficiency, conflict, and waste. The second capability relates to information: the organization must have access to accurate information for planning, such as the number of patients who meet the clinical criteria for receiving the technology. The third capability relates to expertise: the organization must have access to experts who can provide advice about the different brands and any special issues relating to either safety or effectiveness, such as required training programs or a steep learning curve.

Technology Implementation

Successful implementation of a new technology has different faces depending on whether or not the technology meets the agreed-upon criteria for effectiveness and benefit. For technologies that do not yet meet the criteria, the implementation is negative. That is, the organization will need to hold the line and not make the technology available until further research can show that it is effective and beneficial. An alternative approach for an unproven technology is to restrict its general use but allow it to be used on patients if they are participating in clinical trials that are designed to produce the needed information about effectiveness, benefits, and harms. The critical issue is to ensure that the trial is sufficiently well designed to produce an answer and is not just a registry or other halfway design created to provide an excuse and a research cover to buckle to the pressure. Whichever route is taken, it can be supported by a variety of administrative tools that include contractual denials of coverage for investigational or experimental technologies, denials based on lack of medical necessity, negative guidelines (designed to "turn off" the use of the technology), disease management programs and performance measures, exclusion from a drug formulary, and use of alerts.

If a technology meets the criteria for effectiveness and benefit, the organization will want to get the word out to physicians about the specific groups of patients for whom the technology's effectiveness and benefits have been shown. There are a wide variety of tools for doing this. They include affirmative guidelines, disease management programs and performance measures, specification of the technology as a clinical priority or strategic goal, inclusion in a drug formulary, and a wide variety of decision support tools, which can range from plastic pocket cards to the use of reminders in an automated clinical information system.

In addition to getting the word out, the organization will want to monitor the use of a new technology to ensure that the right patients are getting it and the wrong patients are not and to feed that information back to physicians to ensure its appropriate use. The organization might also want to monitor some of the short-term outcomes of the technology to confirm that it is performing as expected.

Whether the assessment of a technology is positive or negative, there are two keys to successful implementation. The first is a good information system. Ideally, the information system should work in two directions. It should be able to send information out—to guide physicians about the appropriate use of the technologies and support their decisions through reminders and alerts. It should also be able to get information back—to monitor which patients are actually getting the technology, as well as some of the outcomes that are occurring to them. The second key is the support of physicians. This is needed because the physicians must agree to accept the conclusions of the assessment and deployment teams, which often requires setting aside their personal preferences. The importance of this aspect of implementation is documented by the voluminous literature on physician practice variations.

Theory: Should Prepaid Group Practices Be Expected to Excel at Technology Processes?

To paraphrase the Preface to this volume, the critical components of prepaid group practice include the following:

- A multispecialty group practice
- Any hospitals or other facilities owned by or affiliated with the multispecialty group practice
- A voluntarily enrolled population that contracts with the PGP through a sponsor or as individuals
- Comprehensive health care services provided or arranged for by the PGP
- Per capita prepayment
- Usually, a mutually exclusive arrangement between the delivery system and the insurance entity
- Accountability for the quality and cost of the care that is delivered

Of these characteristics, three have special importance for the assessment, deployment, and implementation of technologies. The first is the provision of care to a defined population, which both motivates and enables the PGP to plan the most efficient ways to provide the population access to new technologies. This is especially important for technologies that involve expensive equipment or large outlays of capital, require extensive training and quality control, or require close coordination across health care providers.

The second characteristic is the use of prepayment, which strongly affects physicians' incentives to use technologies. Most important, in a PGP, there is no incentive to use investigational technologies prematurely or to overuse established technologies. The fact that some medical groups have bonuses that are linked to the amount of budgeted funds left over at the end of the year might be an incentive toward underuse of technologies. However, the actual magnitude of the incentive experienced by any particular physician to underuse a technology is trivially small (because in large medical groups it is spread out over hundreds or thousands of physicians) compared to the financial incentive experienced by a physician practicing under fee-for-service to overuse a technology (where the financial gain is one-to-one).

The third feature of PGPs that can potentially affect the use of technologies is the close relationship between the delivery system (including the physician group) and the health plan. For convenience, I will call this "integrated management" (see Chapter One). One effect of integrated management is that the health plan and the physician group have a shared contractual responsibility—they are both in the same boat—with respect to cost and quality. Another effect is that the health plan and the medical group can share control over management decisions. A third effect is that through its hierarchical structure—medical directors, specialty chiefs, cross-specialty care coordinators, unit heads, guidelines champions—a medical group is in a much better position than other types of practices to ensure that a decision made at the top is actually implemented by the physicians who make the patient-by-patient decisions. The use of guidelines, clinical priorities, and strategic goals are examples of the types of tools medical groups can use to achieve this third effect of integrated management.

In contrast, with fee-for-service insurance or carrier HMOs, there is usually a large gap between the health plan and the physicians. One aspect of the gap is the difference in incentives; the physicians typically are incented to do more, charge more, or overdescribe what they do (because they want to be paid more), while the health plan wants them to do less, charge less, and be accurate when describing what they do. Another aspect of the gap is that there are no organizational links that tie the physicians to the health plan (the only link beyond the contract is the exchange of money for services). Indeed, there are rarely any organizational links that connect physicians to one another beyond the loose bonds of small group practices or independent practice associations.

In nonintegrated organizations, a health plan can decide whether or not it will pay for a service, but it will typically make that decision unilaterally and will have few, if any, mechanisms at its disposal to influence what physicians actually do. In turn, physicians who are paid through fee-for-service insurance or by a carrier HMO will have no direct influence on the payment policies made by the insurer or carrier, and if they disagree with those policies, their only real recourse is to seek ways to undermine them (for example, use fraudulent codes to inflate their reimbursement).

There is a feature of some PGPs that could put them at a theoretical disadvantage compared to non-PGPs with regard to new technologies. Because they are prepaid, PGPs do not have the same inherent need to keep track of every procedure that is done, as organizations that are paid fee-for-service do. While this lowers administrative costs, it also means that PGPs do not have the same need for claims data. This can affect their ability to detect the inappropriate use of a technology, which is an important part of implementation. This said, some PGPs do have claims data—HealthPartners in Minnesota is an example—and others are investing in the information systems that can produce such data.

In addition to these general observations about the theoretical advantages and disadvantages of PGPs, there are theoretical issues that pertain to each part of the technology process.

Technology Assessment

In theory, there is no reason to expect that PGPs should be able to perform technology assessments better than other types of organizations. Any insurer, government agency, or HMO can create a centralized process, put together the necessary team, and teach the principles of formal technology assessment to the members of the team. Large organizations have an advantage because technology assessments are expensive and can benefit from economies of scale. However, the advantage of size does not give any theoretical advantage to PGPs: many PGPs are relatively small, providing care to only a few hundred thousand people, and even a large PGP may choose to forgo the economies of scale and decentralize the technology assessment process to individual regions or medical centers. It is also pertinent that any organization, large or small, can purchase technology assessments from the Blue Cross Blue Shield Association program or other health research and technology assessment companies such as ECRI (formerly the Emergency Care Research Institute) and Hayes, Inc. As for the ability to withstand the pressure that accompanies unpopular decisions, there are no inherent reasons that PGPs should be more willing or able to do so than non-PGPs; the press and juries are "equal opportunity" critics, and all types of organizations want to avoid bad press and high plaintiffs' awards.

The lack of any theoretical advantage for PGPs is illustrated by the fact that the best technology program to date is run by the Blue Cross Blue Shield Association, which is not a PGP. One PGP, Kaiser Permanente, has been a partner with the Blue Cross Blue Shield Association in its Technology Evaluation Center (TEC) program since 1993. Kaiser Permanente holds two seats on the TEC's Medical Advisory Panel, which makes judgments about whether new technologies meet the TEC criteria. In return, the TEC program receives the benefit of reviews by Permanente physicians and technology experts. However, the TEC program was originally developed by the association, which ran the program alone for about a decade before the partnership with Kaiser Permanente.

Technology Deployment

In theory, PGPs should be able to do a better job than other types of organizations at deploying a new technology: selecting the best brand; estimating the need; determining how many units to buy; determining the best places to put them; deciding whether to buy, lease, or contract out; and negotiating the best deals. The reason is that these decisions are usually made locally, by individual hospitals, clinics, and physicians. The integrated management of the PGP means that whatever parts of these decisions are made by physicians can be coordinated with the management of the health plan. The parts of these decisions that are made by hospitals may or may not be under the control of the PGP, depending on whether the hospitals are owned by or under exclusive contracts with the PGP (vertical integration). In other types of organizations, the insurer or carrier will contract with hospitals and physicians but will usually have little direct control over what care they deliver or how they deliver it. In those types of organizations, the selection, purchase, and location of equipment is usually made at the local level by individual medical centers, hospitals, and clinicians.

The practical implications of these distinctions are illustrated by the deployment of "cutting-edge" imaging machines such as PET scans. When acting on their own, each hospital wants its own machine to establish its reputation as the leading-edge center, irrespective of the needs in the population it serves. This creates powerful incentives to overuse and overcharge for the technology. Vertical integration and coverage over wide geographical areas can control this type of waste.

Technology Implementation

For implementing new technologies—whether that means holding the line on technologies that do not yet meet criteria for effectiveness or benefit or promoting the use of technologies that do meet the criteria—the story is mixed. On the one hand, the fact that PGPs have integrated management should mean that a management decision about a new technology, and the guidelines designed to implement that decision, should have strong physician support. On the other hand, organizations that use claims-based reimbursement systems may be in a better position to detect, and therefore control, both appropriate and inappropriate uses of a technology.

Theory Versus Practice

Some of these theoretical advantages and disadvantages of prepaid group practices are fixed and will be experienced by all PGPs. Examples are the advantages of defined populations, with their implications for population-based planning, and the very important differences in financial incentives between PGPs and fee-for-service insurers and noncapitated carrier HMOs.

However, the theoretical advantages of integrated management are not fixed. Most important, even if a health plan and a physician group are in the same contractual boat, they can still have very different philosophies about the best ways to take care of patients. For example, health plans are typically run by businesspeople who are used to top-down planning, quantitative thinking, and trade-offs. In contrast, many, if not most, physicians are used to focusing on individual patients, prefer qualitative thinking (for example, "If it might help this particular patient, we should do it"), and tend to find top-down planning intrusive and trade-offs obnoxious. Their idea of good management is likely to be "Leave us alone to take care of our patients." These differences do not necessarily disappear just because a medical group signs an exclusive contract with a health plan. The internal culture of physician decision making—they were all taught in the same medical schools, were trained by the same mentors, read the same journals, belong to the same societies, and go to the same professional meetings—can easily cause physicians in PGPs to identify more with their fee-for-service colleagues than with the senior management of their own organizations.

In the tradition of fee-for-service, some medical groups may insist on decentralization of deployment-type decisions, and some individual physicians may insist on a right to make their own decisions, independent of whatever the health plan or even their physician colleagues might have in mind. To the extent that any of these differences turns into suspicion, distrust, or overt friction between the health plan and the physician group, the theoretical advantages of integrated management can easily be destroyed. There is a joke that "PGPs are the last bastion of fee-for-service medicine."

In the other direction, the theoretical disadvantage PGPs face because they lack claims data for monitoring appropriate and inappropriate uses of technologies can be corrected and even reversed if the PGP develops an automated clinical information system. Here the PGPs have an advantage. It is far easier for a PGP to install an automated clinical information system that spans its physicians, services (pharmacy, lab, and so forth), and delivery sites (offices, clinics, hospitals) than it is for other types of organizations. Outside of PGPs, the fact that each physician can have contracts with a dozen or more insurers and carriers and may use a variety of clinics, services, and hospitals can make the design of an integrated clinical information system very difficult, if not impossible.

The Practice: Three PGP Examples

The types of programs used by PGPs to assess, deploy, and implement new technologies are well illustrated by three PGPs: Kaiser Permanente, Group Health Cooperative in Washington state, and HealthPartners in Minnesota.

Kaiser Permanente. An important feature of Kaiser Permanente that affects its approach to technologies is that it is organized as eight regions, each with its own legally and often culturally distinct medical group. Whatever its beneficial effects, this relative autonomy can have an important negative effect on attempts to coordinate decisions about technologies, achieve economies of scale, and avoid inconsistencies. Another important feature of Kaiser Permanente is that at various times in its history, there has been friction between the management of the health plan and the physician groups. As just described, this can dampen the potential benefits of integrated and vertical decision making.

As might be expected from this organizational and geographical diversity, Kaiser Permanente currently has several programs that perform technology assessment. At the highest level is the Interregional New Technology Committee (INTC). Its membership includes at least one representative from each of the geographical regions. It is composed of physicians, health plan managers, and specialists in such areas as public affairs, law, medical ethics, and analytical methods.

Technologies are selected for assessment based on (1) the importance of the condition addressed by the technology (for example, the burden of morbidity, mortality, and cost), (2) the potential effect of the technology on that burden, (3) the degree of uncertainty about or potential variability in the use of the technology, and (4) the perceived need for a policy or guideline to reduce variability and inappropriate use and to ensure the appropriate use of the technology.

For each technology that is selected for assessment, the staff prepares a summary of the available evidence on the technology's safety and effectiveness. The information for the summary is either drawn from assessments done by other organizations or generated internally by the technical staff of the committee. External sources include other parts of Kaiser Permanente, the Blue Cross and Blue Shield Association's TEC program, the Evidence-Based Practice Centers of the federal

Agency for Healthcare Research and Quality, ECRI, and Hayes, Inc. Each assessment summarizes the evidence, position statements from professional associations, the opinions of clinical experts inside and outside of the organization, and any applicable regulatory decisions. After studying the information, the committee makes a recommendation and disseminates it to the senior management in each region. Each region maintains its own local group or committee that is responsible for communicating with the Interregional New Technology Committee.

Most of the regions use the recommendations of the INTC to develop their coverage policies and benefit structures. However, a few regions have their own programs for assessing technologies and on rare occasions can come to different conclusions. The regional programs and their integration with programwide decisions about deployment and implementation of a technology are well illustrated by the New Technology Management Process in the Southern California region. The committees involved in this process include people with expertise in virtually every department that might be affected by a new technology.

The process consists of three main committees that illustrate the different functions that have to be performed to ensure that new technologies are introduced into the system appropriately. The process begins with the New Technology Assessment Team, which is responsible for conducting the formal, evidence-based assessments of the new medical technologies and making recommendations regarding their appropriateness. A second committee, the New Technology Deployment Strategy Team, is responsible for determining how best to deploy the new technology. For new technologies that are deemed to be appropriate, the deployment committee also defines the target population, forecasts the demand for the technology, arranges for its deployment, and develops any operational or business plans that might be required. The Regional Product Council is then responsible for supporting the selection, acquisition, delivery, standardization, and utilization of the actual materials and services a new technology might involve or require. The Southern California region also has a Regional Pharmacy and Therapeutics Committee, which evaluates existing and new pharmaceuticals for inclusion in the Regional Drug Formulary, and a Regional Biotechnology Committee, which evaluates biologics (see Chapter Six).

Although committees like those just described can ensure that new technologies are carefully evaluated and that decisions about such things as coverage, formularies, guidelines, and disease management programs are based on the best available evidence, a committee process cannot address all the day-to-day questions that might be asked by the twelve thousand or so physicians taking care of more than 8.3 million members. To meet that need, Kaiser Permanente Southern California has created the Technology Inquiry Line. This is a "hotline" that physicians can call to receive rapid, evidence-based answers to questions about the appropriate use of technologies. The inquiries can be general in nature—for example, about the effectiveness or diffusion of a new technology—or can be specific to particular patients. By drawing on the work of the Interregional New Technology Committee and other sources or by performing their own assessments if necessary, the staff of the inquiry line can typically provide answers within hours. The hotline does not provide a specific recommendation about the management of a specific patient; it leaves those decisions up to the patient's personal physician. But it does ensure that the physician is armed with the latest and most accurate information. In turn, topics of inquiries often fuel the agendas of the regional and national technology assessment committees.

Finally, at Kaiser Permanente, the implementation of new technologies is well supported by programs that design guidelines and disease management programs. They include guideline programs in several of the regions as well as the interregional Care Management Institute and the Interregional Guidelines Steering Group. Another important feature of the Kaiser Permanente system is the organization's very large investment in an automated clinical information system. When fully deployed, this will enormously increase the organization's ability to both implement and monitor new technologies and guidelines.

Group Health Cooperative. At Group Health Cooperative in Washington state, the technology assessment process involves three main committees. The Medical Technology Assessment Committee is responsible for deciding whether there is sufficient evidence to determine that a new technology improves health outcomes. The committee membership includes clinical leaders, epidemiologists, and representatives from specialty services, care management, the legal department, and contracts and coverage. A medical librarian conducts literature searches, and clinical epidemiologists critically appraise and summarize the best available evidence, which is presented at the committee meetings.

Following a structured discussion, the committee votes to determine if the technology meets the five Blue Cross and Blue Shield Association's TEC program criteria. A modified set of criteria that includes diagnostic accuracy, risks, diagnostic impact, and therapeutic impact is used for the evaluation of diagnostic tests.

The assessment committee then passes its judgments to the Health Plan Medical Directors Group, whose primary role is to recommend coverage of new technologies by the health plan. The medical directors consider the assessment committee's decision, as well as other factors, including legal issues, community standards, and implications for the delivery system.

Any recommendations of the Health Plan Medical Directors Group that represent a significant cost increase or require changes in contract language are reported to the Cooperative Benefits Committee for coverage approval. This committee is responsible for approving modifications to coverage contracts and developing a consistent package of benefits for the various local markets.

The technology assessments are then forwarded to a department called the Clinical Review Unit (CRU), which is responsible for the implementation and dissemination of the various committees' recommendations. If the Medical Directors Group decides that Group Health should cover the new technology with limits, the Clinical Review Unit develops clinical review criteria for that technology. The CRU is also responsible for posting assessment committee summaries on Group Health's internal Web site and reviewing individual referral requests to determine if the appropriate clinical review criteria are met.

Group Health Cooperative also has a Statewide Pharmacy and Therapeutics Committee, which evaluates existing and new pharmaceuticals for inclusion in the drug formulary.

HealthPartners. The technology assessment program at HealthPartners in Minnesota is closely aligned with the Institute for Clinical Systems Improvement (ISCI), which is an independent, nonprofit collaboration of health care organizations in Minnesota. It was founded in 1993 and is governed by a seventeen-member board consisting of the physician group leadership in Minnesota. It was funded for its first eight years by HealthPartners but is now sponsored by five Minnesota health plans. The primary sponsors are Blue Cross and Blue Shield of Minnesota, HealthPartners, and Medica. Associate sponsors are PreferredOne and UCare Minnesota. The institute provides health care quality improvement services to thirty medical groups ranging in size from eight practitioners in Willmar, Minnesota, to more than one thousand physicians and medical scientists at the Mayo Clinic in Rochester. The combined medical groups represent more than 4,500 physicians.

The ISCI program has four main elements: commitment to improvement, scientific groundwork for health care, support for improvement, and advocacy for health care quality. To date, representatives from the member medical groups have developed and continually review almost fifty technology assessment reports.

The process begins when the institute's Technology Assessment Committee selects a topic. Institute staff then recruit medical professionals from across the participating medical groups to serve in the work group that develops the report. After researching the topic, the institute's health care evidence analysis manager prepares a critical review of the scientific information about the technology. The work group reviews and revises the report, and once consensus is reached, the work group leader presents the report to the assessment committee for approval. After approval, clinicians from all the medical groups review the report. When the revised report is approved by the assessment committee and the work group, it is sent to all the participating medical groups. The report is reviewed by the work group leader within two years to determine if an update is needed.

HealthPartners itself has a well-defined process for reviewing new technologies and determining if they should be added to the benefit package. Three areas in the organization participate. One is the Medical Directors Committee, which consists of ten medical directors as well as representatives from other key areas within HealthPartners, such as medical policy, member services, and the Benefits Committee. The Medical Directors Committee reviews reports to determine if the scientific evidence shows the technology to be safe and effective. Reports by the Institute for Clinical Systems Improvement and other organizations, such as Blue Cross and Blue Shield Association's TEC, ECRI, and Hayes, are used when possible. If necessary, the medical policy staff will research the topic and develop their own assessment.

The Medical Directors Committee makes a recommendation about coverage of the technology in question and submits its conclusions to the Benefits Committee for a decision on whether to include the technology in the benefits package. The Benefits Committee has representation from all administrative areas within the organization, as well as from the Medical Directors Committee. Finally, the Benefits Implementation Group is responsible for ensuring the smooth implementation of new benefits and policies.

Common Features

Although each of these programs is different, they share some common features. First and foremost, they all illustrate one of the main benefits of integrated management. In each of the three organizations described, decisions about new technologies are made by a coordinated set of committees that include representation from both health plan management and the physician groups, along with other pertinent fields. Together these committees address the needs of the new technologies from the initial judgments about their effectiveness and benefits to their deployment and implementation. These types of decision-making structures are very rare and exist in only a handful of larger organized delivery systems across the country.

The second common feature is a commitment to the use of evidence to determine the effects of a technology on health outcomes. A third is the methods the organizations use to ensure that the evaluation of evidence is unbiased. One of the most important is a committee structure that separates the evaluation of evidence from financial, legal, political, contracting, and marketing considerations. It is quite legal and ethical to consider these factors, but it is very important that they not shade or bias the evaluation of the evidence. After the true effects of a technology on patients have been established, these other factors can be considered. Another technique that helps ensure impartiality is the broad membership of the committees. For all three of the programs described here, the committees include practicing physicians, experts from many different specialties, methodologists, and people with expertise and responsibilities in a wide variety of other fields such as administration, law, and ethics.

A fourth common feature of these programs is the orderliness of the processes. All of the committees have clearly defined responsibilities and relationships with other committees. A fifth common feature is the attention to the implementation of a technology. The processes do not end with a determination of the effect of the technology; they go on to address such issues as forecasting need and utilization, defining review criteria to monitor appropriate use, setting standards for equipment, selecting vendors, and other activities that are important to the orderly deployment of the technology. A final common feature is that all of the programs have formal schedules for updating the assessments to ensure that physicians and administrators have the latest and most accurate information.

Comparisons with Other Types of Organizations

It is difficult, if not impossible, to draw firm conclusions about how well PGPs assess, deploy, and implement technologies compared to other types of organizations. No systematic studies have been performed, and the only "evidence" is anecdotal—stories of successful programs. However, the value of even this type of information is limited by the facts that there are also stories of successes in other types of organizations and stories of failures in PGPs, and there is no way to determine the true frequency of any of them.

With those limitations in mind, a few observations can be made. As already stated, the leader in performing technology assessments is the Blue Cross and Blue Shield Association's TEC program, which is not a PGP. Several PGPs have very good programs, but they cannot claim to be unique in this respect, much less to be leaders. Indeed, many PGPs rely heavily on the Blue Cross Blue Shield program for leadership and assessments. It is not possible to determine with certainty the reason that the Blue Cross and Blue Shield Association developed its program faster and further than the PGPs, although a possible answer could be the stronger physician culture in PGPs—the physicians may initially have been more comfortable with the informal approach described at the beginning of this chapter and may not have felt the need for a formal approach. However, with this said, there is no reason that PGPs cannot develop programs that are as strong as the one at the Blue Cross and Blue Shield Association.

With regard to holding the line and restricting the use of a new technology until its effects are known, in practice there is no evidence that PGPs do this any better than other types of managed care organizations or fee-for-service insurers. If being sued is accepted as evidence for holding the line, it is pertinent that other types of HMOs and indemnity insurers held the line quite well against the premature use of the most visible and most important new technology of the last decade, high-dose chemotherapy and bone marrow transplantation in late-stage breast cancer. Several big indemnity insurers were also in the lead in providing financial support for the government-sponsored randomized controlled trials that eventually showed that technology to be ineffective.

With respect to consistency in technology assessment, the results are mixed. While there are many examples of good top-down decision making in PGPs, where a single committee has evaluated a technology and its recommendation has been followed consistently throughout the organization, there are also many examples where, even within a single PGP, different regions or medical centers have conducted their own assessments and come to different conclusions. There are also examples of this type of inconsistency for the guidelines that are developed out of technology assessments.

As for economies of scale, there are examples of successes, with all parties agreeing to coordinate their work and follow agreed-upon methods, but there are also examples of exceptions. For an example of a success, Kaiser Permanente has made important strides toward coordinating its technology assessment programs and taking the greatest possible advantage of assessments done by other organizations. Another example of progress toward economies of scale and consistency is the Interregional Guidelines Steering Group created by Kaiser Permanente to organize collaboration across the different regions. On the other hand, one of the largest regions in Kaiser Permanente has chosen not to participate in that very program, either because it did not want to abide by the agreed-upon evidence-based methodology or because it did not think that the coordinated, programwide effort was worth the resources.

As for monitoring the implementation of new technologies and guidelines, there are certainly examples where this type of monitoring has been implemented in a systematic way by PGPs. The clinical review criteria developed at Group Health Cooperative is one such example. The tracking of pharmaceutical costs is another. However, there are many counterexamples where new technologies and guidelines are not monitored at all.

There is, however, good evidence that PGPs perform well with respect to deploying new technologies. This was illustrated by all three of the PGPs described in this chapter. It is very difficult for a decentralized system that lacks integrated management to perform this type of planning. Though it may not be done perfectly within PGPs and there may be failures, it appears that PGPs can and do perform this function better than most other types of organizations.

Conclusions

In summary, both the theoretical advantages and the performance of PGPs versus non-PGPs are mixed. With regard to technology assessments, there are no theoretical reasons to expect that PGPs should be able to perform better than other types of organizations, and the best assessment program to date is not in a PGP. As for deployment of new technologies, there are good theoretical reasons to expect PGPs to achieve greater efficiencies than other types of organizations. Those theoretical advantages appear to be borne out by the well-developed programs found in at least three PGPs, but there is no direct evidence of greater efficiencies in practice. For the implementation of new technologies, the story is also mixed. The claims data used by many non-PGPs make it easier for them to monitor the use of many technologies. On the other hand, PGPs have a theoretical advantage in the potential for a close alignment of physician practices with management decisions. However, this potential advantage can be muted to the extent that there is suspicion, distrust, or friction between management and physicians, or to the extent that physicians insist on autonomy.

To achieve their full potential, PGPs must maximize their coordination between physicians and management, between various physician groups within the same PGP, and among physicians within those groups. Failure to do this leads to inefficiencies and inconsistencies that make PGPs look more like nonintegrated organizations. Coordination could give PGPs great power in integrating physician practices with good management decisions and implementing the results of assessments appropriately, whether the results are positive or negative.

The most important development on the horizon is the advent of automated clinical information systems. Their ability to enhance vertical integration puts PGPs in a better position to implement automated systems. Group Health Cooperative has had a clinical information system for several years, and Kaiser Permanente is committing billions of dollars to developing a system. As these systems are installed, and to the extent that they are installed sooner by PGPs, they should greatly improve the ability of PGPs to implement and monitor decisions about new technologies.

Appendix: Examples of Technology Assessment in Prepaid Group Practice

This appendix presents two examples of technology assessments in a prepaid group practice, one with a positive conclusion and the other with a negative conclusion. Both are narrative summaries of assessments by Kaiser Permanente's Interregional New Technology Committee, based on evidence reviews conducted by the Blue Cross and Blue Shield Association's TEC program.

Capsule Endoscopy for the Small Intestine

Performed October 2002.

Background. A miniature video camera (M2A) is swallowed by the patient and, with the aid of peristalsis (the natural movement of the bowel), the capsule moves smoothly and painlessly through the gastrointestinal (GI) tract. As the capsule passes through the GI tract, it transmits video signals, which are stored in the receiving unit. These signals also enable the system to trace the physical course of the capsule's progress. The capsule is excreted naturally out of the body.

A wireless recorder worn on a belt around the patient's waist receives signals transmitted by the capsule through an array of antennae placed on the patient's body. The ambulatory belt, which can be worn comfortably, permits users to continue their daily activities. A computer workstation, equipped with Given Imaging's proprietary RAPID (Reporting and Processing of Images and Data) software, processes the data and produces a short video clip of the small intestine together with additional relevant information from the digestive tract. The RAPID workstation permits physicians to view, edit, and archive the video and save individual images and short video clips.

Patient Indications. The potential target population for capsule endoscopy includes patients who have symptoms of chronic abdominal pain or chronic or unexplained rectal bleeding in the absence of small bowel obstruction, but in whom other procedures, including upper GI endoscopy, colonoscopy, "push" enteroscopy (in which a tube is "pushed" through the small bowel), and enteroclysis have been done and failed to discover the cause.

FDA Approval. Capsule endoscopy is available from only one vendor (Given Imaging, Ltd.) and was approved by the Food and Drug Administration (FDA) through the 510 (k) process on August 1, 2001. The FDA approval specified that the capsule was being approved for use "along with—not as a replacement for—other endoscopic and radiological evaluations of the small bowel."

Evidence. A comprehensive review of the published literature revealed two clinical studies. One was a study by Lewis and Swain in which twenty patients who had obscure GI bleeding were given both capsule endoscopy and push endoscopy.[3] Fourteen of the patients had negative examinations by push endoscopy. In those fourteen, capsule endoscopy found the cause of the bleeding in five (or 36 percent). In each case, the finding led to a change in treatment, with a presumption of an improvement in outcomes.

The other study, by Ell and colleagues, involved thirty-two patients who had chronic GI bleeding and had received "complete conventional diagnostic workup" with other tests.[4] In this group, twenty patients had negative examinations by push endoscopy. Of those twenty, capsule endoscopy found causes of the bleeding in thirteen (66 percent).

Conclusions About the Evidence. Despite the fact that the total published experience with the use of capsule endoscopy for patients who have negative examinations by other methods, including push endoscopy, was limited to two studies, the evidence was considered sufficient to conclude that capsule endoscopy does improve patient outcomes.

Other Considerations. It was noted that the adverse outcomes that were initially anticipated have not occurred, and the device appears to be quite safe. It was also noted that the Northern and Southern California regions of Kaiser Permanente were currently involved in a pilot study of the technology. Additional issues to consider are that the length of time to interpret the images is expected to be much longer than the thirty to ninety minutes quoted by the manufacturer, that there might be pressure to expand the potential uses of the technology beyond the bounds of FDA approval and the evidence, and that a system for locating the capsule after it comes out in the stool is currently under review by the FDA.

Conclusion. The Interregional New Technologies Committee recommended that capsule endoscopy is a medically appropriate diagnostic option for selected patients with chronic, obscure occult bleeding when standard diagnostic imaging techniques have failed.

Percutaneous Intradiscal Radiofrequency Thermocoagulation for Chronic Low Back Pain Caused by Disc Damage

Performed June 2002.

Background. Approximately 20 percent of the U.S. population (or about 57 million people) suffers from low back pain. The North American Spine Society estimates that in approximately one million of these, the pain is caused by disc damage. Percutaneous intradiscal radiofrequency thermocoagulation is an arthroscopic treatment that permits the controlled delivery of electrothermal heat to the intervertebral disc by way of a thermal resistive coil embedded within a catheter. The catheter is passed through the skin (it is "percutaneous") and placed within a symptomatic disc under fluoroscopic guidance and local anesthesia. Thermal energy is then conducted into the annular wall at temperatures from 80 to 95 degrees Celsius. This causes contraction and thickening of the collagenous structure and coagulation of the neurovascular tissues.

One system for delivering this radiofrequency thermocoagulation is called intradiscal electrothermal therapy (IDET) and uses a catheter called SpineCATH marketed by ORATEC. At least two other systems are being marketed for the same purpose: the Radionics RF Disc Catheter System and the ArthroCare System 2000.

Percutaneous intradiscal radiofrequency thermocoagulation is an outpatient procedure performed by an orthopedist, anesthesiologist, physiatrist, radiologist, general surgeon, or neurosurgeon. The procedure typically takes one hour for each disc that is treated, and the patient recovers in forty-five minutes to a few hours. Postoperative recovery, including physical therapy, may require four months, with restrictions on physical activity. According to ORATEC, approximately twenty-five hundred spine physicians are trained to use IDET, and thirty thousand IDET catheterization procedures were performed between 1997 and 2000, the majority after mid-1999.

FDA Approval. All three systems have received 510(k) clearance from the FDA.

Evidence. The published evidence consists of two comparative trials and three case series. One of the comparative trials is a randomized double-blind placebo-controlled study by Barendse and colleagues that compared radiofrequency thermocoagulation with a sham procedure in a total of twenty-eight patients.[5] The results showed no significant differences between groups in any outcomes after a follow-up period of eight weeks.

The second trial, by Karasek and Bogduk, was not randomized. It compared radiofrequency thermocoagulation with rehabilitation.[6] The authors did not control for potential differences in groups on baseline characteristics, and the assignment of patients to the different treatments may have been biased. Patients who received radiofrequency thermocoagulation reported greater relief of pain after three months on a visual analogue scale (VAS). However, there is no way to determine if the difference in pain relief was due to the treatment or due to initial differences in the patients who were assigned to receive the different treatments, such as differences in severity or duration of disc disease.

The three case series do not provide useful information about whether radiofrequency thermocoagulation is more effective than a placebo or other treatments.[7]

Conclusions About the Evidence. The evidence is considered insufficient to determine if percutaneous intradiscal radiofrequency thermocoagulation improves patient outcomes.

Other Considerations. It was noted that although there have been no published reports of adverse events directly related to the IDET procedure, there are some possible complications including transient worsening of symptoms, diskitis, neurological injury, and catheter breakage. One case of *cauda equina* syndrome resulting from IDET was reported.

According to ORATEC, there are at least two ongoing clinical trials. One is a double-blind, randomized placebo-controlled trial being conducted at St. Andrew's Hospital in Adelaide, Australia. The other is a placebo-controlled, double-blind randomized study being conducted at East Texas Medical Center in Tyler, Texas.

Conclusions. The Interregional New Technologies Committee recommends that there is insufficient evidence to conclude that percutaneous intradiscal radiofrequency thermocoagulation is a medically appropriate treatment option for chronic low back pain due to disc damage.

Notes

1. Blue Cross and Blue Shield Association's Technology Evaluation Center, "TEC Assessments," 2003 [http://www.bluecares.com/tec/tecassessmentvols.html].
2. Blue Cross and Blue Shield Association's Technology Evaluation Center, "TEC Criteria," 2003 [http://www.bluecares.com/tec/teccriteria.html].
3. B. Lewis and P. Swain, "Capsule Endoscopy in the Evaluation of Patients with Suspected Small Intestinal Bleeding: The Results of a Pilot Study," *Gastrointestinal Endoscopy*, 2000, *56*, 349–353.
4. C. Ell and others, "The First Prospective Controlled Trial Comparing Wireless Capsule Endoscopy with Push Enteroscopy in Chronic Gastrointestinal Bleeding," *Endoscopy*, 2002, *34*, 685–689.

5. G. A. Barendse and others, "Randomized Controlled Trial of Percutaneous Intradiscal Radiofrequency Thermocoagulation for Chronic Discogenic Back Pain: Lack of Effect from a 90-Second 70C Lesion," *Spine*, 2001, *26*, 287–292.

6. M. Karasek and N. Bogduk, N., "Twelve-Month Follow-Up of a Controlled Trial of Intradiscal Thermal Annuloplasty for Back Pain Due to Internal Disc Disruption," *Spine*, 2000, *25*, 2601–2607.

7. R. Derby and others, "Intradiscal Electrothermal Annuloplasty (IDET): A Novel Approach for Treating Chronic Discogenic Back Pain," *Neuromodulation*, 2000, *3*, 82–88; J. A. Saal and J. S. Saal, "Management of Chronic Discogenic Low Back Pain with Thermal Intradiscal Catheter: A Preliminary Report," *Spine*, 2000, *25*, 382–388; J. A. Saal and J. S. Saal, "Intradiscal Electrothermal Treatment for Chronic Discogenic Low Back Pain: A Prospective Outcome Study with Minimum 1-Year Follow-Up," *Spine*, 2000, *25*, 2622–2627.

CHAPTER SIX

MANAGING THE PHARMACY BENEFIT IN PREPAID GROUP PRACTICE

William H. Campbell, Richard E. Johnson, and Sharon L. Levine

The past three decades have witnessed a pharmacological revolution in health care. Prescription drugs have accounted for an increasing proportion of total health care expenditures, in recent years outstripping the average annual growth in personal health care expenditures. Between 1990 and 2002, total health care expenditures in the United States increased by 5.6 percent per year, while spending on prescription drugs increased by 12.0 percent per year.[1] Between 1994 and 1999, outpatient prescription drug costs grew from 6.7 percent of total U.S. health care spending to 9.4 percent.[2]

Some 22 percent of this increase in drug spending can be attributed to price increases, 36 percent to "change in mix" (the replacement of older drugs with newer, more expensive drugs), and the largest proportion, 42 percent, to increased utilization.[3] This latter increase appears to be the result of drug therapy moving in two directions simultaneously: drug therapy as *treatment substitution* (the use of drug therapy to avoid or delay other—sometimes more expensive or intensive—services, such as hospitalization), and drug therapy as *treatment expansion* (the use of drug therapy earlier in the course of an illness or condition or to treat previously untreatable conditions).[4]

This pharmacological revolution and its impact on prescription drug expenditures raise a number of questions. Are these increased expenditures producing commensurate increases in health? How well are health care organizations integrating the new pharmacotherapies and approaches into the overall delivery of medical care to effect optimal health and economic value? Are consumers receiving greater value from a dollar spent on prescription drugs than from any alternative use of that dollar in health care?

This chapter explores the promise, performance, and potential of prepaid group practices (PGPs) in creating value for consumers through integration and management of pharmacy benefits. It also examines and highlights differences between pharmacy benefits managed and delivered by prepaid group practices and pharmacy programs operated by network-model Health Maintenance Organizations (HMOs), or "carrier HMOs," as they are termed in this volume. The chapter examines five processes necessary to the integration of pharmacy benefits, analyzing them from the perspective of the known and theoretical opportunities that arise from horizontal and vertical integration. Next, the chapter describes the five processes in empirical terms, reviewing the published literature regarding carrier HMO versus prepaid group practice performance relative to pharmacy benefit management. The chapter concludes with the results of a survey of pharmacy leaders in PGPs.

Pharmacy Benefits in PGPs and Carrier HMOs

Confusion about the costs and benefits of drug therapy is a long-standing hallmark of U.S. health care policy. When the legislation creating Medicare and Medicaid was signed in 1965, it did not include a prescription drug benefit under Medicare, and prescription drugs were listed as an optional benefit in Medicaid (although all states have chosen to provide a Medicaid pharmacy benefit). Almost forty years later, Medicare still did not include prescription drug coverage as a basic benefit. However, as this volume went to press, Medicare drug coverage had just been signed into law.

The Carrier HMO Pharmacy Model

In the Preface, Alain Enthoven and Laura Tollen discuss the "carrier HMO" versus the prepaid group practice or "delivery system HMO" as a framework for understanding differences in organized health care systems. Carrier HMOs usually require (with some exceptions) the services of a separate organization, generally a pharmacy benefit management (PBM) company, to deliver and manage a drug benefit. Exhibit 6.1 illustrates how the PBM contracts with an insurer (for example, a Blue Cross plan) or a self-insured payer (for example, a state or municipal government) to define a pharmacy benefit for a group of beneficiaries. The PBM also contracts with the insurer or payer to manage the benefit and negotiates

EXHIBIT 6.1. CARRIER-PBM MODEL OF PHARMACY BENEFITS.

	Entity	Examples	Function
	Insurer or payer	Blue Cross Blue Shield, state government	Defines the health care benefit available to beneficiaries
	Contract A		
Pharmaceutical industry	Pharmacy benefit manager	Advance-PCS, Medco	Defines the prescription benefit available to payers and beneficiaries
Contract B			
	Contract C		
	Pharmacy provider network	Walgreen's, CVS	Provides prescription services as specified by contract

individual contracts with a provider network of chain and independent community pharmacies to dispense prescriptions.[5]

The PBM operates through three sets of contracts, one (A) with its insurers and payers, the second (B) with pharmaceutical companies, and a third (C) with its pharmacy providers.[6] In this structure, it is often unclear who is "in charge" of decisions about benefits (for example, whether a drug is on or off the formulary or to which tier it belongs), the PBM or the payer. One of the greatest frustrations with the carrier-PBM model is this lack of clear accountability—to both beneficiaries and providers—for decisions about the pharmacy benefit.

The ability of the PBM to require specialized services from its pharmacy providers is limited by the terms of its contracts with payers and insurers. Requiring pharmacies to modify their standard practices can be difficult because the number of beneficiaries under a specific insurance plan is a small percentage of any pharmacy's customer base. More important, it is nearly impossible for a PBM to integrate pharmacy services with physician, hospital, or other services because the latter are covered under separate contracts independent of the PBM.

The PBM generates revenue by a combination of administrative fees from sponsors and rebates from pharmaceutical companies, which are often associated with efforts to "switch" patients from one brand of drug to another. In these situations, the PBM may have to choose between the goals of adding revenue through rebates or providing balanced information to support evidence-based drug therapy—goals that may or may not be compatible, depending on the nature of the rebate and the particular drug involved. The PBM may also generate revenue by selling drug utilization data or prescriber information to pharmaceutical companies, which use such data for marketing purposes. These practices are coming under closer scrutiny by private and public groups concerned about their ethical and legal ramifications.[7]

The PGP Pharmacy Model

At first glance, the delivery of a pharmacy benefit in the prepaid group practice model (see Exhibit 6.2) appears similar to the carrier-PBM model, but the differences are substantial. Perhaps the most important difference is that in the PGP model, the pharmacy organization is *part of* the same integrated delivery system as the prepaid group practice, rather than being linked to it merely by contract. The pharmacy organization performs many of the same functions as the PBM in the carrier model, but it does so in partnership with all other parts of the integrated delivery system and with better alignment of incentives. Rebates and discounts negotiated with drug manufacturers accrue to the benefit of, and are shared by, the enrollees of the prepaid group practice. The pharmacy benefit is an

EXHIBIT 6.2. PREPAID GROUP PRACTICE MODEL OF PHARMACY BENEFITS.

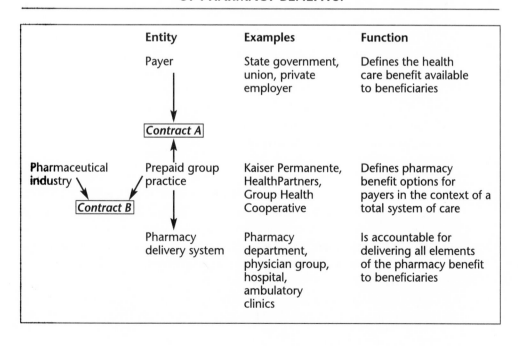

Entity	Examples	Function
Payer	State government, union, private employer	Defines the health care benefit available to beneficiaries
Prepaid group practice	Kaiser Permanente, HealthPartners, Group Health Cooperative	Defines pharmacy benefit options for payers in the context of a total system of care
Pharmacy delivery system	Pharmacy department, physician group, hospital, ambulatory clinics	Is accountable for delivering all elements of the pharmacy benefit to beneficiaries

Pharmaceutical industry

Contract A

Contract B

essential component of a comprehensive package that includes hospital, physician, laboratory, and other services organized and provided by the medical group and its affiliated hospitals.

Five Essential Elements of Pharmacy Benefit Integration

To understand how integration makes a difference in the pharmacy benefit, we focus on five basic processes that must be performed for patients to receive prescription services: pharmacy administration and management, drug selection, drug prescribing, drug dispensing, and drug use and monitoring. We will compare these processes in the carrier-PBM model, which relies on a pharmacy benefit management company, and the prepaid group practice model, which relies on an integrated delivery system.

Pharmacy Administration and Management

Pharmacy administrative policies and procedures in a prepaid group practice are coordinated both vertically and horizontally. *Vertical* integration connects all organizational components from "top to bottom" through unified management and budgeting for the entire system. *Horizontal* integration connects pharmacy facilities of different types, such as outpatient, off-site (mail service), satellite, specialty, and other facilities.

Information integration is a critical capability of care management. Because pharmacies, medical offices, and laboratories in a PGP are part of the same organization, barriers to information exchange are reduced. As a result, pharmacy, laboratory, and other kinds of medical information are more likely to be available to practitioners at the point of care. An integrated information system provides real-time prescription data for purchasing and inventory control and supports negotiations with suppliers based on the ability to promise and deliver market share.

Perhaps the form of integration that most differentiates the prepaid group practice from the carrier-PBM model of pharmacy benefit management is the cooperation between health care professionals and management, facilitated by their shared responsibility for organizing and delivering effective and efficient care, including pharmacy care. Such integrations are generally not possible in the carrier model, as the PBM does not have access to up-to-date clinical information or encounter data.

More important, the PGP's level of accountability to its membership is greater than that found in the carrier-PBM model because the PGP is responsible for providing all elements of health care. The confusion earlier noted about who is in charge of the pharmacy benefit exists to a much lesser degree in the PGP model. In the PGP, providers and patients understand the organization and can address concerns through multiple points of contact. Similarly, a prepaid group practice has an established consultative relationship with its members and providers and can regularly contact them to determine their satisfaction with the pharmacy services they receive and provide, respectively.

Drug Selection

The U.S. pharmaceutical armamentarium consists of all prescription and non-prescription (over-the-counter, or OTC) drugs approved by the federal Food and Drug Administration (FDA). Despite advertising claims, each of the many thousands of proprietary products does not represent a significant advantage over all other competitors. Many products are inferior therapeutic choices. Many have equally effective but less costly alternatives, and many are simply duplicative.

Pharmacy benefit management companies are reluctant to impose direct controls on physician prescribing because the carrier HMO model relies on a network of physicians who are not accustomed to, and may resist, efforts to restrict their choice of drugs. The PBMs are more likely than prepaid group practices to employ indirect controls on physician prescribing, such as disincentives (reducing pharmacy payments for some drugs) and patient financial incentives and coverage restrictions (for example, prior authorization—although it should be noted that many PBMs are giving up this practice in favor of tiered cost-sharing arrangements).[8] This strategy of coverage manipulation is inherently inefficient, reactive, and frustrating for all concerned. In surveys of pharmacists, physicians, and beneficiaries, the time required for dealing with PBM administrative procedures, such as explaining a change in refill policy or why a drug previously covered is no longer covered, is by far the most common complaint.[9]

In a prepaid group practice, the pharmacy benefit can be designed to optimize drug selection based on therapeutic efficacy, efficiency, and value for money. Rather than including thousands of different products in the formulary, the focus is on inclusion of the drugs deemed most appropriate for prescribing. Using criteria such as quality, safety, and value, drugs are chosen by a committee of health care professionals (often a "pharmacy and therapeutics committee"). The final list of drugs makes up the formulary. The formulary in a PGP, however, is more than a list of drugs. It is also a system of policies and procedures to guide the choice and prescribing of drugs. Evidence-based programs to promote drugs of choice for certain conditions, practitioner prescribing profiles, and dosing guidelines and other information can be provided to physicians for education and to support quality improvement. These and other support activities substantially extend the value of a formulary beyond simply a list of drugs.

Formularies and pharmacy and therapeutics committees are also present in PBM operations, but substantial differences exist between them and the prepaid group practice model in terms of integration of care and the participation of practicing physicians. The first and perhaps most important difference is that in a prepaid group practice, the physicians in the medical group create the formulary. They do so through broad participation of clinical experts representing all specialties. These experts are accountable to their peers and have frequent and substantive interaction with them. This formulary development process takes place in partnership with pharmacy administrators and practitioners, and it blends with the broader web of clinical policies, education, and prescribing guidelines to support clinician decisions and therapeutic choices.

In contrast to this, providers contracting with insurers and health plans who use a PBM to manage drug benefits are almost always practicing with multiple formularies, each of which is plan-specific or carrier-specific. Physician involvement in and ability to influence drug selection are much more limited. Whereas drug selection and formulary decision making in the PGP model precede and drive the contracting process with drug manufacturers, in the PBM, contracts with manufacturers often drive drug selection and formulary creation.

Drug Prescribing

The physician's role in prescription drug therapy is that of a "learned intermediary"—one possessed of specialized knowledge and having responsibility for translating complex information about therapeutic alternatives into meaningful information for patients. This occurs in the context of a practice environment that is fast-paced, sometimes stressful, and often overloaded with information.

A particular challenge to the role of learned intermediary is the relative lack of unbiased information available to physicians about the comparative efficacy and cost effectiveness of drugs. New single-source, patent-protected drugs are aggressively promoted by pharmaceutical manufacturers, with little head-to-head comparison of these drugs to older, effective, and often less expensive drugs. This has led to calls for a national commitment to provide more balanced information to physicians and other prescribers.[10]

In the carrier HMO environment, pharmaceutical sales representatives make themselves available to physicians as a convenient and easily accessible source of drug information, seeking time with physicians in medical offices to promote the use of their employers' drugs. Little counterbalancing information is available to physicians outside organized systems of care. When PBMs do provide drug information to network physicians, these efforts are often represented by the PBMs as "disease state management programs," but they have earned widespread skepticism among physicians as marketing strategies rather than as quality-of-care improvements.

The prepaid group practice is a more conducive environment for providing timely, objective, and balanced information to physicians about prescription drugs. The promotional efforts of the brand-name pharmaceutical industry are tempered by policies and procedures that limit the industry's access and influence through restriction or outright elimination of free samples, unscheduled sales visits, "detailing" (promotion) of nonformulary drugs, on-site displays, and other promotional efforts. Some PGPs and large integrated medical groups have learned from and adapted the successful practices of industry, instituting generic sampling programs, gifts (pens, coffee cups, notepads) and reminders to promote formulary choices, and continuing education programs related to optimal drug use management.

The PGP is in fact organized to take advantage of multiple information channels to support quality, economical prescribing. For example, in the Kaiser Permanente system in California, physician prescribing is supported by the following information channels:

- Clinical practice guidelines developed by clinical experts, which incorporate prescribing guidelines
- A drug information service (which serves all the Permanente medical groups) staffed by pharmacists who review the literature, develop monographs for drugs being considered for formulary inclusion, and staff a toll-free number to provide real-time consultation to clinicians
- Drug education coordinators in every medical center who provide academic detailing of preferred therapeutic alternatives and work with individual clinicians
- Continuing medical education programs developed in-house, which incorporate formulary recommendations
- Information systems that integrate diagnosis, lab, X-ray, and pharmacy data to enable point-of-care reminders, alerts, and prompts to reinforce evidence-based prescribing in real time

Some of these methods are also employed in carrier HMOs and PBMs. In a prepaid group practice, however, the methods originate entirely within the organization and are developed by practitioners in the context of a self-governed, self-managed medical group practice. Their rationale and methods represent a professional consensus of physician peers. It is this ownership of both content and process that results in physician cooperation and participation in prescribing improvement programs, rather than reluctant compliance with externally applied controls.

Drug Dispensing

To fill a prescription, the carrier-PBM model requires a beneficiary to present an identification card to a pharmacy. The pharmacy must verify that it is part of the provider network authorized to provide services to the beneficiary, and it must also confirm that the beneficiary is eligible to receive services. Next, the pharmacy must determine the specific characteristics of the benefit (copayment amount, days' supply, product restrictions, and so on). If allowable, the pharmacy will dispense the requested drug product to the beneficiary. However, in approximately 30 percent of "card system" encounters, some administrative problem must be adjudicated or additional information obtained.[11] With the carrier-PBM model, a pharmacy does not have access to other health information about the beneficiary, the specific drug product may not be in the pharmacy's inventory, contact with the prescriber will routinely be difficult, and specialty pharmacy services are likely to be nonexistent. If the prescription order cannot be dispensed, it will be up to the beneficiary to identify a different participating pharmacy and begin the process anew.

The process of drug dispensing is quite different in the prepaid group practice, in which integration enables the collection and sharing of information about the demographics and health status of the membership, which in turn informs the development of a plan for drug distribution. Pharmacies are often placed in proximity to medical offices so that beneficiaries can fill prescriptions at the point of care. Refill prescriptions for longer-term maintenance drugs can be ordered online or by mail, prepared at an off-site fulfillment center, and sent to an outpatient clinic pharmacy or to the member's home. In a horizontally integrated system with integrated prescription databases, the member is not locked into a single pharmacy but can be served at multiple sites.

Various technologies can be used to integrate pharmacies, such as automated dispensing systems linked to management information systems that generate purchasing and inventory control requests. Automated dispensing systems not only fill prescription orders but also can print drug information leaflets that advise the patient of appropriate use and warnings about a particular medication.

Integration of the drug dispensing process also means that regardless of where the prescription order is dispensed, it is possible for a pharmacy to access information about other services. For example, in dispensing a statin drug as maintenance medication for lowering serum cholesterol, practice guidelines may require monitoring of blood cholesterol. Rather than being subjected to unnecessary physician office visits to manage this requirement, the patient may be contacted by the pharmacy under a physician-directed protocol before the prescription is due to be refilled. Then a lab test can be ordered and the results posted in the automated record. The information is available to the pharmacist dispensing the prescription refill, who can proceed with dispensing the order if the lab results fall within the parameters of the protocol.

Prepaid group practices also have the ability to implement specialty pharmacist or pharmacy services, such as geriatric, oncology, coagulation, pain management, HIV, and pediatric services. These and other specialized services can be provided by the pharmacy department (horizontal integration) or through medical, home care, or other departments (vertical integration). In either case, the integration of administrative and clinical data to achieve optimum pharmacotherapy is uniquely possible in a prepaid group practice and virtually impossible in a carrier-PBM model.

Drug Use and Monitoring

The desired outcome of providing a pharmacy benefit is compliance with therapy and, ultimately, improved health status. The carrier-PBM model and the prepaid group practice use common methods to facilitate appropriate prescription drug use, but the degree of integration varies markedly between the two models.

An important aspect of ensuring compliance with drug therapy is consistent patient education and counseling. Every PBM network pharmacy has a computer system for displaying a beneficiary's current medication record. However, the pharmacies use different commercial software systems and have different capabilities and protocols, such as the criteria for drug-drug interactions, dosage errors, noncompliance, and other "signals" that are sent to the pharmacist. Consequently, a prescription filled at different network pharmacies may result in different warnings and interventions by the pharmacist, as prompted by their different computer systems. However, a prescription filled at different pharmacies of a prepaid group practice will have uniform warnings and interventions because there is a single standard of practice and a single computer system.

Unlike the PBM-affiliated network of pharmacy providers, the PGP has the ability to define an organizational standard of practice above and beyond minimum legal standards. These standards are supported through formal criteria and definitions of patient counseling, performance standards for evaluating pharmacists, physical design and layout specifications to ensure privacy and maximize effectiveness of counseling, and adequate staffing and other support. The end result is that each pharmacy must deliver care that not only complies with legal standards but also meets organizational standards designed to meet the unique needs of the patient population.

In addition to member counseling and member drug profiling, PGPs may use several other services designed to improve drug utilization by members. (It should be noted that health plans that use PBMs may also employ some of these methods. However, the difference is that in the case of the PGP, these processes are "owned" by the medical group, rather than by the health plan or the PBM.) A monthly or quarterly general health information brochure is commonly mailed to members, including information about drug therapy. Topics range from pharmaceutical issues of timely concern (for example, market removal of a drug for adverse effects) to discussion of a current controversy (for example, hormone replacement therapy) to a review of a newly released drug heavily promoted through direct-to-consumer advertising. Targeted newsletters to groups (for example, members with diabetes or hypertension) can offer information and encouragement about the benefits of long-term compliance with drug therapy.

Other avenues for members to obtain drug information and advice may include on-call consulting nurse and pharmacist services and direct integration of ambulatory care pharmacists into care teams. The unique value of these services is that the complete prescription drug profile is available to the health professional offering advice. Advice on continuing or discontinuing a prescription drug due to a suspected adverse effect (one of the most common questions in an on-call drug information service) can be promptly and accurately provided, based on the patient's specific clinical and prescription information, which is readily available.

While the prepaid group practice has distinct advantages in implementing methods for influencing drug use, it has even greater advantages in using its full clinical database to understand what drug use problems should be addressed and what interventions should be used in particular situations. In contrast, the carrier-PBM model of pharmacy benefits relies on the prescription as its only database for identifying and correcting problems. The prescription generates five information elements: (1) identification of the specific drug product (for example, "ciprofloxacin 500 mg"), (2) identification of the prescriber ("Dr. Myron Smith"), (3) identification of the patient ("Ms. Carolyn Jones"), (4) identification of the pharmacy ("ChainRite #439"), and (5) chronicity of the prescription (date, number of refills, and so on). Limited additional information can be linked to this information. For example, using the National Drug Code, it is possible to add information about the specific drug product, such as manufacturer, cost, dosage form, and therapeutic category. Similarly, the identity of the prescriber can be expanded to include address, specialty, and other characteristics. Patient information can be linked to age, sex, eligibility status, and insurer.

The information from millions of prescriptions can be useful to a PBM in measuring program operations and managing resources. A PBM can aggregate data across many prescriptions and analyze how prescription drugs are being used. Common measures include total number and cost of prescriptions per year and average cost per prescription. These and other, more detailed measures are aggregated for large numbers of prescriptions and used by PBM administrators and drug manufacturers. The information, however, measured and available at an aggregate level, has little utility in clinical quality improvement efforts because it is not linked to other clinical databases, such as diagnoses or encounter data.

Far more useful in terms of patient care is information about the total number of prescriptions issued in accordance with clinical practice guidelines and the outcomes and costs of care associated with different patterns of drug use and with differing conditions. It is nearly impossible to obtain this type of information within the PBM environment but is quite feasible within a PGP.

In contrast to the carrier-PBM model, the PGP relies on an integrated system of care as its source of data, with the capability of linking each element of information to all other elements, thus creating clinically useful data. This makes it possible to analyze the care received by a person with a particular diagnosis and to study retrospectively the outcomes associated with different treatment patterns. The linked database becomes a powerful tool for health outcomes research (turning every clinical encounter into a potential data point in a clinical research inquiry), as well as for interventions aimed at health status improvements in individuals or populations.

Very complex analyses of this type are possible and in fact are routinely conducted in mature PGPs. Standard reports to professional and administrative staff help identify practice patterns and practitioners who are prescribing outside recommended boundaries. Interventions to modify physician practice patterns can be implemented by peer experts employing a range of options, from continuing education to feedback through peer comparison reports. The ability to measure and analyze care in a PGP is greater than in the carrier-PBM model due to the quantity, quality, and linkage of pharmacy data with clinical data.

An example of the application of integrated databases to measure and improve pharmacy care is the campaign in one of Kaiser Permanente's regions to reduce antibiotic use in the treatment of viral infectious illnesses. An educational program was directed at both patients and providers. Progress was monitored by matching office visits for common viral respiratory illnesses with prescriptions for antibiotics written in association with these visits. Over two winter respiratory illness seasons, antibiotic use for viral illnesses was significantly decreased (about 25 percent), with no associated increase in doctor office visits or hospitalizations. The success of the campaign resulted largely from the ability to link prescription and office visit data, a feature not found in the carrier-PBM model.

Further Observations

Overall, the difference between the PGP and the carrier-PBM model in each of these five key areas is largely one of incentives. The PBM is an independent, profit-maximizing entity, not a part of a system that seeks to maximize overall health outcomes and value for money. Pharmacy benefit management companies' decisions may be influenced by the size of the rebates and discounts they obtain from manufacturers. They may be concerned about the total health and cost impacts of different drugs, but they are insulated from those impacts. The PBM's assignment from employers is to assist in holding down *drug* costs, regardless of whether the use of a specific drug results in an increase or decrease in the *total* cost of care.

Physicians' and other providers' incentives also differ between the two models. In most cases in the carrier-PBM model, the providers on the formulary committee are not the same as those treating patients. The former see only the pharmacy budget. They have little information and little reason to care about the impact of drug choices on, for example, hospital days. Furthermore, prescribing physicians have little information about costs versus benefits of specific drugs. Each physician's base of experience is too small to allow him or her to make cost-benefit comparisons. In addition, physicians in the carrier-PBM model often deal with dozens of different formularies associated with the different carriers, none of which is of his or her own making and the specifics of which change, depending on the latest discounts or rebates the PBM has negotiated.

By contrast, the providers and pharmacies in the PGP are part of an integrated system whose goal is to achieve better health outcomes at lower cost. The PGP can structure itself so that incentives are aligned throughout the organization. Formulary decisions are made by the individuals who are treating the patients, and there is only one formulary, developed by treating physicians and their colleagues. The incentive is to consider total costs and benefits of prescribing decisions because the costs of poor quality are borne by all parts of the integrated delivery system, as well as the patients themselves.

Finally, the pharmacies themselves face different incentives in the two models. In the carrier-PBM model, the pharmacy (often a drugstore or supermarket) that dispenses the drugs is rewarded financially only for selling more, not for in-depth counseling or for seeking out and documenting drug interactions. In the prepaid group practice model, pharmacists are a part of the system and are paid for counseling patients, checking for unfavorable drug interactions, and in effect for *not dispensing* a prescription drug when that is the appropriate therapeutic decision.

Literature Review and Interviews with Pharmacy Leaders

To complement the conceptual analysis presented here, we conducted both a literature review and a series of interviews with pharmacy leaders in several prepaid group practices.

Literature Review

We conducted a Medline review of English-language articles published in U.S. journals on pharmacy benefits in prepaid health care. For the period 1960 through 2002, a total of 177 articles were selected for in-depth review.[12] A preponderance of the published literature (85 percent of the reviewed articles) is of a descriptive nature. The two largest groups of descriptive articles concern drug utilization ($n = 71$) and formulary operations ($n = 54$). Only five articles reported patient care outcomes following interventions, and no articles compared the performance of pharmacy operations in an integrated health care setting to other settings, such as prepaid group practice versus the carrier-PBM model.

There is a paucity of evidence in the published literature linking drug use management approaches to improvements in patient care (five articles). One could speculate that marketing and market research data exist that could shed light on these important topics, but such data are missing from the published literature. Therefore, we are forced to rely on conceptual models to assess the potential versus realized economic and patient care performance of a pharmacy benefit in prepaid group practice. There is an obvious need for health services research and applied clinical research to guide policy and practice in this area.

Interview Findings

In an attempt to validate the theoretical advantages of PGP pharmacy benefit management, we interviewed pharmacy executives in several prepaid group practices, two of which also had some contractual relationships with networks of physicians.[13] The interviews focused on the extent to which pharmacy systems in prepaid group practices have been integrated into the delivery system and may perform as we have theorized. In the summary to follow, we do not distinguish between "pure" and "mixed" model experience because in all cases the pharmacy management and operations activities conformed to the "pure" PGP model (even when other parts of the delivery system may have been mixed). The interviews were structured around the five processes listed earlier in this chapter: pharmacy administration and management, drug selection, drug prescribing, drug dispensing, and drug use and monitoring. Two additional topics emerged from the interviews and are reported: research, and barriers to achieving greater efficiency and effectiveness of the pharmacy benefit.

Pharmacy Administration and Management. Pharmacy leadership operates at the second (vice president) or third (director) level of management in the settings surveyed. The pharmacy organization has a voice in the planning of pharmacy benefit packages through administrators and practitioners or pharmacists. Almost all comprehensive benefit packages include a prescription drug benefit.

Drug Selection. Although physicians make up a majority of membership on the formulary committees, pharmacists participate as voting members or as staff to the committees or through a drug information service. As part of such a service, pharmacists may create monographs for drugs under consideration or provide information from operational prescription drug data to support the deliberations of the pharmacy and therapeutics committee regarding adding or deleting drugs from the formulary.

Drug Prescribing, Dispensing, Use, and Monitoring. Rather than discussing these processes separately and in detail, we summarize the executives' comments. Development of these processes is assigned a high priority, as reflected by the attention of the executive and the allocation of personnel and capital resources. All executives emphasized the importance of integrating these processes horizontally and vertically, as, for example, the linkage of formal drug use monitoring activities with physician prescribing.

Most of the surveyed organizations have or are in the process of developing computerized physician order entry systems to facilitate prescribing and information transfer. In some, prescription refill activities have been centralized in locations remote from outpatient pharmacies. In addition, some of the PGPs have centralized repackaging programs. In some, dispensing pharmacists have access to patients' medical records at the point of service, while in most, pharmacists have access to patients' medication and laboratory data.

Either individual pharmacists serving in nondispensing roles or disease state management programs with pharmacists as a part of the team review and in some instances assist in managing patients with a variety of high-risk conditions. In addition, all the pharmacy systems have either specialty pharmacies or specialty pharmacists that participate in the treatment and monitoring of elderly patients and patients with specific diseases and conditions.

Research. The surveyed organizations conduct pharmacy-related research to address questions of interest to the organization, as well as questions of interest at the national level. Sponsorship (funding) of research may include internal allocation as well as extramural support through private and public sponsors. Pharmacists with research skills and interests participate in many of these projects.

Barriers to Greater Efficiency and Effectiveness. One concern of the interviewed executives was the continuing escalation of drug copayments, reflecting both increasing drug costs at the manufacturer level and the need to respond to competitors selling products with more limited drug benefits. All pharmacy executives were concerned about the prospect of shifting more drug costs to patients, potentially resulting in reduced access to or compliance with drug therapy and adverse health outcomes. Of particular concern is the direct-pay Medicare population, a group in need of pharmacy benefits and yet with few viable options. A related concern was maintaining a comprehensive benefit that included prescription drugs in the face of the risk that healthy members may choose to migrate to less comprehensive, lower-premium benefit programs.

It appears from the interviews that pharmacy systems in prepaid group practices are capitalizing on many opportunities unique to their integrated delivery system environments. While they are involved in most of the activities we indicated in our discussion, they also appear to be entering new areas we did not anticipate, particularly where there are collaborative practice opportunities and where drug therapy can play a significant role in patient outcomes.

One example comes from Henry Ford Health System (HFHS) and involves an intervention to improve use of statin therapy to manage patients with high serum cholesterol levels (particularly those with a history of coronary heart disease). HFHS developed a lipid clinic on a trial basis for eight hundred patients that allowed pharmacists, without direct physician involvement, to track patients' lipid levels, modify dosage, provide behavior modification counseling, and encourage patients to exercise and reduce fats in their diet. About 84 percent of patients in the pilot project achieved desired levels of blood lipids, at a short-term annual cost increase of $145 per patient. However, the long-term benefit-to-cost ratio was projected to be 2:1. This example illustrates the ability of integrated delivery systems to organize resources to achieve improvements in quality and efficiency of care, but it also illustrates the dilemma of short-term versus long-term costs and benefits. Although the lipid clinic demonstrated clear patient benefits, in a competitive market, HFHS might well find itself paying to reduce cholesterol levels in patients who would no longer be its patients by the time their averted heart attack would otherwise have occurred.[14]

Conclusions

We started this chapter by describing the factors that have had a major influence on drug expenditures. Drug therapies are now available to treat an increasing number of clinical conditions, and some of these therapies may replace or reduce the need for other health care services, though the evidence to support this claim is limited. Furthermore, concerns about the cost and effectiveness of, and need for, prescription drugs cause insurers and consumers to question whether they are receiving commensurate health value for these rapidly growing expenditures.

To shed light on these concerns, we compared five pharmacy-related processes in prepaid group practices and carrier-PBM settings: pharmacy administration and management, drug selection, drug dispensing, drug prescribing, and drug use and monitoring. Relying on current knowledge and a conceptual framework, we postulated that the prepaid group practice enjoys many potential advantages over the carrier-PBM model for delivering an efficient and effective pharmacy benefit. Our interviews with pharmacy executives strongly supported this conclusion, revealing a high degree of integration of pharmacy into prepaid group practice. The executives' organizations are developing an impressive array of initiatives and programs to deliver health benefits more efficiently and more effectively through the use of prescription drugs. A major gap in knowledge is the absence of published data comparing pharmacy management and operating procedures in prepaid group practices versus other systems.

Our analysis of the potential advantages in administrative procedures, drug selection, drug prescribing, drug dispensing, and drug use leads us to conclude that in each of these processes, PGPs offer an improved health outcome, a less costly approach, or both. When physicians can agree on a single drug of choice, where more than one option exists in a class of drugs, it is likely that the organization will obtain a lower price for the product, thus reducing total treatment costs. When, after rigorous review, a limited number of drugs have been accepted by physicians as the most cost-effective alternatives, the result is reduced inventory costs and improved outcomes of treatment. Dispensing a large proportion of prescription orders using an automated refill system with close to zero dispensing errors ensures safety in dispensing and capitalizes on economies of scale. Having drug use management and disease state management programs that integrate pharmacists' drug knowledge with the perspectives of other providers is likely to optimize the health and economic value delivered.

The key to achieving such results appears to be the integration of pharmacy with all other parts of the delivery system. One critical factor is the integration of health professionals, particularly the close partnership between physicians and pharmacists. Another important factor is the integration of clinical and management information. Complete, timely, and accurate information helps physicians discharge their role as "learned intermediary" and helps pharmacists provide technical support. Integrated information systems also provide the opportunity to track and review the performance of all participants (prescribers, pharmacists, pharmacy technicians, and others) in the system.

In Chapter One, Stephen Shortell and Julie Schmittdiel described the "promise, performance, and potential" of prepaid group practice. As we look at pharmacy benefit management and operations, the promise is clear. We believe that to date, PGPs are outperforming carrier HMOs in providing a pharmacy benefit that delivers health and economic value to beneficiaries. It is true some differences exist in the degree to which pharmacy activities are integrated into the delivery systems, and differences also exist in how activities such as formulary creation and management, drug selection guidelines, prescribing guidelines, dispensing initiatives, and drug use initiatives are organized and implemented across delivery systems. Still, little of this is even possible in the carrier-PBM model, where disparate people and organizations are connected primarily through contracts for reimbursement. In the Kaiser Permanente system, for example, integration is evolving rapidly across many fronts, with pharmacists and physician leaders from each region meeting monthly by teleconference and face-to-face twice a year to share performance data, learn from one another, and undertake new quality, safety, or drug use management efforts. Although this type of interaction may seem unremarkable in a large, multistate, integrated delivery system, it would be unthinkable (and probably illegal due to competitive and confidentiality concerns) among pharmacy providers in a PBM network.

When we think about potential and look to the future, a number of issues emerge, and the picture is less clear. Can the lessons learned from prepaid group practice be translated to broad networks of physicians, who contract with multiple health plans that in turn contract with PBMs? What is the likelihood of the fragmented prescriber community outside organized systems of care coming together to critically assess their practices, create guidelines and formularies, and negotiate effectively with pharmaceutical manufacturers? Is state or federal legislation likely to make that easier or more difficult?

One area in which federal legislation is likely to produce important outcomes is that of Medicare reform. On the basis of 2003 legislation, it appears that a prescription drug benefit will be implemented in 2006, with discretion granted to regional PBMs for delivering the benefit to Medicare beneficiaries. Given the complex web of potentially conflicting incentives among PBMs, their providers, and beneficiaries, it seems essential that extraordinary efforts be made both to predict the practices and performances of PBMs and to develop objective criteria and methods for monitoring the performance of PBMs in delivering a Medicare prescription drug benefit.

Another area that should be of concern to policymakers is the ability of PGPs to maintain the comprehensiveness of their pharmacy benefits and services in a market moving rapidly toward overall benefit reductions and shifting costs to consumers. The efficiencies of purchasing and the effectiveness of formulary-compliant, evidence-based prescribing in PGPs have so far enabled these organizations to maintain relatively comprehensive prescription drug benefits, minimize cost shifting to members, and reduce obstacles to access when compared to what is happening with PBMs and the rest of the market. But their ability to continue to do so while competitors pursue more direct cost-cutting strategies is questionable. Even if the two approaches—integrated pharmacy management and benefit reductions—achieve similar cost savings, the outcomes on quality of care could be very different, and so could the cost burden on consumers. Furthermore, there is a very real risk of adverse selection against the products with more comprehensive drug benefits.

Will the comprehensive nature of pharmacy benefits in PGPs and other "delivery system HMOs" cause integrated systems to become victims of their own success? Will they attract sicker patients, drawn to more comprehensive drug benefits, and will this be a threat to maintaining a balanced risk pool? Delivery system HMOs provide high-quality, coordinated care for the chronically and acutely ill, as well as maintain and improve the health of members. Their continued success may well depend on robust risk adjustment, based on the disease burden of the member population, if they continue to compete against health plans that segment risk.

Notes

1. Authors' calculation based on data presented in B. C. Strunk and P. B. Ginsburg, "Web Exclusive: Tracking Health Care Costs: Trends Stabilize but Remain High in 2002," *Health Affairs*, June 11, 2003 [http://www.healthaffairs.org/WebExclusives/Strunk_Web_Excl_061103.htm].

2. Centers for Medicare and Medicaid Services, from *Annual Reports of the Office of the Actuary* (Baltimore: National Health Statistics Group, 2000).

3. National Institute for Health Care Management, "Prescription Drug Expenditures in 2000: The Upward Trend Continues," May 2001 [http://www.nihcm.org/spending2000.pdf].

4. D. M. Cutler and M. McClellan, "Is Technological Change in Medicine Worth It?" in J. K. Iglehart, ed., *The Value of Rx Innovation: A Primer from Health Affairs* (Millwood, Va.: Project HOPE, 2001).

5. G. Jay, "Pharmacy Benefit Managers and Unique Customer Segments: Large Employers," *Journal of Managed Care Pharmacy*, 2000, *6*, 342–353.

6. A. Cook, J. Kornfield, and M. Gold, "The Role of PBMs in Managing Drug Costs: Implications for a Medicare Drug Benefit," report prepared for the Henry J. Kaiser Family Foundation, Jan. 2000.

7. B. Martinez, "Two Hats: Firms Paid to Trim Drug Costs Also Toil for Drug Makers," *Wall Street Journal*, Aug. 14, 2002, p. A1.

8. Cook, Kornfield, and Gold, "The Role of PBMs."

9. National Association of Chain Drug Stores, "Pharmacy Activity Cost and Productivity Survey," conducted by Arthur Anderson LLP, Nov. 1999 [http://www.nacds.org/user-assets/PDF_files/arthur_andersen.pdf].

10. R. Califf, "The Need for a National Infrastructure to Improve the Rational Use of Therapeutics," *Pharmacoepidemiology and Drug Safety*, 2002, *11*, 319–327.

11 B. Svarstad and J. Mount, "Evaluation of Written Prescription Information Provided in Community Pharmacies: A National Study," report prepared for the Food and Drug Administration and presented to the Drug Safety and Risk Management Advisory Committee, Gaithersburg, Md., July 17, 2002.

12. The initial search parameter was for all articles having "drug," "pharmacy," or "pharmacy benefit" as a keyword, yielding a total of 348,041 articles. Searching for the keywords "formulary," "dispensing," "prescribing," or "utilization" reduced the total to 6,898 articles. Further searching for the keywords "HMO," "managed care," and similar terms used to describe organized health care setting yielded a total of 177 articles. A further search on "cost effectiveness" or "quality" yielded too few articles (20), with numerous null cells, to conduct a meaningful analysis.

13. Participating in interviews for this chapter were Albert L. Carver, vice president of pharmacy strategy and operations, Kaiser Permanente California Regions; Michael E. Kinard, regional pharmacy manager, Kaiser Permanente Northwest Region; Barbara Zarowitz, vice president for pharmacy care management, Henry Ford Healthcare System, Detroit; Denise A. Clark, manager of pharmacy benefits and support services, Kaiser Permanente Colorado Region; and Sue Cooper, pharmacy director, HealthPartners, Minneapolis.

14. S. Leatherman and others, "The Business Case for Quality: Case Studies and an Analysis," *Health Affairs*, 2003, *22*(2), 17–30.

CHAPTER SEVEN

PREPAID GROUP PRACTICE AND MEDICAL WORKFORCE POLICY

Jonathan P. Weiner

The characteristics of the United States health care workforce have profound clinical and economic implications for consumers, delivery organizations, and society at large. Accordingly, the approach that Kaiser Permanente and other prepaid group practices (PGPs) use to deploy their physicians, nurses, and associated medical professionals is central to their mission. It also goes a long way toward explaining their accomplishments and challenges. For most patients served by PGPs, the provider workforce *is* the organization.

This chapter documents the approach used to staff eight large PGPs that provide care to more than 8 million enrolled consumers. A major objective of

This project would not have been possible without the full cooperation of the eight PGPs that freely opened their books for the purpose of this analysis. The leadership of both the medical groups and health plans at the Kaiser Permanente, Group Health Cooperative, and HealthPartners organizations are thanked for this unprecedented support. Thanks are also given to the very knowledgeable and cooperative staff at these organizations that provided administrative data from many parts of their organizations. These include Glen Hentges at Kaiser Permanente, Philip Mealand at Group Health Cooperative, and Maureen Peterson and Tammie Lindquist of HealthPartners of Minnesota. Jennifer Neisner of the Kaiser Permanente Institute for Health Policy and Cheryl Kaplowitz at the Johns Hopkins University also played very important roles in facilitating this chapter at many levels. The editorial assistance of Tracy Lieberman at Johns Hopkins is also gratefully acknowledged.

this analysis is to identify the unique approaches that each PGP has taken in developing its clinical staff and to offer potential lessons for other health care systems in the United States and elsewhere. To better accomplish this, this study documents the current staffing at the eight PGPs and compares them with the current U.S. medical workforce.

The strategies that early PGPs used to organize their physician panels were not only unique; they were also at odds with the more common mode of American medical practice: solo and small group fee-for-service (FFS). Prepaid group practices developed highly structured, multispecialty delivery settings that emphasized primary and preventive care. The physician group was reimbursed on a capitated, prepaid basis, and individual providers derived most of their income from a salary. PGPs were among the first to welcome nonphysician clinicians such as nurse practitioners and physician assistants (jointly referred to here as "nonphysician providers," or NPPs).

Many of these early workforce innovations have since been disseminated widely within the more traditional and mainstream health care system. However, other facets of these staffing and organizational approaches still set PGPs apart.

Since their inception, health care managers and policymakers in the non-PGP arena have looked to the established PGPs as models for how best to "staff up" to provide care for defined populations, be they enrolled in an insurance plan or residing in a defined geographical catchment area. Many consider the self-contained PGP as a microcosm that exemplifies how human resources should ideally be deployed in the pursuit of the optimal balance between affordability and quality. In our disaggregated American health care system, there are few other instances where a "numerator" of providers and a "denominator" of consumers or patients are so clearly demarcated.

Over the past four decades, policymakers, workforce and labor planners, and clinic managers have used staffing in PGPs as an important benchmark to determine whether the given number and type of providers in a particular geographical area are "adequate."[1] Also, PGPs have served as important incubators and test beds for workforce innovations. For example, in the 1960s and 1970s, much of the seminal work documenting the cost and quality implications of innovation with nurse practitioners and physician assistants was done in PGPs.[2] Furthermore, significant work comparing the relative roles of different types of physician care has been based at PGPs.[3]

In addition to these areas of inquiry, national and regional health care workforce planners have assessed the potential impact of PGPs as organizations patterned to some degree after them (such as Independent Practitioner Association (IPA)-model Health Maintenance Organizations (HMOs)) have become more widespread. Specifically, in the late 1980s and early 1990s, when national health care reform based on competitive integrated delivery systems was being seriously considered, there was intense interest in staff and group-model HMOs as a forerunner of these proposed delivery organizations.[4]

Although such government-led reform did not come to pass, another type of change did occur: corporate-controlled "managed care" became ubiquitous. But after a decade of dominance by these mainly for-profit, loosely organized plans, a widespread backlash resulted, and policymakers and consumers are now seeking alternatives. PGPs, with their very different roots in the social welfare and cost containment movements, represent a unique alternative model for the future of U.S. health care.

Against this backdrop, and in keeping with the intent of this volume, the goal of this chapter is to provide a detailed case study describing how Kaiser Permanente and two other well-regarded, large PGPs have chosen to structure their physician and nonphysician provider workforces. This chapter focuses on allopathic and osteopathic physicians, physician assistants, nurse practitioners, and other nurse specialists (such as midwives and nurse anesthetists) who can be viewed, at least to some extent, as "physician substitutes." To a more limited degree, this chapter will also document the PGPs' employment of certain non-M.D. and non-D.O. doctors (for example, optometrists, psychologists, and podiatrists) and other "independent" providers (for example, mental health therapists).

Because of the unprecedented nature of the data provided by the participating PGPs, this chapter significantly extends previous work in this area. For example, this is the first time this type of analysis has provided detailed staffing information for both ambulatory and hospital-based physician specialties, out-of-group contracted care, and nonphysician providers broken down by specialty.

Study Sites and Methods

This chapter provides information derived from six large geographical regions of Kaiser Permanente, plus Group Health Cooperative in Washington and HealthPartners in Minnesota. In total, these eight PGPs include providers practicing at more than 350 clinic sites and 33 PGP-staffed hospitals serving a population of more than 8 million consumers residing in nine states and the District of Columbia.

An unusual degree of information regarding inpatient and tertiary care specialties is available at the two largest Kaiser Permanente regions: Northern and

Southern California. Combined, these regions serve more than 6 million enrollees who obtain care from over 140 ambulatory sites and 28 fully staffed inpatient facilities. In no other geographical area of the country does a medical group (prepaid or otherwise) approach this size and level of comprehensiveness.

The Group Health and HealthPartners organizations also own and staff their own hospitals, but compared to the six Kaiser Permanente regions, they make greater use of nonemployed contracting physicians to care for their members. These two organizations supplied us with detailed aggregate billing information regarding these external providers, and Kaiser Permanente provided estimates regarding out-of-plan services. All PGPs in this study provide mental health services on site rather than contracting with a "carve-out" plan.

The patient populations included in this analysis represent only those enrollees who are registered with primary care sites staffed by the PGP and not those served by the independent physician networks. The percentage of the enrollees thus excluded was fairly modest (less than 10 percent) for Kaiser Permanente and Group Health Cooperative, but for HealthPartners this percentage is significant: about 50 percent of all HealthPartners enrollees are served by contracting group practices in the Twin Cities.

Two of Kaiser Permanente's eight regions (accounting for less than 8 percent of the organization's national enrollment) were excluded from this study because a significant proportion of the services in those locales was provided by independent contract physicians, and the data describing use of these contractors were inadequate for the purposes of this study. For similar reasons, the eastern Washington and Idaho regions of Group Health Cooperative were also excluded from the study, and only the western Washington region was included.

The information used in this analysis was provided by the plans during mid-2002 for a reporting period in late 2001 or early 2002. The statistics in this chapter were developed in close collaboration with expert management and analysis staff from each organization.

Relevant characteristics of the populations served by the six Kaiser Permanente regions included in the study and by Group Health Cooperative and HealthPartners are presented in Table 7.1. This table provides key summary information about the in-scope enrolled population at each site, including size, demographics, and the proportion of those enrolled in Medicaid. The relevant demographic characteristics of the U.S. population are presented for comparison purposes. The table also presents estimates of the percentage of all hospitalizations provided in hospitals owned and staffed by each organization and the proportion of overall covered physician services that are delivered by non-PGP contract providers.

TABLE 7.1. CHARACTERISTICS OF PREPAID GROUP PRACTICE SITES INCLUDED IN THIS ANALYSIS, 2001/2002.

| | Kaiser Total | Kaiser Permanente Sites[a] | | | | | | | GHC[b] | HP[c] |
		S.CA	N.CA	CO	HI	Mid-Atl	NW			
Number of Enrollees Served by In-Scope Providers (thousands)	7,781	3,077	3,132	373	225	526	448	368	215
Percentage under age 16 (U.S. average = 24%)[d]	23.0%	23.4%	23.7%	23.7%	21.3%	22.1%	21.0%	20.2%	21.3%
Percentage over age 65 (U.S. average = 13%)	11.4%	10.1%	13.3%	13.6%	11.0%	7.9%	11.3%	14.0%	12.9%
Percentage female (U.S. average = 51%)	53.6%	51.3%	57.3%	52.2%	50.8%	53.1%	52.1%	53.0%	53.0%
Percentage enrolled in Medicaid (U.S. average = 12%)	2.9%	2.9%	2.8%	1.0%	7.8%	0.7%	5.5%	13.3%	10.8%
Approximate percentage of admissions in HMO-owned hospitals	71%	83%	83%	0%	64%	0%	45%	26%	34%
Estimated percentage of covered care provided by contract and out-of-area providers	6%	5%	5%	5%	5%	10%	16%	13%	20%

[a]Permanente Medical Group Regions: S.CA = Southern California, N.CA = Northern California, CO = Colorado, HI = Hawaii, Mid-Atl = Mid-Atlantic (Maryland, District of Columbia, Virginia), NW = Northwest (Oregon, Washington).

[b]GHC = Group Health Cooperative Medical Group (Washington).

[c]HP = HealthPartners Medical Group (Minnesota).

[d]U.S. average figures from Department of Health and Human Services, *Health, United States, 2002,* DHHS Publication no. 1232 (Rockville, Md.: National Center for Health Statistics, 2002).

Results

Table 7.2 presents a comprehensive, specialty-specific description of the employed physicians at each PGP. The rates are expressed in terms of full-time equivalent (FTE) patient-care medical doctors (M.D.'s) and doctors of osteopathy (D.O.'s) on the employed staff per 100,000 consumers enrolled at each site.

To enable a comparison with the current overall U.S. medical workforce, the most recent data on the availability and characteristics of physicians were obtained from published and unpublished sources. Totals for nonfederal, nontrainee providers actively involved in patient care in the United States are also provided. (Note that about 18 percent of the current active U.S. physician supply—approximately 280 M.D.'s and D.O.'s per 100,000 population—is thus excluded from the comparison, even though most are serving the health care system in one capacity or another.)

The eight sites included in this analysis are very large and established, with the majority of care provided by physicians employed by the group. However, for the tertiary specialties and those that are traditionally hospital-based, the staffing rates in Table 7.2 may be incomplete outside of the two California Kaiser Permanente sites. The implications of care provided by nonemployed physicians are discussed later in some detail.

At some PGPs, medical directors and other administrative physicians actively involved in the care management process are reported within their respective medical specialty, while other organizations include these individuals in a separate "medical director" category. At all sites, the proportion of employed physician time that is spent on nonclinical activities (for example, research) was excluded from the reported staffing rates.

Table 7.3 presents a breakdown of nonphysician providers (NPPs) who deliver services that typically (in other settings) are delivered by physicians. For each PGP, Table 7.3 offers information for four distinct NPP cohorts: nurse practitioners (NPs) and two other types of advanced practice nurses (APNs)—midwives and nurse anesthetists; physician assistants (PAs), non-M.D. and non-D.O. doctors, such as doctors of optometry (O.D.'s), doctors of podiatry (D.P.M.'s), and doctors of psychology (Ph.D.'s); and "other" providers, which for this analysis includes mental health therapists with various non-Ph.D. backgrounds. The rate of each of these four classes of NPPs is reported per 100,000 enrollees by ten separate specialty designations.

Some of the sites (notably Group Health Cooperative and a few of the Kaiser Permanente regions) made considerable use of nurses (generally registered nurses without nurse practitioner training) to staff triage "call centers" around the clock. Although an innovative use of clinicians, these nurses—along with other

TABLE 7.2. SPECIALTY DISTRIBUTION OF PHYSICIANS EMPLOYED BY PGPs COMPARED WITH U.S. SUPPLY, 2001/2002.

Specialties	Total Kaiser	Kaiser Permanente PGPs[a]							HP[c]	U.S. Supply[d]
		N.CA	S.CA	CO	HI	Mid-Atl	NW	GHC[b]		
Total	138.9	138.2	139.6	140.6	160.7	132.4	135.5	144.3	176.7	228.9
Primary Care Specialties	57.1	55.6	55.5	62.1	74.4	66.7	54.6	67.1	89.9	92.7
Family practice[e]	12.7	6.1	19.1	16.7	19.0	7.6	14.4	47.2	31.0	30.2
Urgent care	0.8	0.2	—	0.2	1.4	7.5	2.5	—	2.5	—
General internal medicine	27.6	32.8	21.0	31.4	28.1	33.3	25.4	11.7	40.9	43.5
Geriatric medicine	—	—	—	—	1.2	—	—	—	—	—
Hospitalist	0.7	—	—	—	9.3	6.2	—	—	—	—
Pediatrics—Total	15.3	16.5	15.3	13.7	15.4	12.1	12.4	8.2	15.5	19.0
Pediatrics—General	11.9	13.7	10.4	11.5	13.4	12.0	9.5	7.8	15.5	18.5
Pediatrics—Subspecialties[f]	3.4	2.8	4.9	2.1	2.0	0.0	2.9	0.4	—	0.5
Medical Subspecialties	16.2	15.7	17.4	14.1	17.1	14.0	15.6	14.3	25.1	23.7
Allergy and immunology	1.0	1.0	1.0	1.2	0.8	1.1	1.2	1.1	1.3	1.2
Cardiology	2.9	3.3	2.7	2.8	3.6	1.5	2.7	3.0	5.4	6.6
Dermatology	2.4	2.5	2.5	1.8	2.8	2.2	2.5	1.5	3.0	3.1
Endocrinology	1.2	1.0	1.5	1.1	0.7	1.1	0.6	0.2	1.0	1.2
Gastroenterology	2.1	2.0	2.4	2.2	2.7	1.9	1.7	2.0	3.0	3.4
Genetics	0.2	0.3	—	—	—	—	0.3	0.1	—	0.1
Hematology and oncology	2.0	1.8	2.3	1.9	1.8	1.3	2.0	1.9	3.1	1.1
Infectious disease	0.9	0.7	1.1	0.5	1.1	1.2	1.2	0.5	1.3	1.2
Nephrology	1.3	1.1	1.7	—	2.0	1.4	1.1	1.1	2.6	1.7
Pulmonary disease	0.9	0.3	1.3	1.5	1.2	1.0	1.6	1.8	2.8	2.5
Rheumatology	0.9	1.0	0.8	0.8	0.4	1.2	0.8	1.1	1.6	1.1
Other specialties[g]	0.3	0.6	0.2	0.3	—	—	—	—	—	0.5
Surgical Specialties	31.0	30.3	31.5	30.8	35.6	31.2	29.8	27.7	30.3	49.8
Cardio-thoracic surgery	0.8	1.0	0.9	—	0.9	0.2	0.2	—	—	1.7
General and other surgery	5.8	5.6	6.3	5.3	6.5	4.3	5.7	5.8	9.9	10.6
Neurosurgery	0.8	0.6	1.0	1.1	1.2	—	1.1	0.9	—	1.5
Obstetrics and gynecology	10.1	9.9	9.7	9.7	12.0	13.6	9.0	6.6	12.1	13.1
Ophthalmology	3.6	3.8	3.4	4.7	3.7	3.2	2.7	3.3	5.0	6.2
Orthopedics	4.1	3.8	4.1	5.0	5.1	4.8	4.8	6.0	—	6.9
Otolaryngology	2.5	2.5	2.3	2.4	2.7	2.5	2.9	2.6	0.7	3.0
Plastic surgery	1.0	1.0	1.1	1.1	0.9	0.2	0.4	—	2.6	2.1

Urology	2.5	2.2	2.7	1.5	2.7	2.7	3.1	2.6	—	3.4
Other	—	—	—	—	—	—	—	—	—	1.2
Hospital-Based Specialties	15.2	17.0	14.3	12.9	13.7	11.1	15.3	16.9	3.0	27.2
Anesthesiology	6.4	6.8	6.6	7.6	3.5	4.5	5.1	6.4	—	11.6
Pathology	2.3	2.5	2.3	1.6	2.3	1.3	2.4	1.8	3.0	4.1
Radiology	5.3	4.9	5.4	3.7	6.6	5.4	7.8	8.6	—	9.5
Intensive and critical care	1.2	2.8	—	—	1.3	—	—	—	—	0.7
Other	—	—	—	—	—	—	—	—	—	1.2
Other Specialties	19.5	19.6	20.8	20.6	19.9	9.5	20.1	14.5	28.4	35.6
Psychiatry and mental health	5.7	5.7	6.1	5.0	3.4	4.4	5.0	5.2	9.7	13.5
Emergency medicine	7.2	9.5	6.8	6.1	6.8	—	3.9	5.1	10.9	6.9
Neurology	1.7	1.7	1.8	1.6	2.0	1.7	1.5	1.8	4.1	3.6
Occupational medicine	2.0	1.5	2.7	1.4	—	0.3	4.3	1.1	2.2	1.1
Physical medicine and rehabilitation	1.3	1.2	1.8	0.3	1.8	0.4	1.3	0.2	1.5	1.9
Administrative and medical directors[h]	—	—	1.6	4.6	3.2	2.3	2.9	4.9	—	5.7
Other specialties[i]	0.3	—	—	1.8	2.6	0.4	1.2	—	—	2.8

Note: All PGP figures represent FTE physicians per 100,000 population.

[a] 2001 data from six Kaiser Permanente Group model HMOs with total membership of 7,780,049 and individual memberships of 3,130,384 (N.CA), 3,077,457 (S.CA), 373,102 (CO), 225,455 (HI), 525,801 (Mid-Atl), and 447,840 (NW); Glen Hentges, Department of Finance, Permanente Federation, Oakland, Calif., personal communication, Oct. 2002.

[b] 2001–2002 data from Group Health Cooperative, with membership of 367,778; Philip Mealand, Department of Delivery Systems Management Services, Group Health Cooperative, Seattle, personal communication, Oct. 2002.

[c] 2002 data from HealthPartners of Minneapolis, staff model HMO with membership of 227,485; Tammy Lindquist, Department of Health Services Analysis and Reporting, HealthPartners, Minneapolis, personal communication, Oct. 2002.

[d] 2000 and 2001 data; includes nonfederal, patient care, and administrative M.D.'s and D.O.'s; residents and fellows excluded. Numbers represent active full-time providers and not FTEs. M.D.'s = approx. 588,000; D.O.'s = approx. 41,600. Those not classified by specialty are proportionally distributed across specialty categories. Data from American Medical Association, Physician Characteristics and Distribution in the United States, 2002–2003 ed. (Chicago: American Medical Association, 2002), and American Osteopathic Association, personal communication, 2002.

[e] GHC includes urgent care and walk-in clinic with family practice; the other sites separate them.

[f] Pediatric subspecialties may include adolescent medicine, neonatology, perinatology, surgery, cardiology, endocrinology, gastroenterology, hematology and oncology, rheumatology, intensive care, and cytogenetics.

[g] Other specialties not defined by Kaiser: nonprimary care by D.O.'s, practice focus unknown.

[h] Kaiser N.CA and HP include medical directors and other administrative physicians within their respective specialty.

[i] Other specialties may include aerospace medicine, travel medicine, continuing services, contemporary and alternative medicine, epidemiology, and public health medicine; other nonprimary care by D.O.'s, practice focus unknown.

TABLE 7.3. DETAILED NONPHYSICIAN PROVIDER (NPP) SUPPLY BY PGP, 2001/2002.

	Kaiser Total					GHC[a]				HP[b]				
	All NPP	NP + APN	PA	Non-M.D./D.O.[c]	Other[d]	All NPP	NP + APN	PA	Non-M.D./D.O.[c]	All NPP	NP + APN	PA	Non-M.D./D.O.[c]	Other[d]
Primary care	13.0	8.3	3.4	0.7	0.5	22.9	—	22.9	—	8.7	8.3	0.4	—	—
Adult or family medicine	11.1	6.7	3.2	0.7	0.4	20.9	—	20.9	—	5.7	5.3	0.4	—	—
Pediatrics	1.9	1.6	0.2	—	0.1	2.0	—	2.0	—	3.0	3.0	—	—	—
Specialty Care	41.2	14.7	3.6	11.0	10.2	29.9	10.0	4.9	15.0	39.0	18.0	—	10.2	10.8
Medical specialties	1.7	1.2	0.4	0.1	—	1.6	—	1.6	—	3.0	3.0	—	—	—
Obstetrics and gynecology	5.3	5.2	0.1	—	—	6.1	4.6	1.5	—	9.9	9.9	—	—	—
Ophthalmology and optometry	5.1	—	—	5.0	—	12.6	—	—	12.6	6.4	—	—	6.4	—
Other surgical	4.0	0.7	2.0	—	—	1.8	—	1.8	—	—	—	—	—	—
Psychiatry and mental health	16.5	0.5	0.1	5.7	10.2	2.4	—	—	2.4	19.7	19.7	—	3.8	10.8
Anesthesiology	6.8	6.7	—	—	—	5.4	5.4	—	—	—	—	—	—	—
Other specialty	1.8	0.4	1.0	0.2	—	—	—	—	—	—	—	—	—	—
Total	52.4	23.0	7.0	11.7	10.7	52.8	10.0	27.8	15.0	47.7	26.3	0.4	10.2	10.8

Note: Rates reflect providers per 100,000 population.

[a]The NP + APN column includes midwives and anesthetists only; the PA column includes NPs and PAs combined. No practitioners at GHC were in the "Other" category.

[b]Staff providers at HP serve a significant number of non-HMO enrollees. The rates in this table reflect a downward adjustment for this factor. The adjustment factors for M.D.'s and D.O.'s described in Table 7.7 were applied.

[c]Includes O.D.'s, D.P.M.'s, and Ph.D.'s.

[d]Includes mental health therapists.

ambulatory care nurses, such as "clinic nurses" or "case managers," and other inpatient nurses—were excluded from this physician-services-oriented analysis.

Table 7.4 provides a site-specific summary of the rate of overall employed providers, including both M.D.'s and D.O.'s and nonphysician providers (including only nurse practitioners, advanced practice nurses, and physician assistants). The physician figures are broken down by primary care and specialty care.

As noted, over the past several decades, workforce planners have used PGP staffing rates as an important national benchmark. But before doing so, a series of adjustments are generally appropriate to account for differences between the PGP context and the national situation.[5] Three types of important adjustments are made, based on information provided by the study sites: adjustments for enrollee demographics, the extent to which covered care is provided by nonemployed physicians, and the proportion of provider time spent on patients not enrolled with the PGP.

Table 7.7 in the appendix to this chapter offers estimates of these three sets of "adjustment factors" for each PGP. (For Kaiser Permanente, the non-California sites are combined.) All of the factors noted in this table are "multiplicative," meaning they should be multiplied by the employed provider rates presented in previous tables in order to derive estimates of the total number of full-time equivalent (FTE) providers (both employed and contracted) that would be required to serve a benchmark population.

Table 7.5 provides an overview of the provider supply at the PGPs after applying the three sets of adjustment factors described in the appendix to this chapter. The U.S. rates are also presented as a point of reference. No adjustments have been made to these national rates. The top three rows in Table 7.5 provide estimates of physician supply per 100,000 enrollees after the "outflow" (associated with nonemployed providers) and "inflow" (associated with nonenrolled patients) are taken into account. The remaining rows in Table 7.5 also incorporate demographic adjustment and respectively summarize the supply rates for M.D.'s and D.O.'s, nonphysician providers, and total providers.

These figures represent this chapter's "bottom line" in terms of how overall PGP medical provider staffing compares to the current U.S. provider supply, once demographic adjustments are taken into account.

Reflecting the long-term interest in the issue of PGP workforce staffing, an analysis similar to this one was published in 1989 using 1983 data.[6] Using these data, with augmentations from other sources for nonphysician providers,[7] it was possible to do an eighteen-year trend analysis for Kaiser Permanente. These 1983-to-2001 trends are then compared to the underlying U.S. supply trends during approximately the same time period (1980–2000). Table 7.6 presents these two sets of figures by specialty class and separately for physicians, nonphysician providers, and both combined. The Kaiser Permanente data in this table have not

TABLE 7.4. EMPLOYED FTE PROVIDERS AT PGP SITES COMPARED WITH NATIONAL SUPPLY, 2001/2002.

| Staff Providers | Total | Kaiser Permanente Sites | | | | | | | | | U.S. Supply[a] |
		S.CA	N.CA	CO	HI	Mid-Atl	NW	GHC	HP	
Physicians (M.D. and D.O.)	138.9	139.6	138.2	140.6	160.7	132.4	135.5	144.3	176.7	228.9
Primary care	57.1	55.5	55.5	62.1	74.4	66.7	54.6	67.1	89.9	92.7
Specialty care	81.8	84.01	82.6	78.5	86.3	66.6	80.9	77.2	86.8	136.2
Percentage in primary care	41%	40%	40%	44%	46%	50%	40%	48%	51%	40%
Nonphysician Providers	30.0	30.4	25.6	30.2	35.2	30.4	56.7	37.8	26.3	41.0
Nurse practitioners[b]	23.0	20.9	23.5	14.1	26.2	N.A.	38.4	N.A.	25.9	24.6
Physician assistants	7.0	9.5	2.1	16.1	9.0	N.A.	18.3	N.A.	0.4	16.4
Total Providers	**168.9**	**170.0**	**163.8**	**170.8**	**195.9**	**162.8**	**192.2**	**178.3**	**203.0**	**269.9**

Notes: Rates reflect providers per 100,000 population. Rates do not include any adjustments, such as for contracted out-of-plan care, nonenrolled patient inflow, or demographic differences. N.A. = not available.

[a]Reflects nonfederal, nontrainee patient care M.D.'s and D.O.'s, nurse practitioners, and physician assistants in active practice. Data from American Medical Association, *Physician Characteristics and Distribution in the United States, 2002–2003* ed. (Chicago: American Medical Association, 2002), and American Osteopathic Association, personal communication, 2002.

[b]Includes nurse midwives and nurse anesthetists.

TABLE 7.5. ESTIMATED PRIMARY CARE AND SPECIALTY CARE PROVIDER SUPPLY AT EACH PGP COMPARED WITH U.S. SUPPLY AFTER ADJUSTING FOR INFLOW AND OUTFLOW OF PATIENTS AND DEMOGRAPHICS, 2001/2002.

	Kaiser Total	GHC	HP	United States
With Inflow and Outflow Adjustment Only				
Physicians (M.D. and D.O.)	143	166	178	229
Primary care	58	69	81	93
Specialty care	85	97	97	136
Percentage in primary care	41%	42%	46%	41%
With Inflow, Outflow, and Demographic Adjustments				
Physicians (M.D. and D.O.)	144	166	176	229
Primary care	58	69	80	93
Specialty care	86	97	96	136
Percentage in primary care	40%	42%	46%	41%
Nonphysician Providers[a]	30	38	26	41
Primary care	12	23	9	15
Specialty care	18	15	17	26
Percentage in primary care	40%	60%	35%	37%
Total Providers	174	204	202	270
Primary care	70	92	89	108
Specialty care	104	112	113	162
Percentage in primary care	40%	45%	44%	40%

Notes: PGP rates reflect FTE providers per 100,000 population, and U.S. rates reflect nontrainee patient care providers per 100,000 population. Inflow and outflow adjustments compensate for covered physician services provided by out-of-plan contracting physicians and services provided to nonenrolled patients by staff doctors, respectively. (The latter is estimated to be 80 percent specialty care.) Demographic adjustments compensate for differences in age distribution between PGPs and the U.S. population; see Table 7.7 for the specific adjustment factors used.

[a]Includes nurse practitioners, nurse midwives, nurse anesthetists, and physician assistants. Only demographic adjustment was applied to NPPs, except at HP, where inflow adjustments were applied previously in Table 7.3.

been adjusted and reflect employed FTEs. To account for the slightly different number of years included in the two data points, per annum trends are presented in the last row.

Discussion

The following section summarizes key findings, discusses data limitations, highlights workforce innovations at the PGPs, and identifies a series of implications for American workforce policy.

TABLE 7.6. STAFFING TRENDS, 1983–2001, AT KAISER PERMANENTE (KP) COMPARED WITH U.S. WORKFORCE SUPPLY TRENDS.

| | Physicians | | | | | | Nonphysician Providers[b] | | | | | | Total Providers | | | | | |
| | Total | | Primary Care | | Specialty Care | | Total | | Primary Care | | Specialty Care | | Total | | Primary Care | | Specialty Care | |
Year[a]	KP	US	KP	US	KP	US	KP	US	KP	US	KP	US	KP	US	KP	US	KP	US
1983[c]	111	170	54	60	57	110	20	18	12	11	8	7	131	190	66	72	69	117
2001[c]	139	229	57	93	82	136	30	41	12	15	18	26	169	270	69	108	100	162
Trend (%)																		
Period[d]	25	35	6	55	44	17	50	127	0	36	125	271	29	42	5	50	45	38
Per year[e]	1.4	1.7	0.3	2.8	2.4	1.2	2.8	6.4	0.0	1.8	6.9	13.6	1.6	2.1	0.3	2.5	2.5	1.9

[a]U.S. comparison rates are for the twenty-year period 1980–2000 and reflect estimated nonfederal, nontrainee patient care M.D.'s and D.O.'s. U.S. data from American Medical Association, *Physician Characteristics and Distribution in the United States, 2002–2003 ed.* (Chicago: American Medical Association, 2002); American Osteopathic Association, personal communication, 2002; E. Salsberg and G. Forte, "Trends in the Physician Workforce, 1980–2000," *Health Affairs,* 2002, 21, 165–173; and J. P. Weiner, "Forecasting the Effects of Health Reform on U.S. Physician Workforce Requirement: Evidence from HMO Staffing Patterns," *Journal of the American Medical Association,* 1994, 272, 222–230. Kaiser Permanente data from R. Mulhausen and J. McGee, "Physician Need: An Alternative Projection from a Study of Large Prepaid Group Practice," *Journal of the American Medical Association,* 1989, 261, 1930–1934; and Glen Hentges, Department of Finance, Permanente Federation, Oakland, Calif., personal communication, Oct. 2002. Includes Kaiser Permanente employed providers only. No adjustments applied.

[b]Nurse practitioners, midwives, registered nurse anesthetists, and physician assistants. Note that the 2001 split between NPP primary care and specialty care is based on detailed information. The 1983 primary and specialty care split is an estimate based on the following sources: R. Hooker, "The Roles of Physician Assistants and Nurse Practitioners in a Managed Care Organization," in D. Clawson and M. Osterweis, eds., *The Roles of Physician Assistants and Nurse Practitioners in Primary Care* (Washington, D.C.: Association of Academic Health Centers, 1993); R. Mulhausen and J. McGee, "Physician Need: An Alternative Projection from a Study of Large Prepaid Group Practice," *Journal of the American Medical Association,* 1989, 261, 1930–1934; and R. Hooker and D. Freeborn, "Use of Physician Assistants in a Managed Health Care System," *Public Health Reports,* 1991, 108, 90–94.

[c]Provider FTEs per 100,000 population.

[d]Trend over the time period used for each data set.

[e]Annualized trend.

Summary of Findings

Across the eight PGPs, the overall physician staffing ratios (before adjustment) range from about 132 to 177 per 100,000 enrollees, compared with a national supply of about 229 per 100,000. The ratios for nurse practitioners and physician assistants range from about 26 to 57 per 100,000 enrollees, compared with about 41 nationally. When both physicians and NPPs are combined, the overall (unadjusted) supply ranges from about 164 to 203 per 100,000, which compares with about 270 providers per 100,000 nationally.

Once the various adjustments, including contracting physicians and demographic mix, are taken into consideration, the total provider supply across the three organizations ranges from 174 per 100,000 at Kaiser Permanente to 202 at HealthPartners and 204 at Group Health. In terms of clinicians per member, this is equivalent to about one provider per 490 enrolled persons at Group Health, one per 495 at HealthPartners, and one per 575 at Kaiser Permanente. This compares to a national (nontrainee, nonfederal) provider-to-consumer ratio of about one to 370 Americans.

The overall workforce staffing at the three PGPs, including the six regions within Kaiser Permanente, fall within a fairly tight range. But beyond this aggregate level, a number of interesting variations are noteworthy and show the alternative approaches these organizations have taken to staffing in order to best meet the needs of their populations.

The proportion of physicians at each site who are in the primary care specialties ranges from about 40 percent to 48 percent after adjustments are made for contracting providers. This compares with about 41 percent of M.D.'s and D.O.'s in the primary care specialties nationally. However, focusing just on percentages may be misleading: The U.S. primary care supply ratio is about 93 per 100,000 population, whereas the adjusted PGPs primary care supply ranges from 58 to 80 per 100,000 population. With reference to primary care, Group Health and HealthPartners make considerable use of family practitioners. But in most of the Kaiser Permanente regions, internists are most common among adult primary care physicians. At HealthPartners, 10 percent of the primary care providers are nurse practitioners or physician assistants; at Kaiser Permanente, the non-M.D., non-D.O. proportion is 17 percent; and at Group Health, it is 25 percent. Nationally, about 14 percent of primary care providers are non-M.D.'s.

Nurse practitioner and physician assistant staffing, in total, ranges across the PGPs from about 26 to 38 per 100,000 (compared to approximately 41 per 100,000 nationally). It appears that the nonphysician practitioners (which for this analysis includes midwives and nurse anesthetists) are concentrated in the specialty care areas at HealthPartners and Kaiser Permanente (65 percent and 60 percent, respectively). In contrast, the NPP focus at Group Health is predominantly (60 percent) primary care. When other types of nonphysician providers beyond nurse practitioners, advanced practice nurses, and physician assistants are taken into consideration (such as non-M.D. and non-D.O. doctors and mental health therapists), the deployment at the three groups is fairly similar across all participating PGPs, ranging from 48 to 53 providers per 100,000 enrollees (see Table 7.3). No comparable national rates are readily available for this expanded NPP definition.

Although a discussion of staffing patterns for each of the forty physician subspecialties documented in Table 7.2 is not feasible, a few comments at this level of detail are appropriate. For many subspecialties, the rates across the eight PGP sites are surprisingly similar, particularly when the HealthPartners' 0.70 outflow adjustment factor is considered. (As described in the footnote to Table 7.7, it is suggested that most of the HealthPartners specialist ratios in Table 7.2 be discounted by 30 percent to account for services the PGP physicians provide to nonenrollees.)

It is suggested that the rates at the two very large Kaiser Permanente regions (Northern and Southern California) be viewed as the most "stable" set of ratios in Table 7.2; these PGPs are by far the largest in the analysis and represent the locations with the least use of nonemployed contracting providers (given that most hospital-based specialists practicing at the PGP staffed facilities are included in the FTE statistics).

As noted, the rates in Table 7.2 reflect employed FTEs and do not include any adjustments. However, since the overall site-specific adjustment factors for specialists described in Table 7.7 are modest or nil for the two California sites (1.03 and 1.00 for Southern and Northern California, respectively), the FTE figures in Table 7.2 can be viewed as representing reasonable estimates of the total (including both on-staff and contracting) supply at these sites for a population with the approximate demographic makeup of the nation as a whole. With this in mind, it is interesting to note that the specialty-specific rates for a few subspecialties at the Kaiser Permanente California regions are comparable to or higher than the national rates, but for most, the supply levels are lower.

The eighteen-year trend analysis at Kaiser Permanente suggests that the PGP's rate of annual growth in the overall physicians-to-population ratio (1.4 percent) is not dissimilar to the national increase of 1.7 percent during roughly the same period. However, this global trend obscures a noteworthy finding. Unlike the national situation, most of Kaiser Permanente's growth has been among nonprimary care physicians; there was a 2.4 percent annual increase in specialist supply at Kaiser Permanente and only a 0.3 percent per annum growth for primary care physicians. This compares to 1.2 percent for specialists and 2.4 percent for primary care at the national level.

For Kaiser Permanente nonphysicians, the specialist-oriented trend was even more pronounced. There was a 6.9 percent annual growth for nonprimary care nurse practitioners and physician assistants and no growth for primary care. But this lopsided situation does to some extent mirror the national situation, which experienced a 13.6 percent annual increase for specialty care NPPs and a 1.8 percent rate of increase per year for primary care NPPs.

Limitations and Generalizability

The workforce statistics presented in this chapter may be the most comprehensive and most accurate ever compiled, and they are certainly the most up-to-date available in the public domain. However, a number of limitations should be noted, particularly as they relate to the generalizability of these workforce levels beyond the PGP setting.

When collating these workforce data from the multiple study sites, common definitions and data collection frameworks were used whenever feasible. But of necessity, there was considerable reliance on local definitions and existing management databases at the PGPs. For example, each local group used its own operational definition of specialty, FTE status, and clinical versus nonclinical duties. Also, somewhat different approaches were used by each plan to document or estimate out-of-plan contracting and nonenrollee inflow.

When considering the implications of the reported staffing patterns, it is important to acknowledge the context from which they were drawn. That is, the physician and NPP rates must be understood from within the framework of the overall organization, its administrative support staff (beyond that described here), and practice philosophies. The other chapters in this volume provide much of that context. Although many aspects of PGP practice, including approaches to medical staffing, can be emulated in non-PGP health care organizations, in certain instances it may be difficult to adopt just part of the "package."

Comparability Issues. Kaiser Permanente and the other large PGPs provide care to a broad cross section of members, but their enrolled populations are not completely representative of all Americans. In addition to the empirical adjustments described earlier, there are a series of other comparability issues that have been recommended for consideration before PGP staffing ratios, such as those presented in this chapter, should be extrapolated to other organizations or locales.[8]

One issue that needs to be considered for national planning purposes is the degree to which persons enrolled in an HMO choose to receive care outside of the plan (from neither PGP-employed nor contracting providers). Because services at these eight PGPs are so comprehensive, this external use rate is not expected to be very high. Estimates have suggested that the out-of-plan use level is less than 5 percent.[9]

Another interesting issue, the impact of which is difficult to measure, is the degree to which PGPs experience adverse or favorable selection bias. That is, are their enrollees sicker or healthier than non-PGP patients, and therefore should they be expected to require a greater or lesser number of providers? The national studies on this issue are mixed, but those documenting selection bias at the PGPs have suggested that the assumption that PGP populations are less sick than community-based patients is not necessarily valid.[10]

Adding to this national observation was a local analysis at HealthPartners, which has been a leader in applying risk-adjustment and case-mix strategies for care management and financing. For the denominator of enrollees included in this study, HealthPartners was able to identify case-mix differences between the PGP component of the plan relative to the network component. This analysis suggested a morbidity burden among the PGP patient cohort that was approximately 10 percent greater, in terms of diagnosed morbidity status based on the Ambulatory Care Group (ACG) case-mix system.[11] This suggests a degree of adverse selection bias, perhaps due to the urban location and comprehensiveness of the PGP sites relative to the more suburban network practices.

Another issue of comparability relates to the potential need for socioeconomic adjustments. These PGPs have Medicaid memberships that range from 0.7 percent to 13 percent of their populations. Their enrollees include no uninsured patients. This compares to 11 percent and 13 percent, respectively, for these special-need population cohorts in the United States overall. The evidence is mixed on whether an upward or downward adjustment would be needed if the PGP populations included a proportional representation of these special-need patients.[12]

The issue of geographical distribution is also worthy of comment. The PGP study sites are among the largest in the nation and serve consumers in nine states and the District of Columbia, but they are based primarily in the West and Midwest and do not have a significant presence in rural areas. Practice patterns in the study site locales could be different than in the nation overall, although there is no evidence that the needs of the populations in the underrepresented geographical areas would be higher or lower than consumers enrolled in these PGPs.

Concepts of Productivity. As much a conceptual issue as one of comparability is the controversy over how to define provider "productivity" and "full-time equivalency." That is, does one FTE physician at the PGP equal one FTE outside of the PGP? Further adding to the controversial nature of this question is its relationship to the provider's gender.

American Medical Association (AMA) surveys and other sources have documented significant differences in terms of number of patients seen per year by "private practice" physicians and PGP-employed physicians. Fee-for-service doctors, on average, see 15 to 20 percent more patients annually than those in more structured settings, such as PGPs.[13] Therefore, some have suggested that it takes fewer FFS physicians to provide comparable amounts of care. These surveys do not attempt to assess comparability or efficiency associated with the patient-physician interactions but simply the number of hours per year spent seeing patients in different settings.

Another related issue is the number of individuals it takes to constitute one "full-time equivalent." Because of the structure of PGPs, it is believed that a significant proportion of physicians work in such settings on a part-time basis. For example, Kaiser Permanente-Northern California reports that 20 percent of all physicians on staff work less than 90 percent of what they consider to be a full-time schedule.[14] Although comparable national data are not available, the AMA reports that based on a 2000 national survey, the number of physicians working fewer than twenty hours per week, along with those describing themselves as not fully active, represented less than 10 percent of all licensed physicians.

The PGP staffing levels documented in this chapter are presented in terms of "full-time equivalents." But one FTE does not necessarily represent one employed physician. That is, it can be estimated that for every FTE reported, approximately 1.1 to 1.2 individuals are employed. Nationally, it can be estimated that the comparable rate falls in the 1.05-to-1.10 range. This full-time equivalency and PGP-versus-non-PGP productivity issue should be the subject of further inquiry.

Being able to balance professional life with personal life is an issue of increased importance to all physicians and especially to women physicians, who now represent about 40 percent of today's medical school graduates. To reach this balance, there has been a documented tendency for women physicians to work fewer hours per year than their male counterparts. Some workforce analysts have cited this as being a significant factor in understanding national supply and requirement patterns.[15] As it relates to this analysis, PGPs appear to appeal to women physicians, possibly because of the supportive and flexible nature of the practice environment. For example, across the six Kaiser Permanente sites included in this study, the proportion of physicians who are female ranged from 31 percent to 47 percent of the total number of M.D.'s and D.O.'s on staff. This compares to approximately 22 percent of physicians (posttraining) in the United States.[16] The proportion of physicians who practice part-time at Kaiser Permanente is not available by gender category, but it is believed to be higher for women.

A full discussion of productivity (patient contacts per provider per year) and gender goes beyond the scope of this chapter, but the bottom line is that the nature of the physician stock serving the PGP enrollees and the manner in which they provide care are different than in the non-PGP setting. It appears that today's PGP practices may be indicative of what the future U.S. physician cohort may look like ten to twenty years hence, given the current gender mix of medical school graduates.

Workforce Innovations

The main goal of this chapter was to present a comprehensive, empirical description of PGP staffing levels. Embedded within these numbers are many unique approaches and innovations that, taken together, are indicative of each PGP's unique "staffing signature." While it is not possible to describe every facet of the many clinical areas across the PGPs, a number of workforce-related innovations are highlighted here.

All three of the PGP systems included in the study have nationally regarded health services research and development centers that have made workforce issues one of their priorities over the years (see Chapter Eight). Much of the seminal work on the role of nurse practitioners and physician assistants as members of an integrated clinical team was performed in these and other PGPs. This research and development has had a real impact on the care of patients and has provided the foundation for considerable innovation regarding the role of NPPs in many areas of PGP practice.[17] These innovations include the use of nurse practitioners as case managers for disease management programs and as geriatric case managers.[18] It should come as no surprise that the locations that have most carefully documented the benefit of these types of clinicians (Group Health and the Kaiser Permanente-Northwest Region) have a considerably higher supply of NPPs in primary care.

Bucking the tide of "carving out" mental health services to an external organization, all eight of the study PGPs provide mental health care to members in an integrated fashion, with psychiatrists, primary care physicians, psychologists, and other therapists all playing vital roles. They have also developed models for making use of the most efficient level of provider or therapist appropriate to the patient's mental health needs. Finally, they all spend considerable time attempting to integrate primary care and other types of somatic care with psychiatric services.[19]

At each of the PGPs, there have been programmatic innovations that have offered new structural approaches for the delivery of care. These have had direct implications on workforce staffing. One example at Kaiser Permanente is the "group medical visit," which focuses on major chronic problems, often among the elderly. These "drop-in group medical appointments" (known as "DIGMAs" or "cluster visits") were patterned to some extent after the group therapy visits long common in mental health. They have proved to be quite popular and effective, particularly among older enrollees.[20]

Unlike most other models of "managed care," the PGPs are truly integrated delivery systems that cut across care settings. Kaiser Permanente, Group Health, and HealthPartners all own, operate, and staff inpatient facilities in addition to their owned and operated multispecialty ambulatory clinics. The use of full-time inpatient primary care physicians or "hospitalists" in providing care to admitted medical patients was pioneered at these and other PGPs.[21] Even though the FTE supply figures in Table 7.2 do not show PGPs reporting hospitalists separately at most sites, all locations make considerable use of this approach, and the providers are reported within their respective specialty (usually internal medicine). This approach to providing inpatient care by doctors already on site is one explanation for the efficiency of the PGP staffing levels.

Implications for Workforce Policy

The PGP staffing ratios presented in this study are likely to have direct implications for human resource planners in other large integrated delivery systems in the United States and abroad.[22] In addition to providing staffing benchmarks, the data may suggest novel approaches for staff deployment, such as significant use of nonphysician providers, full-time inpatient hospitalists, and specialized disease and case management support staff. Such implications may apply not only to other PGPs but also to integrated physician-hospital organizations, large nonprepaid group practices with geographically defined patient bases, government providers such as the military, and the structured delivery systems found in many other nations.

For example, given the fairly rigid demarcation between ambulatory-based generalists and hospital-based specialists in many other nations, the PGP staffing described here offers one approach for using a multispecialty ambulatory group practice to develop better care integration without considerable expansion of staffing levels.

What are the implications of the provider staffing rates described here for the majority of Americans who do not receive care from PGPs or other organized delivery systems? It is not a goal of this study to evaluate the adequacy of the current or projected U.S. physician supply. Rather, the intent is to offer fresh information to support the formal workforce planning activities now under way in both the public and private sectors (for example, the government-sponsored Council on Graduate Medical Education and the efforts of the America Association of Medical Colleges).

Primary Care and Specialist Distribution. This study provides evidence that organized, prepaid group practices in urban and suburban areas can and do provide high-quality, cost-effective care to a diverse insured population with considerably fewer physicians than in other practice environments. After adjustments are made for differences in demographics and use of non-PGP providers, the physician-to-population ratios at the eight PGPs is approximately

28 to 37 percent lower than in the United States overall. When nurse practitioners and physician assistants are added to the mix, the PGP total provider supply rate is about 24 to 36 percent lower than national levels.

When these supply differences are assessed separately for primary care and specialty care, an interesting situation comes to light. Two of the PGPs' primary care provider staffing levels are closer to the national average than their specialty care rates are. At Group Health and HealthPartners, the primary care provider rate is 15 to 18 percent lower than national rates, and their specialty rate is about 30 percent lower. At Kaiser Permanente, both the primary care and specialty supply are about 35 percent lower. It is also interesting to note that the proportion of providers in the primary care specialties at Group Health and HealthPartners (45 percent and 46 percent, respectively) is higher than that for the nation as a whole (40 percent). The proportion of providers in primary care at Kaiser Permanente is comparable to the national rate.

The trend analysis at Kaiser Permanente suggests that this organization (and potentially other PGPs) has been playing catch-up with regard to national specialist staffing. Ironically, this PGP specialist growth seems to have occurred at roughly the same time the national supply of generalists has approached the relatively high proportion seen in PGPs a few decades earlier. Although the causes and consequences of these obverse trends are not entirely clear, they do lend support to the premise that the nation must carefully reassess the appropriate balance between primary and specialty care. However, the data here offer little support to those who believe that the U.S. population's medical needs or demands should be met with a higher rate of specialists than are available today. PGPs appear to function well with considerably fewer specialists per population than the national average.

Provider Satisfaction. The lower level of PGP staffing relative to the national supply raises the question of whether this tighter provider-to-population ratio has an impact on professional satisfaction among PGP practitioners. A recent survey of practicing physicians in California compared the perceptions of Kaiser Permanente physicians to their non-PGP office-based colleagues.[23] The results clearly indicate that whether due to actual differences in practice or provider self-selection, Kaiser Permanente physicians had significantly higher levels of satisfaction than non-PGP providers. This observation held for both specialists and generalists. For example, when asked if they felt their practice organization represented an "advantage" or "disadvantage" with regard to quality of care for their patients, 59 percent of generalists and 64 percent of specialists answered positively, while only 14 percent and 5 percent, respectively, answered that the setting detracted from quality.

The comparable responses from non-PGP, office-based practitioners in California were dramatically different. When responding to the query of how they viewed their IPA and insurance plan's infrastructure in terms of their effects on the quality of patient care, only 16 percent of office-based generalists and 8 percent of specialists responded that such structures offered "advantages." Fully 52 percent and 57 percent, respectively, viewed the support infrastructure as a "disadvantage" in terms of quality.[24]

Conclusions

In recent years, interest in assessing the "adequacy" of the U.S. medical workforce has increased dramatically. Key parties are calling for a reappraisal of our current and future national physician and nonphysician provider workforce. A high-profile article has suggested that due to the aging of the population and the expansion of economic and social expectations, there will be significant increases in consumer demand for physicians, particularly for specialists.[25] Accordingly, there is a growing call for an expansion in medical training programs.

Other analysts believe that the future will involve not so much a provider shortage as an inappropriate distribution of what by many yardsticks will be an adequate or even abundant supply of providers.[26] The PGP trend over the past two decades does point toward a higher proportion and number of specialists and a growing overall supply of providers. This offers some support for the premise that workforce patterns are changing and moving more toward increased specialization. It is possible that this trend is associated with increased expectations by enrollees who are "aging in place" (in other words, staying enrolled in their HMO as they get older).

However, an important implication of this chapter is the fact that the PGP supply of both primary care physicians and, particularly, specialists is significantly lower than the current national provider-to-population ratio. Given the PGP model's achievement in terms of quality and cost efficiency, it is evident that the PGP represents a viable approach for making use of valuable medical professionals more efficiently than is generally the case in the United States.

Although the PGP staffing levels may not translate directly into benchmarks for the nation, the findings of this chapter do indicate that policymakers should deliberate carefully before encouraging the costly expansion of medical training programs. Another potential implication of this chapter for workforce planners is the finding that a significant proportion of nonphysician providers at the PGPs are practicing outside of primary care. This suggests that the commonly accepted notion that PGPs rely on nonphysician providers mainly for primary care is not necessarily accurate. This analysis suggests a need for increased attention to the role of NPPs and their impact on both patients and physicians.

On the surface, workforce planning appears to be largely a statistical undertaking. But at its heart, the process is not a technical enterprise. Rather, determining what a medical workforce should, could, or would look like in the future is fraught with conceptual, political, and even moral challenges and choices. Thus it is essential that analyses such as this one provide private and public policymakers with information that supports rational decision making.

When policymakers select from among the many alternative approaches to medical workforce staffing, it is essential that the benefits to society at large are maximized, whatever the desired (or feasible) level of resource commitment. Prepaid group practices have devoted considerable energy to the pursuit of this delicate balance between benefits and costs. Therefore, it seems only fitting that we look to PGPs as a source of guidance as we chart the course toward a more optimal medical workforce.

Appendix: Adjustment Factors for Extrapolating PGP Staffing Rates as Benchmarks

The first row in Table 7.7 presents an approximate "demographic" adjustment. This is based on a comparison of the demographic characteristics of the plan with the U.S. population characteristics as of 2000. For example, if the members at a site are younger and less likely to use services than a more nationally representative population, the staff rates reported here will need to be adjusted upward to take these differences into consideration. The demographic factors in this table are based on an indirect standardization method using ambulatory physician contacts reported from an HMO survey.[27] Note that all eight PGPs have a significantly higher proportion of elderly enrollees than the U.S. HMO average and thus have age distributions that make them very similar to the national U.S. population distribution. Therefore, very little adjustment of the reported staffing rates is needed to account for demographic mix.

Even though the PGPs in this study are among the largest and most comprehensively staffed delivery systems in the nation, community-based physicians not employed by the plan deliver a portion of their members' physician care (these rates are summarized in the bottom row of Table 7.1). Outside providers are reimbursed primarily on a fee-for-service basis, so by using these utilization data, it is possible to approximate the full-time equivalency of the contract providers serving the in-scope enrollee populations. Two of the sites (Group Health Cooperative and HealthPartners) were able to share specialty-specific information on contract care. Patterned after a method developed at Group Health Cooperative, national information on average per-physician billing rates at large group practices was used to estimate contracting FTEs on a specialty-specific basis.[28] Kaiser Permanente, which makes less use of nonemployed providers, offered estimates based on historical experience.

As might be expected, nonemployed physician services vary significantly by specialty category. For example, the proportion of contract care is much higher for emergency room (ER) specialists, as much ER care is delivered out of area. At those sites making less use of PGP-staffed hospitals, a significant proportion of hospital-based specialty care is provided by non-PGP doctors practicing at these contracting facilities. At Group Health Cooperative and HealthPartners, approximately 25 percent of all physician services provided by nonemployees is for ER or hospital-based specialists (radiologists, anesthesiologists, and pathologists).

The "external contract provider" factors presented in Table 7.7 are multiplicative. Using Group Health as an example, if 13 percent of all covered care for

TABLE 7.7. SITE-SPECIFIC ESTIMATED ADJUSTMENT FACTORS FOR USE IN EXTRAPOLATING PGP STAFFING RATES TO THE U.S. POPULATION.

	Kaiser Permanente					
Adjustment Factor	**Total**	**S.CA**	**N.CA**	**Other**	***GHC***	***HP***
Demographic[a]	1.01	1.02	0.99	1.01	1.00	0.99
External Contract Providers (Outflow)						
Total	1.06	1.05	1.05	1.08	1.15	1.25
Emergency medicine	1.21	1.18	1.18	1.35	1.53	1.14
Hospital-based radiology, anesthesiology, pathology (in all settings)	1.10	1.05	1.05	1.25	1.37	4.55
Surgical specialty	1.06	1.05	1.05	1.10	1.22	1.43
Medical specialty	1.06	1.05	1.05	1.10	1.28	1.28
Primary care	1.02	1.02	1.02	1.02	1.05	1.05
Nonenrollee Care (Inflow)	0.98	0.96	0.96	0.99	0.95	0.75[b]

Sources: J. P. Weiner, C. J. McLaughlin, and S. Gamliel, "Extrapolating HMO Staffing to the Population at Large," in M. Osterweis, C. J. McLaughlin, H. R. Manasse Jr., and C. L. Hopper, eds., *The U.S. Health Workforce: Power, Politics, and Policy* (Washington, D.C.: Academic Health Centers, 1996); Tammy Lindquist, Department of Health Services Analysis and Reporting, HealthPartners, Minneapolis, personal communication, Oct. 2002; Glen Hentges, Department of Finance, Permanente Federation, Oakland, Calif., personal communication, Oct. 2002; and Philip Mealand, Department of Delivery Systems Management Services, Group Health Cooperative, Seattle, personal communication, Oct. 2002.

Notes: All figures in the table should be multiplied by the relevant FTE provider figure reported in this chapter in order to account for the "adjustment factor" noted. See the text for discussion of other global adjustments that may also be appropriate before using these figures as national benchmarks.

[a]Demographic adjustment factors for other Kaiser Permanente regions are as follows: CO, 0.99; HI, 1.01; Mid-Atl, 1.04; NW, 1.01. The demographic factor calculation is based on an indirect standardization approach using ambulatory physician contact information from a national survey of HMOs, plan-specific age breakdown for each PGP, and the U.S. 2000 age breakdown; J. P. Weiner, C. J. McLaughlin, and S. Gamliel, "Extrapolating HMO Staffing to the Population at Large," in M. Osterweis, C. J. McLaughlin, H. R. Manasse Jr., and C. L. Hopper, eds., *The U.S. Health Workforce: Power, Politics, and Policy* (Washington, D.C.: Academic Health Centers, 1996).

[b]29 percent of the HP group's services (based on 2001 relative value units) were provided to nonenrollees. After accounting for differential billing rates, this translates to an overall estimated FTE adjustment factor of 0.75. Specialty-specific factors were estimated as follows: primary care, 0.85; emergency medicine, pathology, and psychiatry, 0.55; and other specialties, 0.70.

the in-scope enrollees is provided by community doctors—and 87 percent by the PGP's employed providers—the adjustment factor would be 1.15. This factor is then multiplied by the FTEs employed at the PGP—144 per 100,000—to estimate the combined number of employed and contract FTE physicians that serve the population, in this case about 166 physicians to 100,000 members.

All of the PGPs in this study primarily serve the members of a single health plan. The medical groups are paid a capitated fee for these services. But in certain circumstances, the medical groups care for patients from outside of the PGP's enrollee denominators described in Table 7.1. This might include emergency care to non–plan members, "reciprocal" coverage for members of another HMO, services to members of the partner health plan enrolled with an external network, or care for members insured under a separate policy (for example, workers' compensation). The "nonenrollee" adjustment factors, based on actual recent history at each site, are presented at the bottom of Table 7.7. They indicate the approximate downward adjustment of the employed FTEs that is necessary before the employed FTE provider rates can be used as benchmarks.

This "inflow" adjustment is significant at HealthPartners, and as noted in the footnote to Table 7.7, varies by specialty. There are two reasons for this site's higher rate. First, there are other health plan members not enrolled with the PGP (in other words, served by primary care doctors in the network branch of the health plan) who rely on the PGP providers for a subset of care provided on a fee-for-service basis. Second, the PGP staffs a full-service hospital and outpatient department that was previously run by the local health department. Many patients not enrolled in the PGP use this hospital.

Notes

1. Office of Technology Assessment, *Forecasts of Physician Supply and Requirement* (Washington, D.C.: U.S. Government Printing Office, 1980); D. Steinwachs and others, "A Comparison of the Requirements for Primary Care Physicians in HMOs with Projections Made by the GMENAC," *New England Journal of Medicine*, 1986, *314*, 217–222; R. Kronick, D. Goodman, J. Wennberg, and E. Wagner, "The Marketplace in Health Care Reform: The Demographic Limitations of Managed Competition," *New England Journal of Medicine*, 1993, *328*, 148–152; J. P. Weiner, "Forecasting the Effects of Health Reform on U.S. Physician Workforce Requirement: Evidence from HMO Staffing Patterns," *Journal of the American Medical Association*, 1994, *272*, 222–230; T. Dial and others, "Clinical Staffing in Staff and Group-Model HMOs," *Health Affairs*, 1995, *14*, 169–180; D. Goodman and others, "Benchmarking the U.S. Physician Workforce: An Alternative to Needs-Based or Demand-Based Planning," *Journal of the American Medical Association*, 1996, *276*, 1811–1844; R. Mason, "Manpower Needs by Specialty," *Journal of the American Medical Association*, 1972, *219*, 1621–1626.

2. J. Record and M. R. Greenlick, "New Health Professionals and the Physician Role: A Hypothesis from Kaiser Experience," *Public Health Reports*, 1975, *90*, 241–248; J. Record and others, "New Health Professions After a Decade and a Half: Delegation, Productivity and Costs in Primary Care," *Journal of Health Politics, Policy, and Law*, 1980, *5*, 470–497; R. Hooker, "The Roles of Physician Assistants and Nurse Practitioners in a Managed Care Organization," in D. Clawson and M. Osterweis, eds., *The Roles of Physician Assistants and Nurse Practitioners in Primary Care* (Washington, D.C.: Association of Academic Health Centers, 1993).

3. J. Selby and others, "Differences in Resource Use and Costs of Primary Care in a Large HMO According to Physician Specialty," *Health Services Research*, 1999, *34*, 503–518; K. Grumbach and others, "Resolving the Gatekeeper Conundrum: What Patients Value in Primary Care and Referrals to Specialists," *Journal of the American Medical Association*, 1999, *282*, 261–266.

4. Kronick, Goodman, Wennberg, and Wagner, "The Marketplace in Health Care Reform"; Weiner, "Forecasting the Effects of Health Reform"; A. Tarlov, "HMO Growth and Physicians: The Third Compartment," *Health Affairs*, 1986, *5*, 23–35.

5. Weiner, "Forecasting the Effects of Health Reform"; J. P. Weiner, C. J. McLaughlin, and S. Gamliel, "Extrapolating HMO Staffing to the Population at Large," in M. Osterweis, C. J. McLaughlin, H. R. Manasse Jr., and C. L. Hopper, eds., *The U.S. Health Workforce: Power, Politics, and Policy* (Washington, D.C.: Academic Health Centers, 1996); L. G. Hart, E. Wagner, S. Pirzada, and A. Nelson, "Physician Staffing Ratios in Staff-Model HMOs: A Cautionary Tale," *Health Affairs*, 1997, *16*, 55–70.

6. R. Mulhausen and J. McGee, "Physician Need: An Alternative Projection from a Study of Large Prepaid Group Practice," *Journal of the American Medical Association*, 1989, *261*, 1930–1934.

7. Weiner, "Forecasting the Effects of Health Reform"; R. Hooker, ed., *Physician Assistants, Nurse Practitioners, Certified Nurse Midwives, and Nurse Anesthetists: The Kaiser Permanente Experience* (Portland, Ore.: Kaiser Permanente Center for Health Research, 1994).

8. Kronick, Goodman, Wennberg, and Wagner, "The Marketplace in Health Care Reform"; Weiner, "Forecasting the Effects of Health Reform"; Weiner, McLaughlin, and Gamliel, "Extrapolating HMO Staffing"; Goodman and others, "Benchmarking the U.S. Physician Workforce"; Council on Graduate Medical Education, *COGME Physician Workforce Policies: Recent Developments and Remaining Challenges in Meeting National Goals* (Rockville, Md.: Department of Health and Human Services, 1999).

9. Weiner, "Forecasting the Effects of Health Reform."

10. E. Schaefer and J. Reschovsky, "Are HMO Enrollees Healthier Than Others? Results from the Community Tracking Study," *Health Affairs*, 2002, *21*, 249–259.

11. Tammy Lindquist, Department of Health Services Analysis and Reporting, HealthPartners, Minneapolis, personal communication, Oct. 2002.

12. J. P. Weiner, "The Demand for Physicians in a Changing Health Care System: A Synthesis," *Medical Care Review*, 1993, *50*, 411–449.

13. American Medical Association, *Socioeconomic Patterns of Medical Practice in the United States, 2002–2003* (Chicago: American Medical Association, 2002).

14. Glen Hentges, personal communication, Oct. 2002.

15. P. R. Kletke, W. D. Marder, and A. B. Silberger, "The Growing Proportion of Female Physicians: Implications for U.S. Physician Supply," *American Journal of Public Health*, 1990, *80*, 300–304.

16. Glen Hentges, personal communication, Oct. 2002; American Medical Association, *Socioeconomic Patterns of Medical Practice.*

17. Record and others, "New Health Professions"; Hooker, "Roles of Physician Assistants and Nurse Practitioners"; R. Hooker and D. Freeborn, "Use of Physician Assistants in a Managed Health Care System," *Public Health Reports,* 1991, *108,* 90–94; P. Lairson, J. Record, and J. James, "Physician Assistants at Kaiser: Distinctive Patterns of Practice," *Inquiry,* 1974, *11,* 207–219; J. Record and H. Cohen, "The Introduction of Midwifery in a Prepaid Group Practice," *American Journal of Public Health,* 1972, *62,* 354–360.

18. E. Wagner and others, "Chronic Care Clinics for Diabetes in Primary Care: A Systemwide Randomized Trial," *Diabetes Care,* 2001, *25,* 695–700; E. Wagner, "More Than a Case Manager," *Annals of Internal Medicine,* 1998, *129,* 654–656; C. Sadur and others, "Diabetes Management in a Health Maintenance Organization: Efficacy of Care Management Using Cluster Visits," *Diabetes Care,* 1999, *22,* 2001–2017; T. Von Sternberg, K. Hepburn, P. Cibuzar, and L. Convery, "Post-Hospital Sub-Acute Care: An Example of a Managed Care Model," *Journal of the American Geriatric Society,* 1997, *45,* 87–91; T. Von Sternberg, "The Role of the Geriatrician in Managed Care: Opportunities and Responsibilities," *Journal of the American Geriatric Society,* 1999, *47,* 605–610.

19. M. Baird, "Integrated Primary Care at HealthPartners of Minneapolis: A View from the Deck," *Families, Systems and Health,* 1998, *16,* 159–164; T. Davis, "From Pilot to Mainstream: Promoting Collaboration Between Mental Health and Medicine," *Families, Systems and Health,* 2001, *19,* 34–43; J. A. Feinman, D. Cardillo, J. Palmer, and M. Mitchel, "Development of a Model for the Detection and Treatment of Depression in Primary Care," *Psychiatric Quarterly,* 2000, *71,* 59–78; R. A. Dea, "The Integration of Primary Care and Behavioral Healthcare in Northern California Kaiser Permanente," *Psychiatric Quarterly,* 2000, *71,* 17–29.

20. Sadur and others, "Diabetes Management"; E. Noffsinger, "Will Drop-In Group Medical Appointments (DIGMAs) Work in Practice?" *Permanente Journal,* 1999, *3,* 58–67; E. Noffsinger and J. Scott, "Understanding Today's Group Visit Models," *Permanente Journal,* 2000, *4,* 99–112.

21. D. Craig, L. Hartka, and W. Likosky, "Implementation of a Hospitalist System in a Large Health Maintenance Organization: The Kaiser Permanente Experience," *Annals of Internal Medicine,* 1999, *130,* 355–359.

22. R. Feachem, N. Sekhri, and K. White, "Getting More for Their Dollar: A Comparison of the NHS with California's Kaiser Permanente," *British Medical Journal,* 2002, *324,* 135–143.

23. K. Grumbach and others, *California Physicians, 2002: Practice and Perceptions* (San Francisco: Center for Health Professions, University of California, 2002).

24. Ibid.

25. R. Cooper, T. Getzen, H. Mckee, and P. Laud, "Economic and Demographic Trends Signal an Impending Physician Shortage," *Health Affairs,* 2002, *21,* 140–162.

26. J. P. Weiner, "A Shortage of Physicians or a Surplus of Assumptions?" *Health Affairs,* 2002, *21,* 160–162; K. Grumbach, "Fighting Hand to Hand over Physician Workforce Policy: The Invisible Hand of the Market Meets the Heavy Hand of Government Planning," *Health Affairs,* 2002, *21,* 13–27.

27. Weiner, McLaughlin, and Gamliel, "Extrapolating HMO Staffing."

28. Hart, Wagner, Pirzada, and Nelson, "Physician Staffing Ratios in Staff-Model HMOs"; Philip Mealand, Department of Delivery Systems Management Services, Group Health Cooperative, Seattle, personal communication, Oct. 2002.

CHAPTER EIGHT

PREPAID GROUP PRACTICE AND HEALTH CARE RESEARCH

Raymond Fink and Merwyn R. Greenlick

Until the 1950s, little was known about how noninstitutionalized populations used health services. At a time when chronic disease was becoming increasingly recognized as a major health concern, little was known about how many people were diagnosed with these conditions or how they used health services. While national and local efforts were getting under way to study community health through household surveys, the first estimates of community health status were being reported by researchers in prepaid group practice (PGP) plans working in California and New York, using data routinely collected about their members.

The emergence of PGPs as a source of medical care to large community populations opened research opportunities not available elsewhere, as these institutions assumed the responsibility for both insuring their members and organizing and delivering medical services. This expanding form of medical care organization offered researchers information about the demographic characteristics of insured members, their health problems, the medical services provided for those problems, and the providers of the services. Even before the advent of computerized storage, retrieval, and analysis, data for each of these areas were accessible in centralized locations to PGP administrators and researchers.

The authors thank John Van Steenwyk for his insights into the reasons behind early PGP decisions to collect medical utilization data.

In the half-century since reports based on these PGP data first appeared, the PGPs have grown, their range of services has expanded, and a large and varied body of research has been published. In many ways, this research has influenced how medical services are provided in this country and elsewhere, as well as how these services are financed. Moreover, health researchers at the national and local levels and in other systems of health care have employed some of the research methods introduced by the PGPs and have delved into research areas that had not been examined before PGPs reported on them.

This chapter follows the development and expansion of PGP research from the 1950s, when it provided the first estimates of Americans' health care use and health status, to the present, when research and disease intervention have been integrated into the PGP structure to improve health outcomes. Attention is also given to research among PGPs in health delivery and financing for the poor and the aged as these groups have gained increased access to federally funded health care. These and other PGP research efforts have been and continue to be important guides to national research and policy agendas.

The chapter begins with a discussion of the factors that have enabled prepaid group practices to become leaders in the area of health care research. This is followed by a summary of some of the most important research to come out of PGPs in the areas of utilization, screening, disease intervention, and provision of care to the poor and the aged. Next there is a discussion of the impact of PGP research on the field of health services research in general. The chapter concludes with some thoughts about the role of PGP research in the evolving health care system.

PGP Structure and Its Impact on Research

The strong link between prepaid group practice and health care research has been forged by some of the unique characteristics of the PGP model and the commonalties among PGPs' clinical databases.

Prepayment and Membership

The system of prepayment imposed on newly organized prepaid group practices compels the need to identify, in advance of providing medical care, a list of all eligible members, which becomes the population denominator. Upon enrollment in the health plan, information is obtained about all persons in the PGP contract, including the spouse and other dependents. This information is updated as changes occur within the family. Consequently, at any point in time, the PGP may clearly identify its members and some key demographic characteristics, thus creating a known population that is the base of all reported PGP rates and proportions.

Diversity of membership adds another critical dimension to PGP research capabilities, and this diversity has increased over time through new enrollment, the broadening of geographical boundaries, and inclusion of newly insured population groups such as the poor and the elderly. This expansion has broadened the applicability of research findings over the past fifty years, and the membership of some of the older plans has increasingly come to resemble the communities in which they are located.[1] Moreover, because many members remain in their PGP plans over long periods of time, longitudinal research following member cohorts over time is often possible.

Comprehensive Health Benefits

Central to the concept of PGPs are the notions that (1) medical coverage includes a comprehensive set of health benefits that ensures that members will receive care for nearly all their medical needs and (2) there will be little need to receive care from outside the plan. Out-of-pocket costs, after the premium has been paid, have been historically low among PGPs, and only recently have deductibles been introduced. The comprehensiveness of members' health benefits and the detailed reporting of information about covered services thus results in a nearly complete and continuous record of members' health history and use of services. While there may be some occasional loss of information when covered services are provided by out-of-plan providers, historically fewer than 10 percent of all members use outside services.[2]

Provider Reporting of Health Services

Nearly all health systems require reporting of services received by members, in addition to what is reported in patient medical records, for purposes of payment to providers. While PGP providers are paid largely through capitation or salary, they nevertheless may also be required to report on each service provided. These reports are the heart of PGP outpatient databases.

Because of the expense that would be required in processing information on all services, most PGPs normally use samples of patient cohorts or of services for research and administration purposes. Recent advances in document scanning and computer technology have allowed some organizations to record information on nearly all services.

There is no published research comparing the accuracy of reports of services by PGPs versus other systems. While it may be argued that providers paid on a fee-for-service basis are more likely to report services fully, such providers also have an incentive to "upcode" office procedure reports, an incentive that does not exist among PGP physicians. Moreover, the sample information provided by PGPs may be subject to more robust editing and scrutiny.

Accessibility of Patients and Providers for Research

Evidence from research conducted across various medical systems indicates higher rates of cooperation in research projects from both PGP members and providers (see "Distinguishing Between PGP and IPA Research" later in this chapter). The higher participation rates increase the applicability of research findings to both PGP and general populations. In addition, because clinical data are collected, processed, and entered into the data systems on a routine basis, most data are available to administrators and researchers relatively soon after the service is provided.

PGP Database Systems

Although there is no universally accepted format for PGP databases, there is considerable similarity of content among PGP systems. The information common to most databases was largely codified for all health maintenance organizations (HMOs), both independent practice associations (IPAs) and PGPs, in the Comparative Database (CDB) developed for what was then called the Group Health Association of America, now known as the American Association of Health Plans.[3] The object was to employ common definitions in order to describe activities and performance among all participating HMOs. The common data include the following:

- *Membership information*—a unique member identification code, gender, date of birth, dates of eligibility and termination, source of enrollment (for example, group, individual, Medicare, Medicaid), and a coded entry that identifies the health insurance benefits for which the member is eligible
- *Inpatient information*—admission and discharge dates, facilities (for example, hospital, specialty facility, nursing home), diagnosis or diagnosis-related group, and admitting and attending physicians
- *Encounter and ambulatory care information*—physicians (including specialty), other providers, and site of care (for example, office, hospital, emergency department)

Many also include diagnoses and medical procedures provided to the member.

In general, where PGPs provided services that were not described in the core database, such as prepaid drug benefits, they expanded their reporting to include these. Social HMOs, which bundle long-term care and acute care for chronically ill seniors, expanded diagnostic and procedural codes to include these services.

The resulting PGP data sets and the research programs that depend on them have become the Rosetta Stone of the PGP model, describing and interpreting its operations and portraying its history. More than that, the research has contributed to subject areas almost as broad as medical research itself. These include epidemiological research, analytical studies of health behavior, population health screening, demonstrations in the introduction of new health benefits, introducing new populations to health insurance, interventions in health care delivery, disease management, quality improvement methods, and risk analysis. In what follows, attention is given to only a few topics in this broad spectrum of research. Clinical research among HMOs is discussed here only as it has intersected with epidemiological or health services research.

Most of the studies cited here were conducted by PGP research and clinical staff. Others are the work of university-based researchers associated with the PGPs. Later in this chapter, several studies are discussed in which PGPs were among a number of participating health care systems.

Research on the Use of Health Services

Little more than a decade after the development of the clinical database systems of the Health Insurance Plan of Greater New York (HIP) and Kaiser Permanente in California, a series of articles was published by HIP research staff describing the epidemiology of specific medical conditions and their distribution by the age and sex of HIP members.[4] Theretofore, the only such description of PGP membership and utilization was a 1951 internal publication of Kaiser Permanente.[5] These papers illustrated the uses of PGP data and demonstrated to plan members and the community the variety and volume of services provided by this new system of care.

In "Medical Care Plans as a Source of Morbidity Data" and elsewhere, Densen, Balamuth, and Deardorff presented a tour de force analysis of medical conditions found at different stages in the life cycle and the volume of services provided for these conditions, using HIP data from the years 1948 through 1951. These early HIP studies documented the common but unsupported assumption of that time that a relatively small number of patients tend to use a high proportion of total services. They also described how, for some population groups and medical conditions there was little change over time, whereas for others there were important variations from year to year. Their analysis also provided a first comparison of disease prevalence between two plans, HIP in New York and Kaiser Permanente in Northern California, pointing to higher rates of respiratory disease and asthma among New Yorkers.

At about the same time, in the first of what would be many comparisons of PGP and fee-for-service insurance plans, Densen, Balamuth, and Shapiro reported hospital utilization rates of HIP and New York's Blue Cross.[6] A prime purpose of the study was to explore the relationship between hospital care and the availability of insurance for outpatient medical care at a time when many insurance contracts were written primarily to support the costs of expensive hospital care. Considerable detailed information was presented on age, gender, diagnosis, and procedure that had not been previously available for any large population group. The study was also notable in that it was an early example of close cooperation between HIP and Blue Cross in collecting such information, a forerunner to what was to be required in the future for studies across health care systems. The observation that HIP hospital admissions were 18 percent lower than those of Blue Cross suggested to the authors that where prepaid insurance for physician care was limited, expensive hospital care may be substituted for outpatient care.

Two decades later, using data from PGPs and fee-for-service plans from a number of other communities, Luft called attention to the consistently lower hospital admission rates among PGP patients, noting as well that the length of hospital stay differed little between PGPs and fee-for-service plans except for slightly lower average stays among the handful of PGPs that owned their own hospitals.[7]

Over the next two decades, through the work of the research team at Kaiser Permanente Northwest, in Portland, Oregon, the conceptual framework for describing the dynamics of health care utilization underwent a major revision. The variables of member demographics, disease, and source of care that were employed in the earlier studies of medical care utilization were expanded and integrated with newly created variables and hitherto unused or unavailable sources of information.[8] Analysis of individuals and individual services, for example, was expanded to studies of the family and of health care episodes. Laboratory and prescription drug use data were added to variables such as physician care in and out of the hospital. The use of the data systems containing medical information together with survey interviews conducted among samples of the member population was especially significant. The combination of these data sources permitted reports of patients' background, behavior, and attitudes to be examined in relation to their health behavior as measured through the plan's highly accurate medical records. The comprehensiveness of these data was further augmented by information specifically gathered by researchers for study purposes.

Research findings on utilization and costs observed by these PGP researchers and others found substantial support in the RAND Health Insurance Experiment, which contrasted a PGP (Group Health Cooperative of Puget Sound) with two fee-for-service health insurance plans, one offering "free" care and the other requiring patient cost sharing.[9] Comparisons with two random samples of Group Health Cooperative enrollees (one previously enrolled in the PGP, the other newly enrolled for this research) found little difference in comparison to the fee-for-service subjects in the use of outpatient services but lower overall costs because of lower hospital use among the Group Health Cooperative samples.

Building on the HIP studies of patient cohorts, McFarland, Freeborn, Mullooly, and Pope, with an expanded Kaiser Permanente Northwest database, opened another phase in the developing research aimed at understanding the determinants of health care utilization.[10] By following a cohort of plan members classified according to their utilization patterns (high, medium, or low) over a seven-year period, they observed a persistence in the use of health services over time. In addition, through the combined use of survey questionnaires and the utilization database, patterns of service utilization could be linked to physical and mental health characteristics. These studies demonstrating how patterns of health care utilization could be linked to member demographic and health characteristics were important forerunners of later research efforts to tie patient health risk to health care costs.

Health Screening, Epidemiology, and Disease Intervention

The availability of complete PGP membership lists presents the opportunity to identify population segments for research of special interest associated with basic demographic characteristics, including age, gender, and the geographical area in which members reside. Moreover, the ability to link individuals with their reported medical conditions and their providers through centralized medical records and computerized encounter information offers additional opportunities for targeting plan members who have particular medical conditions or specific characteristics that increase their health risks. At the time this line of research began, linking patients with personal characteristics was impossible in any other health care model in the United States.

The tools of epidemiology have been effectively applied by PGP researchers in a variety of ways. The most straightforward of these has been the use of diagnoses from physician encounter reports to enumerate all patients with a target medical condition. In some studies, cases have been identified through reported symptoms associated with the diagnosis, while in others, such as emotional disorders, prescribed medications, laboratory records, or other sources of ancillary data have been used to identify their presence.

PGP integrated information systems also permit the generation of study and control groups, using member files for randomization based on personal characteristics. In addition, these systems can create matched control groups for members identified with a target illness in order to observe differences between the groups over time or to study the effect of medical interventions.

Screening Asymptomatic Members

The HIP Breast Cancer Screening Study,[11] begun in 1962, and the Automated Multiphasic Health Testing Study of Kaiser Permanente in Northern California,[12] begun in 1970, are among the best-known studies conducted by PGP staff in which membership lists were used to identify specific asymptomatic members and their risk groups. Both are early examples of long-term PGP research that has influenced health care in this country and elsewhere.

Screening with Mammography

More than two decades after it was initiated in 1963, the HIP Breast Cancer Screening Study sought to test "whether screening with mammography and clinical examination of the breast holds substantial promise for lowering mortality in the female population from breast cancer."[13] A randomized controlled trial was conducted in which more than thirty thousand women in the study group were offered a baseline and three annual examinations with mammography and a similar number of control women received their usual care only.

The HIP Breast Cancer Study required that equivalent study and control groups be selected from among women aged forty to sixty-four years enrolled in HIP and that variability and proper representation be achieved through high rates of participation. The HIP information system was used to randomize eligible women from twenty-three participating medical groups through stratification according to age, size of insured family, and employment group through which the family joined HIP.

Sixty-five percent of the study women received the initial examination, consisting of a mammogram and clinical examination. This high rate may be in large part attributable to the close involvement of the medical groups through which the women received their regular care. Response to the annual examinations was also high, with 60 percent of those who had an initial screening completing all three annual screenings, while only 12 percent had the baseline examination only.

Long-term follow-up of study and control subjects was key to determining women's survival and health status at five-, ten-, fifteen-, and eighteen-year intervals. Mail and telephone contact yielded response rates of between 80 and 90 percent at the five- and ten-year intervals and in excess of 75 percent in later years.

In summarizing the findings to the National Cancer Institute in 1986, Shapiro and the HIP study staff reported, "The screening program resulted in about a 30 percent reduction in mortality from breast cancer during the first ten years of follow-up in the total group of study women aged 40 to 64 at entry. By the end of 18 years from entry, the reduction was close to 25 percent. Accordingly, the HIP study provides strong evidence that periodic screening in this trial is efficacious."[14]

Multiphasic Health Testing

In the 1960s, Dr. Morris Collen and other researchers at Kaiser Permanente in Northern California speculated that new approaches to health care delivery would be required in a prepaid medical care system in which members are not deterred by cost from seeking care. Using innovative informatics technology, they introduced Multiphasic Health Care for Kaiser Permanente members, a system of screening asymptomatic members for a large number of conditions. They also conducted evaluative research to test the effectiveness of this approach in reducing mortality from seven conditions or groups of conditions and in bringing appropriate care to individuals with defined medical conditions.

Using membership lists, subjects aged thirty-five to fifty-four years were randomized into study and control groups, each in excess of five thousand persons. Study members were encouraged to seek annual examinations through Multiphasic Health Care; controls were not. (Since asymptomatic physical examinations were a Kaiser Permanente benefit, members in the control group could participate if they chose to, although few did so.) Study members received a physical examination by a nurse practitioner, completed a medical questionnaire, and underwent a battery of tests that generated a broad array of laboratory and physical measurements. Both groups were followed over a period of sixteen years. The screening program resulted in reduced mortality in the study group from colorectal cancer and hypertension. In the case of colorectal cancer, the researchers suggested that it was unlikely that routine sigmoidoscopy alone accounted for the observed difference but that credit might go to the overall screening activity itself.

Despite some national interest in Multiphasic Health Testing during the 1970s, there have been few such programs outside of Kaiser Permanente, and there, too, the program has been discontinued. Efforts by HIP to use this type of screening program to improve health care access to its poverty-level members ended when funding from the plan was discontinued and similar testing programs outside PGPs were also discontinued.

Although research among PGPs on the efficacy of screening programs continues, the major focus has been on the study of members at increased risk for specific conditions or those already diagnosed. The number and range of these studies has been prodigious. Selby and colleagues, for example, reported a case control approach to the evaluation of screening sigmoidoscopy among Kaiser Permanente members in Northern California, using the Bay Area Surveillance Epidemiology and End Results Registry to identify members who had died of adenocarcinoma of the colon or rectum.[15] The medical records of those so identified were reviewed to determine if they had had a sigmoidoscopy and if their condition had been or might have been detected through this procedure. Case controls were matched by age, sex, and date of entry into the plan. Using detailed medical records of study and control patients to adjust for personal and family history of risk factors, the research strongly suggests that sigmoidoscopy is a valuable screening tool.

Improving Medical Care: Diabetes

Over the past decade, PGPs have made increased use of their information systems not only to identify patients with specific medical conditions but also to classify them for the purpose of special attention and care. Diabetes has been a particularly important target because of its relatively high prevalence and the high medical service utilization among patients. In Kaiser Permanente Northern California, the 4 percent of the population with diabetes uses about 12 percent of PGP services. These rates are similar to those of the general U.S. population.[16]

Several PGPs have tested their diabetes registries to track patient care and to stratify patients according to risk as part of quality improvement and research programs. A necessary first step was assessment of the accuracy and completeness of automated data used in identifying patients with diabetes and in describing the nature and seriousness of their conditions and care received. Researchers at Group Health Cooperative, using patient medical records as the validating standard, identified through the automated data system a range of complications associated with diabetes.[17] In general, the automated data were assessed as useful for research and planning needs, although there was some variation in the reliability of early reports of complications. Most of these, however, were more fully verified by later reports.

Research using a diabetes registry based on automated data was expanded in Kaiser Permanente Northern California to develop a prediction rule for identifying diabetic patients at high short-term risk of complications.[18] Two years of data on diabetic patients' care and complications were used to predict complications occurring within the year following. The resulting models of data-based predictors demonstrated the feasibility and also the limitations of applying automated data in the selection of patients for care appropriate to their conditions.

These efforts establishing the value of automated records have become vitally linked to PGP research and demonstration in the improvement of chronic care management generally and of diabetes care in particular. Drawing from a review of the literature on chronic care intervention, research and clinical staff of Group Health Cooperative identified key elements in community and medical organization as well as patient-provider collaboration that yielded evidence of improved patient care and outcomes.[19] Although the principles selected are seen to be applicable in a range of health care organizations and have indeed been tested elsewhere, PGPs appear to offer particularly hospitable sites for testing.

In randomized clinical trials designed to test the structuring of the medical care system in the treatment of diabetes, researchers at Group Health Cooperative[20] and Kaiser Permanente-Northern California[21] used their diabetes registries for selection and randomization. Kaiser Permanente diabetic patients were included only if they had specific laboratory test findings or if they had not had the required test in the past year. Study subjects received additional training from nurses, health educators, behaviorists, or pharmacists in improving self-care and in seeking appropriate medical care. Controls received usual care only, mostly through their primary care physicians. Training was given to patients in groups and in clusters of training sessions over varying periods.

Both studies measured change in behavior and health status through survey questionnaires, and both found among study subjects higher levels of patient satisfaction and physical functioning. The California study included laboratory tests to measure changes in these values and health plan databases to measure changes in the utilization of health services. Changes in laboratory findings were in a favorable direction, as were changes in utilization during the six months following the study period.

The use of information systems and redesigned chronic care clinics is being tested and adopted in several Kaiser Permanente regions and in other PGPs and managed care settings. The Diabetes in Managed Care Work Group at the Centers for Disease Control and Prevention (CDC), for example, tested diabetes surveillance indicators at Group Health Cooperative and two IPAs.[22] Among the three plans, there were important differences in the methods of data collection, disease classification, data storage, and demographic reporting. The CDC Work Group observed that although it was encouraged by the similarities among the groups in rates of prevalence, treatment, and complications, important limitations remained in the ability to compare and track diabetes care across medical care systems.

The chronic care model is clearly adaptable to other organized care settings in addition to PGPs and may be configured to a medical care organization's structure. Bodenheimer, Wagner, and Grumbach discuss four case studies: Kaiser Permanente Northern California, a large traditional private practice, a large IPA, and a community health center.[23] Improvements in care and outcomes were observed in each of these settings. Direct comparisons among them are not presented, but study findings demonstrate the importance of the organization of health care to the chronic care model selected. In a related report, the authors underscore the feasibility of transferring this model across a broad range of medical care organizations; however, there is no information presented that permits an assessment of how differences in structure contribute to improved care or outcomes.[24]

Screening with Questionnaires in Physicians' Offices

In recent years, there has been increased use of screening in primary care physicians' offices using questionnaires to identify patients whose health behaviors, such as smoking and drinking, place them at increased risk of medical problems. Reports of these behaviors are not likely to be found in medical charts, and although questions about risky behaviors have been asked in Multiphasic Health Testing programs, they are seldom asked routinely. In connection with programs aimed at reducing alcohol and drug consumption, researchers at Kaiser Permanente Northwest screened patients for alcohol and drug use while they were waiting for a medical appointment, and the information was given to the physician at the time of the visit.[25] Physicians were trained to provide the patient with a brief message and also refer, where appropriate, for counseling with a behavioral specialist. Randomized controlled trials aimed at reducing smoking and alcohol use have demonstrated reductions in the use of both substances as a result of brief physician interventions during the primary care visit.

Delivering Services to the Poor and the Aged

The introduction of Medicaid and Medicare in 1965 created a subsequent explosion in the number of previously uninsured persons newly entitled to receive medical services through public funding. Prepaid group practices, consistent with the stated goals of the Title XVIII and XIX laws, made an early determination to bring the poor and the aged into the medical mainstream by enrolling and integrating them into their existing system of care.

Some PGPs already had experience in providing care for low-income and older patients through special demonstration programs under the earlier Old Age

Assistance program and the Office of Economic Opportunity. When Medicare and Medicaid were implemented, PGP evaluations of early experiences provided estimates of how services might be provided to these groups, the resources required, and their costs. From that point forward, PGP research and evaluation activities became integral to these programs' operations. Over time, as enrollment in federally funded health programs grew and changes were made in the delivery and financing of these programs, research issues focused increasingly on cost containment, and particularly on equity of payment based on expected utilization.

Early Demonstration at HIP

In 1962, the New York City Department of Welfare enrolled into seven HIP medical groups twelve thousand ambulatory recipients of Old Age Assistance (OAA) who had been receiving their medical care in outpatient clinics of local hospitals.[26] Researchers compared the medical care utilization of OAA recipients enrolled in HIP to the utilization of OAA recipients receiving their usual care at hospital clinics for the one year preceding HIP enrollment and one year following, using OAA and HIP records. In the predemonstration period, overall average visit rates for the HIP and non-HIP groups were about the same. Although they were also about the same during the study period, there were marked differences between them in how medical services were distributed. HIP members were more likely than the others to receive at least one service during the one-year study period, for example. Further, among those receiving the fewest services during the predemonstration period, services increased significantly more for HIP members than for those not in HIP; among those using the highest number of services during the predemonstration period, HIP patients had reduced utilization during the study, while the non-HIP patients did not. Ancillary, nonphysician services increased among HIP members but not among the others. Although mortality rates between the groups did not differ during the study year, mortality was significantly lower among HIP OAA members in the seventeen months following.

Other Pre-Medicaid PGP Demonstrations

In the two years immediately preceding Medicaid legislation, the Office of Economic Opportunity (OEO) enrolled low-income families in four PGPs (Kaiser Permanente plans at Fontana, California, and Portland, Oregon; Group Health Cooperative in Washington; and HIP in New York) with the specific aim of determining if the newly covered families' utilization would reach the same level as that of the plans' privately insured members.[27] Although initially intended to provide information that might be projected to a national population of poor people, selected participants turned out to be at higher risk than most low-income groups. The data systems of the four plans were used to collect information on services provided to OEO families and a sample of non-OEO members, and questionnaire information was also obtained.

Study findings provided early insight into what happens when a newly insured population with unmet health needs is integrated into a system of care already in place. Service utilization of OEO enrollees for six calendar quarters following enrollment was compared with services received by the plans' regular members. In most of the study settings, evidence of previously unmet medical needs was found in the high OEO utilization rates during the earliest period of enrollment. During this time, utilization was also somewhat higher than that of other PGP members. After about a year, however, there was little difference between the two groups in the use of health resources.

Prepayment Demonstrations for Medicare

When Medicare began in the 1960s, it was modeled after the Blue Cross Blue Shield programs, and thus the basic payment form for the medical and hospital services was fee-for-service. Many of the PGP programs of the time wanted to continue to serve their members after they became eligible for Medicare, and they sought a payment method that would be more in line with the PGP model (see Chapter Four).

It was nearly five years before the first PGP Medicare demonstration project was undertaken, by Group Health Cooperative, under a Medicare waiver in 1972. This demonstration, however, did not allow for the plan to use a fully prospective risk model. But beginning in 1980 and 1981, the Health Care Financing Administration (now the Centers for Medicare and Medicaid Services) supported a fully prospective risk payment methodology to be tested at five sites, including Kaiser Permanente Northwest.[28]

The participating plans sought to encourage new Medicare enrollment by offering supplemental coverage paid from the savings generated by the demonstration. At Kaiser Permanente, the enrollment target of 5,500 persons was rapidly met, and their age and sex distribution differed little from that of the Medicare-eligible population in the community. The new enrollees' hospital utilization, while slightly higher than that of Medicare members previously enrolled in the plan, was considerably below that of others in the community, and outpatient utilization was about 25 percent higher among the new enrollees, a difference that persisted for several years.

These programs demonstrated Medicare beneficiaries' willingness to leave their fee-for-service physicians and become "locked into" HMOs if their Medicare benefits were sufficiently augmented. The early success of this program led to the fully prospective risk payment methodology for HMO Medicare members approved under the Tax Equity and Fiscal Responsibility Act (TEFRA) of 1982. Establishing this payment mechanism led to the dynamic growth of Medicare managed care in the United States.

Medicare Payment and Long-Term Care Demonstrations

Two important lines of research followed from the TEFRA demonstrations. The first continues to be a critical line of work to establish an appropriate payment model under Medicare risk, now known as Medicare+Choice. Critics of the demonstrations argued that payments to plans were either too high or too low. At the heart of the matter was the federal payment methodology, which directed that HMOs should be paid 95 percent of what Medicare would have paid for the same people had they stayed in the fee-for-service world. That concept is simple to understand but difficult to calculate, because it requires assumptions about each beneficiary's underlying medical risk. Research starting in the 1990s by PGP researchers such as Mark Hornbrook and by university researchers such as Arlene Ash, Barbara Starfield, and Jonathan Weiner has moved the field forward but has yet to solve the problem definitively, either for Medicare beneficiaries or for commercial members.[29]

The second line of research that quickly followed from the original demonstrations explored the possibility of adding home- and community-based long-term care services to the Medicare benefit package. The two most successful of these programs flowed from a demonstration at the On-Lok program in San Francisco and from the Social HMO demonstrations carried out within PGPs and led by Brandeis University. The On-Lok demonstration has become institutionalized for Medicare beneficiaries nationally as the PACE program ("Program of All-inclusive Care for the Elderly"). The Social HMO demonstration, seventeen years after it began, provides coverage for home- and community-based long-term care for thousands of plan members at four sites around the country, including at Kaiser Permanente Northwest.[30]

Distinguishing Between PGP and IPA Research

In all of the foregoing, it is important to note that crucial distinctions exist between PGPs and the more loosely integrated independent practice associations. PGPs and IPAs do have in common broad health benefits for their members, knowledge of who their members are, and the requirements that all or nearly all services provided be reported. But there is a major difference between them in that PGP physicians are integrated into group practice, while IPAs are mostly made up of solo practices or small, single-specialty groups. In PGPs, the structure of the health system is clear and relatively stable, whereas IPA physicians are often only marginally involved in one or more HMOs. (In their 1993 study of IPA physicians in New York City, Berliner and Nesbitt found that half belong to two or more HMOs.)[31]

One impact of this difference may be found in the Medical Outcomes Study reports of rates of participation in research by physicians and their patients. Among group practice physicians, 92 percent completed clinic background questionnaires and 85 percent contributed patients for research projects. In solo practice settings, 66 percent completed questionnaires and 58 percent contributed patients.[32]

In recent years, we have seen the beginnings of research programs among IPAs that have used their claims data systems to obtain epidemiologic information. United HealthCare has used information from this source in reporting on quality assessment.[33] During the 1970s and 1980s, PGPs and IPAs were frequently compared on hospital utilization. Then and now, however, there are few published comparisons on outpatient utilization. The absence of these comparisons is particularly crucial in the area of Medicaid managed care, where many states have invested in health care for the poor.

The difficulties in obtaining utilization data from IPA-style programs is acknowledged by Hurley and colleagues, who stated, "The underreporting problem in capitated systems has been a source of controversy and embarrassment for providers, sponsors, and evaluators in several programs."[34] A similar assessment of data coming from Medicaid managed care in New York State was given in a 1995 conference report on this subject by the United Hospital Fund of New York.[35]

For the most part, what is known from research about HMOs is what has been learned from PGPs, and in the absence of comparable studies from IPAs, the application of these findings to IPAs must be assessed on a study-by-study basis.

PGP Research and Health Services Research in the United States

The major contribution by prepaid group practices to research in the United States may be the demonstration of the vast potential for learning what can be understood about health and health care with the availability of large and diverse populations, broad databases, and an organizational commitment to research. Though PGP research and research methods are often transferred to and adopted by others, it is frequently difficult to draw direct links between this research and what has followed from it in national studies and in other health care systems. Some of the subject areas where there are clear connections will be discussed here.

Validating Survey Findings

Before the National Health Interview Survey began in 1957, meticulous methodological research tested the accuracy of patient reports of their medical conditions and services received against information from HIP in New York and Kaiser Permanente in Northern California.[36] The results were used not only to validate patient reports but also as guides to the accuracy of reported events over specified periods. (Acceptable accuracy was found in medical visits reported two weeks before the interview and hospital visits one year before.) In later years, national population-based studies, such as the 1987 National Medical Expenditure Surveys, undertook data collection from providers, insurers, and employers to improve on the accuracy of information obtained through patient-based questionnaires on services received, medical benefits, and insurance and medical costs. In contrast, PGP information systems were readily available to validate questionnaire information and did not require support from outside sources.

Research in Health Screening

The ability of PGPs to define a population and subgroups at increased risk for disease has made possible several landmark studies of asymptomatic persons, most notably the HIP Breast Cancer Screening Study.[37] Similar studies have been conducted in nations with universal coverage, broad health benefits, and the ability to identify covered persons (in other words, almost everybody). PGPs are the closest simulation of this in the United States.

Of course, valuable screening studies have been conducted in the United States outside of PGPs, an important example being the National Health Examination Survey (NHES).[38] Like PGP screening studies, the NHES achieves high rates of participation among identifiable population cross sections. But the high cost of the NHES, which selects participants from randomly chosen geographical areas and provides screening sites (often mobile), requires that the most be made of the survey by testing for many conditions at once. The overall costs have limited these studies to years in which federal support can be assured. In contrast, the National Cancer Institute has funded the work of a consortium of PGPs in carrying out a broad range of cancer studies spread over many geographical regions. This research approaches the NHES capabilities, and at far less cost.

PGP Research and National Health Policy

The introduction to the Society of Actuaries' analysis of health risk assessment methods states that "a key component of many recent proposals for health care reform is a system of risk-adjustment payments among health plans."[39] Progress toward such a system is being significantly enhanced by methods for which the data are provided by PGPs and the models by researchers employed or associated with these plans. The Ambulatory Care Group method was initially developed from inpatient and outpatient information about the enrollees of five PGP or PGP-like groups.[40] The addition of thirty thousand Medicaid-covered persons was limited to those who were continuously enrolled in the program, a condition not unlike that of the PGP samples. In their approach to risk assessment, Hornbrook and Goodman have enriched PGP utilization and cost information with measures of patient-reported functional health status from surveys.[41] Both systems of risk assessment hold promise for health care reform that goes beyond the more limiting methods using primarily age, sex, and diagnosis.

Conclusion: Expanding Research to Understand the Influence of Health Systems on Access to Care and Health

In the past fifty years, prepaid group practice researchers have set in motion the research methods and issues they are likely to follow in the future. The research cited here, and other research such as investigations in mental health (not covered here due to space limitations), has significantly influenced health care nationally, and this impact will surely persist. Moving ahead requires an expansion of what has been done before in at least three ways: improved methods for recording and reporting data, broadening the PGP research and population base, and expansion of parallel information from other systems of care. Some examples of these requirements follow.

Improved Methods for Recording and Reporting Data

In a number of PGPs, particularly those with research histories, only samples of services have been electronically coded, due to cost considerations, while others have retrieved information largely as required by research needs. Although the ability to record electronically nearly all information has been available for years, this has not been done in practice, largely due to high costs. Anecdotal evidence of information expansion through these and other means is now supported by the decision of Kaiser Permanente and other PGPs to make medical records available to members online, as well as to provide eventual online access to health care teams.[42] This may not automatically ensure accessibility of data for research purposes, but it is at least feasible.

Broadening the PGP Research Population Base

With their large and diverse population of over 11 million members, PGPs continue to produce a voluminous array of research, and this base is being expanded through cooperative and merged research efforts. Among these is the HMO Research Network, a consortium of seven PGPs and six organizations that include both PGPs and other forms of managed care.[43] This arrangement has expanded research beyond the relatively few PGPs that some years ago institutionalized their own research programs. The result is an increase in population size and diversity that can also increase the range of topics that may be investigated.

Expanding the Database to Include Information from Other Health Care Systems

Even the limited research comparing PGPs with IPA-based HMOs has expanded our knowledge of how the organization of medical care influences service delivery and outcomes. Present trends suggest an expansion of these studies. The Medicare Current Benefits Survey, which cuts across medical care systems and links interviews among Medicare beneficiaries with claims information, will add to this body of work.[44]

In the delivery of care for specific medical conditions, research among PGPs has resulted in significant innovations in terms of reorganizing care and tracking changes in health services and in patient health. During the past decade, much of this research and innovation has been extended to other delivery systems, even though these systems may not be similarly integrated or have comparable information systems. This has been the case in transference of the chronic care model and intervention and research in care for depression.[45]

There is much to be gained by continuing the extension of PGP research and innovation across other systems of medical care. The importance of integrated systems in the delivery of quality care is being tested for a number of medical conditions, including diabetes, heart failure, asthma, and depression, and closer study of systems serves national, as well as PGP, purposes. Further tests are needed, such as those initiated by Rundall and colleagues of the informational and organizational requirements for improvement in diabetes care.[46] Consideration must also be given to the suggestion by Wagner that PGPs may not have fared well in comparative studies of health outcomes because they have not taken full advantage of their integrated systems.[47]

Future Issues

Although there is recent evidence that PGPs, as well as some insurance organizations, may be expanding their research support, the major support and direction will continue to come from government and foundations. Improving and assuring the quality of medical care will surely continue as a national issue, and PGPs, with their integrated systems of care and access to patient, provider, and system information, will be important leaders. In the event of significant growth in PGPs through new organizations, expanded information systems will permit comparisons among groups, and more reliable information may be expected about "best practices" and the impact of innovations.

Finally, in the event that gains are made in providing care for the uninsured and underinsured, it may be expected that the earliest information on their experience will come from PGP research. The history of PGPs and their readiness to explore means of health care delivery to new populations through research and demonstration ensure their future role in the exploration and dissemination of knowledge across the spectrum of health care concerns.

Notes

1. D. K. Freeborn and C. R. Pope, *Promise and Performance in Managed Care* (Baltimore: Johns Hopkins University Press, 1994).
2. Ibid., pp. 85–92.
3. M. Gold, A. Tucker, and S. Palsbo, "The Comparative Database for Managed Care Systems: An Initiative to Develop Uniformity and Consensus on Data for a Maturing Industry in an Uncertain Environment," *Journal of Ambulatory Care Management*, 1989, *12*(4), 38–47.
4. P. M. Densen, E. Balamuth, and N. R. Deardorff, "Medical Care Plans as a Source of Morbidity Data," *Milbank Memorial Fund Quarterly*, 1960, *38*, 48–91.
5. A. Weissman, "A Morbidity Study of the Permanente Health Plan Population: A Preliminary Report," *Permanente Foundation Medical Bulletin*, Jan. 1951, p. ix.
6. P. M. Densen, E. Balamuth, and S. Shapiro, *Prepaid Medical Care and Hospital Utilization* (Chicago: American Hospital Association, 1958).
7. H. S. Luft, "How Do Health-Maintenance Organizations Achieve Their 'Savings'?" *New England Journal of Medicine*, 1978, *298*, 1336–1343.
8. M. R. Greenlick, D. K. Freeborn, and C. R. Pope, *Health Care Research in an HMO: Two Decades of Discovery* (Baltimore: Johns Hopkins University Press, 1988).
9. W. G. Manning and others, "A Controlled Trial of the Effect of a Prepaid Group Practice on Use of Services," *New England Journal of Medicine*, 1984, *310*, 1505–1510.

10. B. H. McFarland, D. K. Freeborn, J. P. Mullooly, and C. R. Pope, "Utilization Patterns Among Long-Term Enrollees in a Prepaid Group Practice Health Maintenance Organization," *Medical Care,* 1985, *23,* 1221–1233.

11. S. Shapiro, W. Venet, P. Strax, and L. Venet, *Periodic Screening for Breast Cancer: The Health Insurance Plan Project and Its Sequelae, 1963–1986* (Baltimore: Johns Hopkins University Press, 1988).

12. G. D. Friedman and M. F. Collen, "Multiphasic Health Checkup Evaluation: A 16-Year Follow-Up," *Journal of Chronic Diseases,* 1986, *39,* 453–463; S. R. Garfield and others, "Evaluation of an Ambulatory Medical-Care Delivery System," *New England Journal of Medicine,* 1976, *294,* 426–431.

13. Shapiro, Venet, Strax, and Venet, *Periodic Screening for Breast Cancer,* p. 3.

14. Ibid., p. 5. Although there were some criticisms raised about the methods of this and other studies on mammography, these have been effectively addressed by other reviewers, and the HIP study findings are widely accepted. See D. A. Freedman, D. B. Petitti, and J. Robins, "On the Efficacy of Screening for Breast Cancer," *International Journal of Epidemiology,* forthcoming, Feb. 2004.

15. J. V. Selby, G. D. Friedman, C. P. Quesenberry Jr., and N. S. Weiss, "A Case Control Study of Sigmoidoscopy and Mortality from Colorectal Cancer, " *New England Journal of Medicine,* 1992, *326,* 653–657.

16. J. V. Selby and others, "Developing a Prediction Rule from Automated Clinical Databases to Identify High-Risk Patients in a Large Population with Diabetes," *Diabetes Care,* 2001, *24,* 1547–1555.

17. K. N. Newton and others, "The Use of Automated Data to Identify Complications and Comorbidities of Diabetes: A Validation Study," *Journal of Clinical Epidemiology,* 1999, *52,* 199–207.

18. Selby, Friedman, Quesenberry, and Weiss, "A Case Control Study."

19. E. H. Wagner, B. T. Austin, and M. Von Korf, "Organizing Care for Patients with Chronic Illness," *Milbank Quarterly,* 1996, *74,* 511–544.

20. E. H. Wagner and others, "Chronic Care Clinics for Diabetes in Primary Care: A Systemwide Randomized Trial," *Diabetes Care,* 2001, *24,* 695–700.

21. C. N. Sadhur and others, "Diabetes Management in a Health Maintenance Organization: Efficacy of Care Management Using Cluster Visits," *Diabetes Care,* 1999, *22,* 2011–2017.

22. CDC Diabetes in Managed Care Work Group, "Development of a Diabetes Surveillance System," *Diabetes Care,* 1998, *21,* 2062–2968.

23. T. Bodenheimer, E. H. Wagner, and K. Grumbach, "Improving Primary Care for Chronic Illness," *Journal of the American Medical Association,* 2002, *288,* 1775–1779.

24. T. Bodenheimer, E. H. Wagner, and K. Grumbach, "Improving Primary Care for Chronic Illness: The Chronic Care Model," *Journal of the American Medical Association,* 2002, *288,* 1909–1914.

25. D. K. Freeborn, M. R. Polen, J. F. Hollis, and R. A. Senft, "Screening and Brief Intervention for Hazardous Drinking in an HMO," *Journal of Behavioral Health Services Research,* 2000, *27,* 446–453; J. F. Hollis and others, "Implementing Tobacco Interventions in the Real World of Managed Care," *Tobacco Control,* 2000, *9*(Suppl. 1), I18–I24.

26. S. Shapiro and others, "Patterns of Medical Use by the Indigent Aged Under Two Systems of Medical Care," *American Journal of Public Health,* 1967, *57,* 784–790.

27. G. Sparer and A. Anderson, "Utilization and Cost Experience of Low-Income Families in Four Prepaid Group Practice Plans," *New England Journal of Medicine,* 1973, *289,* 67–72.

28. M. R. Greenlick and others, "Kaiser Permanente's Medicare Plus Project: A Successful Medicare Prospective Payment Demonstration," *Health Care Financing Review*, 1983, *4*(4), 85–97.

29. M. C. Hornbrook and M. J. Goodman, "Chronic Disease, Functional Health Status, and Demographics: A Multidimensional Approach to Risk Adjustment," *Health Services Research*, 1996, *31*, 283–307; J. P. Weiner, B. H. Starfield, D. M. Steinwachs, and L. M. Mumford, "Development and Application of a Population-Oriented Measure of Ambulatory Care Case Mix," *Medical Care*, 1991, *29*, 452–470.

30. W. N. Leutz and others, "Adding Long-Term Care to Medicare: The Social HMO Experience," *Journal of Aging and Social Policy*, 1991, *3*(4), 69–87.

31. H. S. Berliner and B. S. Nesbitt, "Structural Characteristics of Primary Care Physicians in IPA-Type HMOs in New York City, 1992–1993," final report submitted to the Health Services Improvement Fund, 1995.

32. S. Greenfield and others, "Variations in Resource Utilization Among Medical Specialties and Systems of Care: Results from the Medical Outcomes Study," *Journal of the American Medical Association*, 1992, *267*, 1624–1630; S. Greenfield and others, "Outcomes of Patients with Hypertension and Non-Insulin-Dependent Diabetes Mellitus by Different Systems and Specialties: Results from the Medical Outcomes Study," *Journal of the American Medical Association*, 1995, *274*, 1436–1444; H. R. Rubin and others, "Patients' Ratings of Outpatient Visits in Different Practice Settings: Results from Medical Outcomes Study," *Journal of the American Medical Association*, 1993, *270*, 835–840; D. G. Safran, A. R. Tarlov, and W. H. Rogers, "Primary Care Performance in Fee-for-Service and Prepaid Health Care Systems: Results from the Medical Outcomes Study," *Journal of the American Medical Association*, 1994, *271*, 1579–1586; A. R. Tarlov and others, "The Medical Outcomes Study: An Application of Methods for Monitoring the Results of Medical Care," *Journal of the American Medical Association*, 1989, *262*, 925–930.

33. J. G. Jollis and others, "Discordance of Databases Designed for Claims Payment Versus Clinical Information Systems," *Annals of Internal Medicine*, 1993, *119*, 844–850; L. Quam and others, "Using Claims Data for Epidemiologic Research: The Concordance of Claims-Based Criteria with the Medical Record a Patient Survey for Identifying a Hypertensive Population," *Medical Care*, 1993, *31*, 498–507.

34. R. E. Hurley, D. A. Freund, and J. E. Paul, *Managed Care in Medicaid: Lessons for Policy and Program Design* (Ann Arbor, Mich.: Health Administration Press, 1993), p. 73.

35. M. I. Krasner, *Monitoring Medicaid Managed Care: Developing an Assessment and Evaluation Program* (New York: United Hospital Fund, 1995).

36. National Center for Health Statistics, *Interview Response on Health Insurance Compared with Insurance Records: United States, 1960* (Washington, D.C.: Department of Health, Education and Welfare, 1960); National Center for Health Statistics, *Origin, Program and Operation of the U.S. National Health Survey* (Washington, D.C.: Department of Health, Education and Welfare, 1963).

37. S. Shapiro, "Screening for Early Detection of Cancer and Heart Disease," *Bulletin of the New York Academy of Medicine*, 1975, *51*, 80–95.

38. National Center for Health Statistics, "Plan and Operation of the Third National Health and Nutrition Examination Survey, 1988–94." In *Programs and Collection Procedures*, Vital and Health Statistics, Series 1 (Washington, D.C.: U.S. Government Printing Office, 1995).

39. D. L. Dunn and others, *A Comparative Analysis of Methods of Health Assessment* (Schaumberg, Ill.: Society of Actuaries, 1996), p. 1.

40. J. P. Weiner, "Risk-Adjusted Medicare Capitation Rates Using Ambulatory and Inpatient Diagnoses," *Health Care Financing Review,* 1996, *17,* 77–99.

41. M. C. Hornbrook and M. J. Goodman, "Chronic Disease, Functional Health Status, and Demographics: A Multidimensional Approach to Risk Adjustment," *Health Services Research,* 1996, *31,* 283–307.

42. "Kaiser to Put Patient Records on Line," *Washington Post,* Feb. 5, 2003, p. E3.

43. The members of the HMO Research Network are Kaiser Permanente (Northern California, Southern California, Hawaii, Northwest, Colorado, and Georgia), Health-Partners Research Foundation, Meyers Primary Care Institute/Fallon Healthcare, Group Health Cooperative Center for Health Studies, United Health Care, Harvard Pilgrim Health Care, Henry Ford Health System–Health Alliance Plan, and Lovelace Clinic Foundation. See www.hmoresearchnetwork.org.

44. E. J. Epping and B. Edwards, "Computer Matching of Medicare Current Beneficiary Survey with Medicare Claims," in *Health Survey Research and Methods: Conference Proceedings* (Hyattsville, Md.: Department of Health and Human Services, 1996).

45. Bodenheimer, Wagner, and Grumbach, "Improving Primary Care for Chronic Illness: The Chronic Care Model"; J. Unutzer and others, "Collaborative Care Management of Late-Life Depression in the Primary Care Setting: A Randomized Controlled Trial," *Journal of the American Medical Association,* 2002, *288,* 2836–2845.

46. T. G. Rundall and others, "Chronic Care Management in Nine Leading U.S. Physician Organisations," *British Medical Journal,* 2002, 325, 958–961.

47. E. H. Wagner, "Managed Care and Chronic Illness: Health Services Research Needs," *Health Services Research,* 1997, *32,* 702–714.

CHAPTER NINE

PHYSICIAN LEADERSHIP

"Group Responsibility" as Key to Accountability in Medicine

Francis J. Crosson, Allan J. Weiland, and Robert A. Berenson

Physicians who attend a popular leadership development course sponsored by Kaiser Permanente are sometimes asked, "What does a person need to become a leader?" The simple answer, they are told, is "followers." But that answer only begs the tougher question of how to get a group of naturally independent, self-assured physicians—every one of whom is regarded as a leader or an authority figure by patients and staff—to behave as followers as well as leaders.[1] "I can call spirits from the vasty deep," boasted Owen Glendower in *Henry IV.* "So can I," said Hotspur, "or so can anyone. But will they come when you do call them?"

This chapter addresses two related questions about physicians and leadership: Why is the leadership of physicians relevant to American health care, and how can it most effectively be reaffirmed? And what are the leadership qualities necessary to persuade physicians to act together in fulfilling that role?

In examining these questions, we review some of the reasons why the traditional model of physician organization (fee-for-service, solo practice, or small group practice) seems to be no longer adequate for the demands of health care leadership in the twenty-first century, as those requirements have been defined by

The authors wish to thank Kaiser Permanente's Institute for Health Policy for facilitating their intellectual collaboration and editor Jon Stewart for enabling this exercise in "editorial group practice."

the Institute of Medicine (IOM).[2] We then examine how the concept of "group responsibility," which provides the most basic organizing principle for the large, multispecialty group practice model, drives a broad set of accountabilities for health care quality and efficiency that closely matches the IOM's demands for health care leadership. As we explain, although prepayment adds a powerful dimension to the advantages of group practice, as in the prepaid group practices examined in this book, similar overall results can be achieved by group practices in the mixed-model and fee-for-service environments.

In the second half of this chapter, we examine the related question of what leadership qualities have proved effective in helping physicians work together in large group practices. We conclude with some observations about why this tried-and-true model of physician organization has not been successfully replicated throughout the United States as advocates had once hoped. We close with suggestions for how the country's premier group practices might still seize the opportunity to provide badly needed leadership in the development of a more accountable, collaborative, integrated, and patient-centered health care system for America.

Why Physician Leadership Matters

It was not so long ago that physicians held a God-like sway over the health care universe. After all, it was a universe that consisted, for the most part, of tens of thousands of highly personalized, independent solo practices, each tending to the health care needs of hundreds of individual patients, one at a time. Within that intimate relationship between physician and patient, the physician held all the knowledge, all the power, all the authority. And the physician and patient were indisputably the only actors who really mattered. Even in the relationships between physicians and hospital administrators or, later, physicians and insurers, physician authority—to set policies and to determine the cost for services rendered—was rarely challenged.

That preeminent status over the entire health care environment is today the stuff of nostalgic TV reruns. For the past decade especially, much of the physician community has been in steady retreat in the face of a daunting array of powerful challengers for influence: larger and ever more powerful, for-profit "managed care" insurance companies; megalithic hospital systems (with the capital to buy up, and then break up, unprofitable physician practices); physician practice management firms focused on Wall Street; state and federal regulators responding to populist political agendas; increasingly activist employers and payers motivated by soaring health care costs; and most recently, health care consumers and patients themselves, empowered by the information revolution and their own growing financial stake in the cost of their health care. The result, proclaimed in every medical trade publication, is that physicians, as a profession, have lost more influence more rapidly than any profession in history.

But does it really matter beyond the immediate interests of the medical profession? Is American health care in any way less effective or less valuable because physicians have ceded so much leadership in health care to other actors—insurers, accountants, regulators, purchasers, and patients?

We believe that the void in physician leadership does matter. The evidence can be read virtually every day in newspaper headlines attesting to the growing turmoil, confusion, and public distrust toward health care institutions. Health care costs have soared at double-digit rates, far outpacing overall inflation. Inevitably, the number of uninsured Americans is rising, and even the best-insured are beginning to take notice of their higher out-of-pocket costs as employers shift the growing cost burden to employees via higher deductibles and copays.

The growth of managed care with its cost containment strategies in the 1990s prompted an unprecedented outpouring of consumer resentment and backlash (fed in large part by physician backlash) that tarnished the entire enterprise. At the same time, a series of landmark, well-publicized quality studies by the Institute of Medicine documented widespread failures in the area of patient safety and an alarming "chasm" between the medical quality standards that are routinely delivered and the enormous quality improvements that are possible but have not been widely realized. "Many patients, doctors, nurses, and health care leaders are concerned that the care delivered is not, essentially, the care we should receive. The frustration levels of both patients and clinicians have probably never been higher," said the IOM's *Crossing the Quality Chasm* report. "Yet the problems remain. Health care today harms too frequently and routinely fails to deliver its potential benefits."[3]

In many ways, American health care entered the twenty-first century both bloodied and bowed—and with *no* effective leadership. As others have observed, the contest for influence among physicians, insurers, regulators, politicians, and purchasers that ensued in the 1990s turned into a mass retreat by the end of the century, leaving the field to the de facto and somewhat reluctant leadership of the consumer (for whom retreat is not an option) and a few scattered purchaser coalitions.[4] Since then, the mainstream physician community has failed to step forward and accept responsibility and accountability in the critically important arena of clinical decision making, and no other stakeholder has stepped up to the broader responsibilities for the daunting financial, technological, and other health challenges that have come to full fruition in health care over the past fifteen years.

Given the great and growing complexity of health care over the past half-century, a whole new pluralistic model of leadership is now required, one in which responsibilities and accountabilities are widely shared among players who are willing and able to act as true partners in a health care *system* that is worthy of the name.

Yet even within such a leadership alliance, the physician, together with his or her patients, must inevitably occupy a special place. For no other party has the professional responsibility, dating back twenty-five hundred years, to always place the interests of the patient above self-interest in all forms and to maintain the highest standards of competence, knowledge, and integrity in the interest of patients' welfare. The acceptance of that ancient responsibility, deeply ingrained in the profession, is the basis for the time-honored social contract on which the medical profession has traditionally derived its special status in society and its special claim to leadership in health care.

In exchange for physicians' effacement of personal interests, their commitments to confidentiality and honesty, and their dedication to the best medical knowledge, patients are able to respond with a degree of trust-based openness and intimacy about their bodies and minds without which effective health care is virtually impossible. It is within the narrow confines of this extremely intimate and trusting relationship between the physician (or the physician-led health care team) and the patient that medicine is actually practiced. As long as this exclusive relationship serves the best interests of the patient, it can also serve as the nexus from which physicians can legitimately claim effective leadership over health care— historically through the physician alone (and by extension through professional associations of independent physicians), but more ideally through a dynamic partnership between patients and their physician-led care teams.

A New Leadership Model for a New Medical Landscape

Unfortunately, that social contract no longer obtains in the age of modern medicine. Physicians themselves may bear part of the responsibility for the breakdown by having allowed modern commercial pressures and entrepreneurial opportunities to sometimes compromise the fundamental ethical principles that define medical professionalism. The intrusion of the administrative bureaucracy of many managed care institutions into the patient-physician relationship in the interests of utilization management and other cost containment strategies has also helped undermine the patients' and the public's confidence and trust in their relationships with physicians. But undoubtedly the most powerful force at work has been beyond the influence of either individual physicians or managed care institutions: it is simply the fundamental disconnect between the traditional organizational model of solo practice—independent physician autonomy—and the vast complexity of modern, evidence-based medicine.

Medicine, it is often asserted, has changed more in the past fifty years than in the previous five hundred, and it will change more in the next ten years than in the past fifty. By the turn of the twenty-first century, a proliferating number of scientific journals were annually publishing an estimated ten thousand research articles based on randomized clinical trials (RCTs), the strongest source of new medical knowledge.[5] That compared to about five hundred RCT articles per year as recently as the 1970s—a pace that even then challenged the ability of individual physicians to keep abreast of relevant new clinical knowledge. As David Eddy, an important physician-leader in promoting evidence-based medicine, stated in a recent Kaiser Permanente issue brief, "The complexity of modern medicine exceeds the inherent limitations of the unaided human mind."[6] That is true for all physicians, but it is increasingly true for the isolated, independent practitioner in solo or small group practice, who has minimal institutional supports.

The remarkable pace of the development of new scientific knowledge is only part of the problem. Even if physicians were able to keep themselves adequately informed of the latest research, the traditional, cottage industry model of physician organization offers no systematic means to reliably institutionalize that knowledge as standard practice. Thus despite the availability of information about important, evidence-based advances in clinical care, vast, inappropriate variations in "standard practice" continue to be the rule from community to community and even within communities, meaning that too many patients are not receiving the quality of care that they have every right to assume and expect.[7] The potentially huge gains in clinical quality available through implementation of existing knowledge remain largely unrealized. This is due not only to physician preferences for familiar practices but even more to the fact that few small physician practices currently have access to or can afford the organizational learning tools or clinical information technology and decision support tools that can help hardwire new knowledge into practice.

Thus in a very fundamental way, the traditional, mainstream model of physician organization is not living up to the health care demands of the twenty-first century. It can no longer support physicians in delivering on the professional obligations of competence, knowledge, and best practice on which physician leadership depended in the past and on which it must rebuild its credibility and its right to leadership in the future.

Redefining Leadership Through Group Practice

Physician leadership in the health care industry is needed today to help define and propagate a new model of care for the twenty-first century. That new model must meet each of the six challenges set out in the *Crossing the Quality Chasm* report. Thus, to paraphrase the IOM report, it must help do all of the following:

- Redesign evidence-based care processes to meet the needs of the chronically ill for coordinated, seamless care across settings and caregivers
- Use information technology to automate clinical information and support clinical decision making
- Manage the explosion of new clinical knowledge through processes and tools for lifelong learning and ongoing licensure and credentialing
- Coordinate care across conditions, services, and patients' life spans
- Promote and advance team-based care through appropriate professional incentives and cultural change strategies
- Incorporate accountability for all levels of performance and outcomes into clinicians' daily work and professional expectations

This is a tall order, one that requires a fundamentally different model of care delivery than what many physicians know today. But the good news is that the foundation of the model exists and has in fact been demonstrating an increasing ability to meet exactly the kinds of challenges we are facing. That model is the large multispecialty group practice, especially as it operates in a prepaid environment. Some seventy years after its basic outlines were forged by farsighted physician pioneers at groups such as the Mayo Clinic in Rochester, Minnesota; Ross-Loos in southern California; Group Health Cooperative of Puget Sound in the Northwest; and the forerunner of the Permanente Medical Groups in California's Mojave Desert, the evolved large multispecialty group practice model remains the most fertile basis for the rejuvenation of medical professionalism and a new model of physician leadership.

What is it about large multispecialty group practice that lends itself to meeting the challenges of physician leadership today? The best group practices, whether operating in the fee-for-service or prepaid environments, share a small number of fundamental principles (some refer to them as their DNA, or "genetic code") that shape their culture and drive their performance. These principles also compel members of the group to accept and even demand a range of responsibilities and accountabilities for the care they provide that reach well beyond those of traditional solo practice medicine. Taken together, these accountabilities constitute a credible basis for rebuilding physician leadership, for they respond directly to the IOM's vision for improved quality of care. They include the accountability of the collective medical group for the following aspects of the health care relationship:

- Effective care, as reflected in standardized measures of patients' clinical outcomes

- Patient trust and satisfaction with the cost and quality of the care they receive, as measured by scientific surveys
- A focus on prevention and wellness that looks beyond the traditional boundaries of illness-oriented health care
- Safe care, as defined in the IOM's patient safety report[8]
- Cost-effective care to keep quality as affordable as possible
- Timely patient access to care that meets both patient and provider needs

The Principles That Drive Accountability

What is the conceptual basis that drives such a broad range of accountabilities? The chief underlying principle of group practice is the notion of *group responsibility*, which refers to the responsibility of all the physicians within a medical group, both individually and collectively, for the health of all the patients within the population served by the group—including those who rarely, if ever, appear in a clinic demanding services—regardless of the payment mechanism. It is this dual responsibility to a population of patients, complementing the traditional Hippocratic commitment to every individual patient, that most distinguishes large group practice from the traditional medical mainstream. And it is this principle, more than any other, that accounts for group practice's deep level of clinical collaboration, the coordination of care among specialties, and the sharing of information and knowledge among all clinicians—practices that are increasingly essential to the delivery of quality care.

The core principle of group responsibility includes a commitment to quality care—a cultural characteristic that permeates the entire group structure and philosophy. This commitment underlies the existence in most group practices of a sophisticated quality improvement infrastructure, including effective peer review procedures, processes for the sharing of evidence-based best practices, and routine processes for monitoring and feedback on physicians' clinical performance, as well as the monitoring and reporting of overall group performance. The quality commitment, along with the resource efficiencies that flow from quality, is also the source of the readiness of most large group practices to invest in the clinical information systems and automated medical record technology that can produce quantum leaps in the quality of patient care. Finally, the commitment to quality drives processes to encourage shared decision making that improve quality and patient satisfaction through deeper patient involvement in care.

In sum, group responsibility has been the cultural key to the success these organizations have quietly enjoyed for the past half-century or more. It drives the creation of critical systematic processes and organizational infrastructures that enable the accountabilities noted earlier: quality outcomes, patient satisfaction, prevention and wellness, safe care, cost-effective care, and timely access to care. And it is the establishment and nurturing of group responsibility that is the key imperative for rebuilding effective physician leadership in American health care.

Note that for the most part, this chapter has not addressed the principle of prepayment among the fundamental elements that enable group practices to assume these accountabilities. Though the advantages of prepayment are obvious to many, it seems increasingly likely that group practice can achieve much of its accountability agenda even in the fee-for-service environment. The nature of health care financing is changing in radical ways, with a growing share of the cost burden now being shifted from employers to the individual health care consumer. This cost shift will inevitably prompt a greater concern for cost-effective care among both consumers and their physicians, increasingly providing fee-for-service group practice physicians with incentives to manage costs as effectively as prepaid groups. In the meantime, it is clear to those who practice in a prepaid environment that capitation does in fact reinforce the responsibility of the physician group for both the affordability and the quality of services rendered to patients. Prepayment also creates a powerful force supporting preventive services and such innovations as self-care programs and Web-based care services, which promote affordability.

Translating Group Principles into Practice: The Challenges of Leading Physicians in Group Practice

This chapter began with the observation that physicians tend to make poor followers, having been socialized throughout long years of medical training to think and act as independent and individually accountable leaders. Certainly all physicians perceive themselves as leaders, and all are trained to make life-and-death decisions and to be held accountable for them. But the particular leadership attitudes and behaviors inculcated into young physicians are effective mainly in the clinical environment—in relationships with patients, physician peers, and other clinicians. They are not necessarily effective beyond that special milieu, as when a physician takes off the white coat and is expected to act as a strategist or an administrative and managerial leader. In that situation, traditional physician leadership skills may actually be counterproductive. A whole new set of skills and perspectives is needed—behaviors such as delegating rather than doing, collaborating rather than acting independently, planning rather than acting, and acting proactively rather than reactively.[9] In short, the notion that physicians make poor followers does not imply that they make good leaders in nonclinical situations.

If this is true, then the challenge of promoting a renewal of physician leadership through group practice, which depends on collaboration, group responsibility, stewardship over shared resources, peer review, teamwork, and that mysterious something called "groupness," must confront a two-headed problem: how to lead and how to follow—how to get eagles to fly in formation.

In fact, the problem is really more one of leadership than of followership, thanks to the self-selecting nature of medical practices, whereby more independent-minded, entrepreneurial physicians gravitate naturally to the fee-for-service, solo, or small group practice world, while those who value collaboration, teamwork, and shared learning are attracted to group practice. But even though group practice physicians may be more inclined than their solo or small group colleagues to follow a leader, the particular skills and competencies required of successful group practice leadership remain a work in progress—one being constructed today, with many variations, in large, prepaid group practices throughout the country. The following observations on physician leadership generally, and leadership of prepaid group practices specifically, are drawn in large part from our own personal experiences in group practice leadership.

Leadership Through Vision

To transcend the professional traditions of individual autonomy and independent practice, physicians need, first and foremost, a compelling, motivating vision—an irresistible promise of a better way of working and living. If it is to drive the long-term success of a group of physicians, that promise or vision must also serve as the source of a set of principles and values capable of guiding the everyday activities of the group. In most cases, the source of that motivating vision is an individual—a visionary. And when a visionary is also charismatic, energetic, pragmatic, driven, and committed to the realization of his or her vision, amazing things can happen. Eagles can be made to fly in formation—physicians to practice together.

Sidney Garfield, the founder of the Permanente Medical Groups, was such a leader. Garfield's remarkable ability to articulate his vision of the combined power of group practice and prepayment won over not only one of the most powerful and wealthy industrialists of the mid-twentieth century, Henry J. Kaiser, who would finance his dream, but a core group of young, idealistic physicians who were willing to face the wrath of organized medicine to help him make it a reality. Yet those same physicians would later reluctantly acknowledge that although Garfield virtually created the Permanente model of prepaid group practice, he lacked the skills needed to manage and administer a large, multimillion-dollar medical care program. When Henry Kaiser removed Garfield from his role as medical director of Health Plan and key liaison to the medical group, Garfield's physician colleagues did not object; they recognized, sadly, that the organization needed a new kind of leadership for the phase of development it had reached.

Physician visionaries such as Garfield or Charlie and Will Mayo, founders of the Mayo Clinic, may be needed to launch successful medical groups but not to sustain them once the vision is embedded in a group culture. Rather, leaders of mature groups need to function as the "keepers of the culture," continually explaining and reinforcing the principles that emanate from the vision and modeling in every way possible how those principles guide daily behaviors. They also need to be able to translate the seminal vision into contemporary and future terms. Physicians will follow a leader who can paint a vivid and credible picture of what is coming or is likely to come and then demonstrate the ability to plan for it in a way that conforms to the group's basic principles. Physicians in a group need to know why they are being asked to behave in a certain way or to implement certain policies and procedures. They need to understand how business plans conform to basic medical ethics and to the values that support the group's culture. How do physician incentives, rewards, and performance evaluation procedures conform to group values? In a prepaid group, it is possible for there to be a bias to underserve, underdiagnose, and undertreat to meet budget targets. Do given performance incentives encourage or discourage such behavior? How do the principles of prepayment and group responsibility affect the distribution of revenues? The values that provide the answers to such questions need to be made explicit in the physician recruitment process, as well as in the subsequent orientation and acculturation processes, each of which should involve direct senior leadership.

In short, a powerfully motivating vision articulated by a charismatic and determined leader may be enough to get things started. But to sustain a group, a lot more is required.

Leadership by Influence and Values

A leader whose values are explicit and consistent with those of the group's culture and who consistently behaves and plans in accordance with those values, making it not only possible but easy for colleagues to follow suit, exerts a seemingly effortless influence over peers and subordinates. This is leadership by example and by influence, by ability to plan, by organizational knowledge and its application, and by creation of effective support systems—not by the heavy-handed control of an authoritarian in a hierarchical structure.

Leaders who try to micromanage physician behavior in a group face an impossible, self-defeating task. The wiser course is to set a range of explicit, well-understood expectations about how decisions are to be made and link those expectations to basic values. In a prepaid group practice, this means, for instance, communicating the expectation that physicians will take care of the needs of the individual patient in a way that also considers the needs of the entire patient population for which the group is responsible—and then providing the supporting procedural infrastructure and information tools that make that balancing act possible.

Another way of saying this is to "make the right thing the easiest thing to do," to borrow the slogan of Kaiser Permanente's Care Management Institute. It requires that the leader first of all have a firm sense of what "the right thing" is and then be able to build the support systems and incentives that present "the right thing" in a format that individual clinicians can incorporate quickly and efficiently into their own practice. Quality and performance improvement practices aimed at reducing unnecessary variation, use of clinical guidelines, sharing of equipment, use of common coding—all those opportunities for superior clinical and cost performance that constitute the competitive advantage of group practice—should self-evidently be "the right thing to do" most of the time.

Communication

In a recent discussion about leadership styles among Permanente physicians, one physician commented that "leadership is a storytelling profession." Another physician responded, "That's right, but in the end, the story had better be backed up with data."

Perhaps the most important story a group practice leader can tell is the "creation myth" of one's own group, for it is the source of the group's sustaining values and culture. Leaders of mature medical groups, such as the Permanentes, the Mayo Clinic, the Palo Alto Medical Foundation, Group Health Cooperative, and some of the other very early group practice pioneers, have a significant advantage in this respect—a rich source of stories and examples, drawn from the group's own heritage, that can be told over and over again to illustrate and reinforce the meaning of enduring values. Where that resource exists, it should be carefully documented, preserved, and made accessible to members of the group in every way possible and as often as possible. Such a heritage is one of the group's most valuable assets.

Successful leaders spend more time communicating with their staff and with members of the group than in any other executive activity—and they understand that effective communication requires a balance between *listening* and talking. Effective leadership means conducting a virtual symphony of information interactions between and among all levels of the group hierarchy (and the fewer the better) and between the group and all-important external stakeholders—patients and members, purchasers, regulators, policymakers, the media, and professional colleagues.

In a 2001 survey of physicians in scores of group practices, the leadership area receiving the greatest number of complaints was that of communication—54 percent negative.[10] The low rating suggests that effective leadership communication is not only harder than most leaders think but is also a source of discontent and dysfunction within groups. It also suggests that if physician-leaders need professional training and support in any area—and most leaders probably benefit from it across the board—communication should be at the top of the list.

Strategic Direction

In a large group practice, leaders can be easily overwhelmed by the daunting range of issues that land on their desks. A key attribute of effective leadership is learning to delegate most of those problems to others for resolution and focusing one's own time and attention on the handful of critical tasks that will determine the success or failure of the group. Among that small set of ultimate leadership issues, none is more important than setting the group's long-term strategic direction—the strategy for continued success in a future environment characterized by a mix of probabilities, possibilities, and uncertainties. That strategy must be based on a close, educated reading of the external environment, including likely trends among the competition, regulators, consumers, policymakers, and society at large (the aging of society, for instance, has enormous implications for health care). And almost by definition, it must leverage the competitive advantages of group practice—the population health perspective, superior clinical quality, and the ability to invest in shared technology, for instance—to create added value for the group's customers: its payers and its patients.

The ability to scan current environmental trends and use them to postulate future directions may be more art than science, but the effort is no less necessary for devising strategy. One of the key roles of leadership is to maintain enough environmental connections to detect even potential shifts that might have implications for the group. The threats—and the opportunities—come from many directions, including the regulatory environment, marketplace attitudes about what constitutes value in health care, demographic changes that affect membership or the clinical workforce, and new technologies. These latter two issues deserve special attention.

Demographic Forces. About half of the physicians entering the workforce today are women, many of whom are not interested in full-time work. Many young male physicians are also interested in more balance between their work and personal lives. This trend has long-term implications for how work is organized, the expectations for continuity of care, and interaction with support staff and with colleagues who cover for the absent individual. For the leader, these questions translate into issues of internal equity around pay and benefits. There is the additional challenge of developing new leadership in an environment where much of the workforce is part-time. How do you engage part-timers in complex but necessary quality and performance improvement activities, such as quality assurance, continuous process improvement, risk management, and utilization management?

Another demographic issue medical group leaders must confront is how to meet the needs for culturally competent care in an increasingly diverse patient population. Until the clinician workforce is more representative of the population, the answer must involve increased emphasis on cultural knowledge, sensitivity, and training within the current workforce.

New Technologies. Technological innovation is an important environmental force that can change the nature of medical care. New information technologies, for instance, offer tantalizing opportunities, especially for prepaid group practice, to make great leaps forward in population-based health care. But information systems and the whole range of other medical technologies can involve major capital investments; they are truly strategic decisions and as such must be made in the context of the values and forward-looking vision of the group. Thus the leadership is responsible for the application of a philosophy and explicit policies around the introduction of new technologies: Is the group to be on the leading edge of technology assessment and implementation? A fast follower? A conservative follower? The leader's role is to clarify the values of the group and monitor the consistent application of those values as challenges and opportunities arise.

Leader as Change Agent

As much as the group leader is the "keeper of the culture," he or she must also function to manage major course corrections. When changes in the external environment bump up against group culture, the leader must chart, explain, and model the cultural adaptations that support any needed changes in group behavior. There are, for instance, growing expectations today for health care to become more "patient-centered" by, among other things, enhancing the patient's role in decision making, which may require some adjustments to the traditional patient-physician relationship. New kinds of benefit packages may force adaptations regarding the values that prepaid group practice brings to the provision of "comprehensive" care. Where cultural change has succeeded in the Permanente context, leaders have cultivated extensive physician input and have carefully instilled new values on the basis of the existing group culture, not in contradiction to it. They have also focused as much attention on communicating and explaining the vision behind the adaptation of values as they have on ensuring that the group's systems and policies will support them.

Leading Through Representative Governance

Permanente Medical Groups operate on the principle of self-governance, which means that physicians determine the policies of their own medical group through direct participation and through elected, representative physician leadership. Whether this type of physician leadership is desirable or necessary in all models of practice is a fair question for debate, since some successful group practices are in fact led by appointed physician-leaders and board members. The argument for the appointed leadership model is that such leaders are better able to represent the interests of the entire group and its shareholders because they are not beholden to any particular constituency, whose interests may not be identical to those of the entire group. For instance, leaders and board members elected to represent the interests of physicians in a particular clinic may (and often do) promote those interests over the broader perspectives and longer-term goals of the group as a whole—a familiar problem in a representative democracy.

The challenge of the nonelected model of governance is satisfying the need of bright, assertive physicians to feel that they have an adequate say in the policies of their group. How do you obtain physician "ownership" of policies that physicians have no direct role in creating or even approving?

Sorting out this difficult question, in both elected and nonelected models, is the job of the group leader, and it is a core piece of the related job of leadership development. Instilling that fine balance between constituency representation and group governance involves the promotion of group values through coaching and modeling appropriate behaviors, teaching and mentoring would-be physician leaders, investing in leadership development training, and explicitly articulating the group's leadership norms and expectations to newly elected board members.

Leading Through Physician Development

Where do the leaders with the skills to create the vision and manage a complex organization through change come from? Some of the innate leadership capabilities may be inborn, but creating an effective environment to develop physician-leaders is a critically important activity.

The first characteristic of such an environment is the expectation that all group members should contribute to activities that improve the group. Most large group practices have orientation processes that foster such expectations from the start of employment. As physicians acculturate into the group, it is not difficult to identify those with a knack for strategic thinking and those who possess communication styles that engender trust and respect. Once they have been identified, a systematic approach should be taken to the development of their basic management skills, such as meeting management, personnel evaluation, and conflict management. This approach should provide not only didactic training but also opportunities for more and more complex experiences, with monitoring and feedback by mentors.

Sophisticated groups create individual leadership development plans for those with the most interest and promise. Many large groups avail themselves of university-based leadership development programs for their promising candidates. Kaiser Permanente, for instance, has created its own comprehensive leadership development program in partnership with the University of North Carolina, where both physicians and nonphysicians gather for weeks at a time to examine leadership issues in health care, in general, and at Kaiser Permanente in particular.

Over time, using mentoring and coaching, didactic training, and progressively more complex experiential management challenges, a group can create a "pipeline" of physicians both willing and able to meet the challenges of leadership.

Leadership in Partnership

This final observation regarding effective physician leadership applies emphatically to that handful of large group practices that are fully integrated with health plans, as in the Kaiser Permanente and Group Health Cooperative models. For the most part, the same observations should apply to a lesser degree to any group practice that is even closely associated with a health plan.

The partnership between the Permanente Medical Groups, which care for Kaiser Permanente members, and the regional and national Kaiser Foundation Health Plans, which enroll and collect dues from those members, constitutes a core principle of the groups' practice philosophy, known as Permanente Medicine. The degree of integration and collaboration between medical group physicians and health plan managers and employees in Kaiser Permanente is so close as to constitute what looks from outside the system like a single organization (Kaiser Permanente) rather than separate medical groups and health plans joined through contracts.

Although this integration has been a vital element of Kaiser Permanente's success over the past six decades, it has also complicated the role of leadership at all levels of the system. It is not enough, for instance, for a medial group leader to act like a "shop steward" and hard-nosed contract negotiator for an organized group of physicians selling medical services—as leaders do in some independent practice associations, which exist for just that purpose. Permanente Medical Group leaders (as well as health plan leaders) need to understand the pressures and needs of both sides of the relationship, communicate the "big picture" to the entire group, and then translate that picture into concrete plans by which the medical group can promote the success of the entire organization. In practice, this means that leaders working in partnership have to learn to "fit into one another's shoes" or to represent each other's interests when one's partner is not in the room.

In a closely integrated system, it is not sustainable to have a medical group that is successful and a health plan that is not: premiums would rise, membership would drop, and the group's capitation revenue would shrink. Nor is the opposite sustainable: a strong medical group is necessary to attract and retain top-quality physicians and staff to meet the clinical and service needs of the members, who would otherwise abandon the health plan. Both must be successful, and the medical director must be able to influence the direction of the overall system (including the health plan) to promote the success of the medical group while simultaneously influencing the group to promote the success of the overall system. It is a difficult—but vital—balancing act.

Evolving a Leadership Model Beyond Permanente

In the early 1990s, the prepaid group practice model, derived mainly from the Kaiser Permanente experience, was envisioned by some forward thinkers as the basis for broader health system reform that preserved a core role for physician leadership. In this vision, the model would evolve beyond large multispecialty group practice to include physicians in more traditional small practices, who could be brought together in virtual, if not actual, group practices with the help of information technology. Indeed, some visionaries even thought that an important attribute of the Kaiser Permanente relationship—mutually exclusive contracting between the medical group and the health plan—could be replicated more broadly, with health plans and physician groups of all shapes and sizes getting together to practice collaboratively in an enduring relationship.

Traditional small practices have attributes to which many physicians and patients cling, such as an environment of personal familiarity, attentiveness, and responsiveness, that are reassuring to patients experiencing the loss of control resulting from disease or disability. Theoretically, the objective of developing a group practice sensibility in these environments is to combine the particularly appealing attributes of the relatively small, decentralized medical practice with the attributes of accountable medical groups as described in this chapter. The 1990s witnessed the rise and fall of the at-risk medical group, especially in California. Virtually all practicing physicians participated in one way or another in one or more types of physician-led organizations, largely in response to the burgeoning presence and demands of health maintenance organizations. The objective was to combine the potential economies of scale of the large medical group with the intimacy of decentralized, community-based practices, adding the compelling logic of prepayment. As has been well documented, many of these physician organizations failed as the logic of major expansion in physician-led medical groups and independent practice associations confronted the realities of the marketplace.[11]

The experience of the failed physician organizations is sobering and points to the importance of physician culture and leadership in managing change. James Robinson of the University of California at Berkeley concludes that the most successful physician organizations were those that had evolved over a fairly long period, were able to build out their facilities and to recruit and socialize their physicians, and were able to develop their management capabilities at a moderate and sustained pace.[12]

Robinson also notes that multispecialty medical groups were confronted with the need to mediate major financial and cultural tensions between primary care physicians and specialists. Within medical groups and independent practice associations, certain specialties learned that they had power "to extort greater shares of the overall budget with threats of unified withdrawal."[13] Indeed, while multispecialty physician organizations were foundering in California and elsewhere, many physicians moved to organize into formal, single-specialty groups that have been better able to resist the principle of prepayment and, accordingly, the need to join with other specialists in integrated, risk-bearing organizations. Rather, they have been able to reinforce the prevailing fee-for-service orientation of the health care system, which drives the volume of procedures but does not promote group responsibility for curing disease, managing disability, and maintaining health. In fact, in many communities, multispecialty group practices have not developed at all.

At the same time, many new "integrated delivery systems"—pairing hospitals with collections of physician practices—have risen and fallen in the past decade. Some observers conclude from this experience that horizontal delivery systems are irrelevant to the current marketplace trends, which favor innovations in product and benefit design over innovations in care delivery. But such views ignore the fact that value is achieved for the health care consumer not in insurance redesign but in constant systematic improvement in quality and affordability of health care *delivery*. It is here, in the promise of improved delivery systems, that multispecialty group practice still forms the vanguard of change and the best hope for the future.

What is little noticed is that the nation's largest and oldest group practices—whether prepaid, fee-for-service, or mixed models—have survived the 1990s and are thriving. It is in these groups that *Crossing the Quality Chasm* is taken seriously as a blueprint for successful change. And it is in these groups that innovations in the use of clinical information technology are quietly taking place—innovations that will transform health care quality and efficiency. In fact, a number of these groups, including many of the most prestigious medical groups in the nation, have formed the Council of Accountable Physician Practices (CAPP) under the auspices of the American Medical Group Association to demonstrate the potential of group practice to lead the physician community in improving the quality and affordability of health care.[14]

Conclusion: Seizing the Leadership Opportunity

A historic opportunity exists right now for the leaders of the country's large multispecialty group practices to step up to the challenge of articulating and promoting a vision of health care delivery that will meet the needs of the twenty-first century. A good road map has already been created by the IOM in *Crossing the Quality Chasm*. It remains only for those delivery systems that are capable of moving along that pathway to excellence to show the leadership that has been lacking for so long from American health care.

Seizing the opportunity will require some significant changes in the way group practice leaders have played their part in recent years. Physicians, generally, have been in a defensive mode, more often protecting and shielding the profession from the pressures and demands of a rapidly changing environment than boldly striking out in new directions. By and large, national physician associations have been fighting rear-guard actions against change on behalf of a nervous physician community. The entire industry, including hospitals, insurers, and physician organizations, has been caught up in a largely unproductive state of turmoil without direction.

What will it take for physicians—specifically the leaders of group practice—to break free from this "Brownian motion," as the IOM calls it, and help propel American health care into the twenty-first century?

Our observations on the qualities of effective physician leadership suggest much of what is needed. In fact, nothing is needed more than a compelling vision—and evidence—that a better way is within our grasp. Both patients and their physicians, not to mention the parties who pay for most of the care, are seeking desperately for a care delivery model that preserves the essential intimacy and trust of the patient-physician relationship while adapting to the new opportunities of evidence-based medicine. Yet after more than half a century of documented success, the group practice model that best delivers on that vision is absent in many parts of the country and is poorly understood even where it has flourished in parts of the Midwest and along the West Coast. The greatest challenge for group practice leaders is to find ways to share the vision and reality of group practice more aggressively and more broadly—with opinion leaders, the academic community, political leaders, and the public.

The group practice vision will be best served by promoting its real-world accomplishments in the areas of quality outcomes, wise resource management, and value creation. Group practices have been challenged in demonstrating their success due to the absence of comparable clinical data from the solo practice nonsystem of care. How can organized systems compare themselves to nonsystems? Independent quality-advocacy groups such as the National Quality Forum, the National Committee for Quality Assurance, the Foundation for Accountability (FAACT), and Leapfrog are looking for new approaches to quality measurement at the level of the care delivery system rather than at the health plan level. This presents a potent opportunity for group practice leaders to come together and help define tomorrow's quality agenda in ways that could be far more meaningful to patients and purchasers—and will ultimately demonstrate the superior outcomes of the group practice model.

Finally, the point cannot be overemphasized that the leadership model demanded by these challenging times is a pluralistic one—physicians of all stripes partnering with hospital administrators, insurers, policymakers, purchasers, and especially patients. Within that broad partnership, group practice leaders can play an especially valuable role—not by urging their model on everyone else but by pushing the entire American health care enterprise toward greater clinical collaboration, systematic integration, and patient-centered accountability, whatever the particular organizational model. In the end, quality and affordability are our objectives. That's the challenge, and that's the opportunity, and we believe that physicians as effective leaders can make it happen.

Notes

1. For a detailed discussion of "followership," see J. Silversin and M. J. Kornacki, "A New Dynamic for Medical Group Governance: Enhancing 'Followership' and Organizational Performance," *Group Practice Journal,* 2000, *49*(2), 27–34.

2. Institute of Medicine, *Crossing the Quality Chasm: A New Health System for the 21st Century* (Washington, D.C.: National Academy Press, 2001).

3. Ibid., p. 1.

4. J. C. Robinson, "The End of Managed Care," *Journal of the American Medical Association,* 2001, *285,* 2622–2628.

5. D. Lawrence, *From Chaos to Care: The Promise of Team-Based Medicine* (New York: Perseus, 2002), p. 17.

6. D. M. Eddy, *Issues in Permanente Medicine: Evidence-Based Medicine* (San Francisco: Permanente Federation, 1999), p. 2.

7. J. E. Wennberg and M. M. Cooper, eds., *The Dartmouth Atlas of Health Care* (Chicago: American Hospital Publishing, 1996).

8. Institute of Medicine, *To Err Is Human: Building a Safer Health System* (Washington, D.C.: National Academy Press, 2000).

9. M. Kurtz, "The Dual Role Dilemma," in W. Curry, ed., *New Leadership in Health Care Management: The Physician Executive* (Tampa, Fla.: American College of Physician Executives, 1994).

10. S. F. Messinger and T. Welter, "The Value of the Group Practice Model: Results from a Comprehensive Survey," *Group Practice Journal,* 2001, *50*(2), 11–16.

11. J. C. Robinson, "Physician Organization in California: Crisis and Opportunity," *Health Affairs,* 2001, *20*(4), 81–96; L. P. Casalino, "Canaries in a Coal Mine: California Physician Groups and Competition," *Health Affairs,* 2001, *20*(4), 97–108; M. B. Rosenthal and others, "Scale and Structure of Capitated Physician Organizations in California," *Health Affairs,* 2001, *20*(4), 109–119.

12. Robinson, "Physician Organization in California," p. 89.

13. Ibid., p. 92.

14. See http://www.amga.org/CAPP.

CHAPTER TEN

THE LIMITS OF PREPAID GROUP PRACTICE

James C. Robinson

Rarely in health policy has so much been expected by so many from so few. Prepaid group practice (PGP) has been conceptualized by its sponsors as combining the organizational locus for physician collegiality with the economic incentives for practice efficiency and the marketplace context for informed, price-sensitive consumer choice.[1] Through various methods in various markets, prepaid group practice has achieved these goals, exerting a dramatic effect on the structure and performance of the health care system. It has moderated cost inflation, enhanced coverage for preventive services, focused attention on chronic disease management, and more generally, demonstrated that America can do better than a fragmented system of independent practitioners, piece-rate payment, and uninformed, cost-unconscious consumer choice.[2] Yet without doubt, the penetration and performance of prepaid group practice have fallen short of the anticipations of its advocates and even of the more cautious predictions of purchasers and policymakers.

After rising for two decades, the tide of consumer enrollment, entrepreneurial energy, and political interest has ebbed to the point where textbook PGPs are difficult to locate. Kaiser Permanente maintains a strong position on the West Coast, and hybrid entities that embody some, but not all, of the elements of prepaid group practice are to be found in many metropolitan areas. But the trend in the health care marketplace is toward broad network insurance products divorced from provider systems, retrospective rather that prospective payment, a purchasing framework that emphasizes copayments at the time of service rather than cost-conscious choice at the time of insurance enrollment, and an institutional framework hostile to the principles and practices of managed competition.[3]

Four Core Elements

This chapter will provide a framework for understanding the limits of prepaid group practice by analyzing each of its critical components: multispecialty physician organization, capitation payment, exclusive organizational linkages between health care delivery and insurance, and a market framework that features multiple choice, defined contributions, and open enrollment. Not all four components need be present simultaneously. Group practice can thrive on fee-for-service payment, capitation can be applied to individual physicians outside the group context, medical groups can contract on a nonexclusive basis with multiple insurers, and sponsors can enforce purchasing discipline even when contracting with a single health plan.

In principle, a system of prepaid group practice that combines all four elements will outperform one that embodies only a few. But in practice, the four core elements seem to be separating from one another as employers reduce the number of health plan choices for their employees, health maintenance organizations (HMOs) shutter their staff-model products, provider systems divest their insurance entities, large medical groups fragment into single-specialty practices, and prepayment is applied narrowly to particular episodes of care rather than broadly to the full spectrum of services. To capture the legacy of prepaid group practice and better anticipate the future of American health care, it is important to consider the four components individually as well as in combination. To conceptually peel the onion of prepaid group practice, it is most useful to begin at the outermost layer, with the market framework of managed competition, and then move inward through vertical integration and capitation to arrive ultimately at the core, multispecialty group practice.

The Market Framework of Managed Competition

The market framework of managed competition has been conceptualized by its proponents as the mix of tax, regulatory, and health insurance purchasing policies that would foster growth among the most efficient forms of health care delivery, which were presumed to be vertically integrated prepaid group practices. In this perspective, the public and private sponsors of health insurance coverage were to move from their exclusive contract with a single indemnity insurer to nonexclusive contracts with multiple plans, ensuring that all plans were open to all beneficiaries and that none practiced explicit or covert underwriting to avoid the sickest individuals. Health plans would be permitted to establish their own premiums, but sponsors would contribute a fixed amount that did not exceed the premium charged by the low-cost plan, requiring enrollees to pay the difference. Cost-conscious consumer choice of health plan would be strengthened by capping the tax exclusion of health insurance payment, which otherwise would subsidize with tax dollars consumers selecting high-cost health plans. Sponsors would risk-adjust their premium contributions, paying more for sicker beneficiaries than for their healthier counterparts, thereby ensuring that the contributions made by enrollees varied according to the health plan chosen and not according to the health status of the one choosing. In collaboration with researchers and health care providers, sponsors would develop methods for measuring the quality of care available in different settings, thereby fostering the patient's ability to make informed trade-offs between price and quality. Sponsors would specify a standard benefit package to facilitate apples-to-apples comparisons of health plans and to increase the price sensitivity of demand. Most generally, public and private sponsors would serve as sophisticated purchasers rather than as passive payers, providing the institutional support for the individual who seeks the best value for his or her health care dollar.

Barriers to the Model. Some elements of the managed competition framework were adopted by the various regulators and purchasers of health insurance. But the framework was never adopted in whole in any sector, and even the partial adoption has encountered serious obstacles and appears now to be in retreat. Sophisticated purchasing requires large scale, which in turn requires that individual sponsors coordinate their efforts and amalgamate their purchasing dollars. But the organizational obstacles to the formation of purchasing alliances proved powerful, and the entrepreneurial rewards for their creation proved weak. Only a very small portion of the trillion dollars that annually flows through the public and private health insurance systems ever has been coordinated by alliances.

Corporate paternalism and the vested interests of brokers and consultants kept private purchasers fragmented and inefficient, while bureaucratic lethargy and the vested interests of insurers and providers impeded the ability of public programs to defend their budgets with any but the bluntest of weapons. Medicare has not, as yet, been able to develop a successful purchasing strategy, underpaying health plans in some regions while overpaying them in others. Many state Medicaid programs indulged in a shortsighted strategy of bait and switch, offering generous payment rates to attract health plans and then cutting the rates until the plans dropped out. Administrative costs and adverse selection undermined the willingness of private employers to contract with multiple insurers, and recent years have witnessed the reduction of contractual partnerships even by public employee programs that once trumpeted broad consumer choice.[4] The popular aversion to taxes and enthusiasm for tax loopholes prevented the capping of the open-ended tax exclusion for health insurance. Many consumers proved unwilling to accept the two-step choice process underlying managed competition, according to which they were to choose a multispecialty physician organization at the time of annual insurance enrollment, when they were healthy, and then stay within that system later, when they got sick.

Current Trends. The institutional framework of the U.S. health care system is currently in turbulence and flux, with no obvious direction. Loud calls for renewed regulation mix with equally emphatic announcements of the dawn of a consumer era free of governmental constraints. Depending on the moment, the nation's health care system seems to be moving toward either nonmanaged competition or managed noncompetition but in any event away from managed competition. Private purchasers are abandoning multiple choice and pursuing single-plan contracting strategies and flirting with mechanisms to extricate themselves from the thankless task of monitoring and motivating the health insurance system. Medicare is retrenching to its core as an indemnity insurer with monopsony pricing power (although Republicans in Congress are attempting to reverse this trend), while Medicaid programs in many states are abandoning the effort to mainstream their beneficiaries in favor of a renewed reliance on safety net providers. Public regulation and private litigation impose ever greater burdens on any entity that promotes provider integration or capitation payment. There are huge short-term political benefits to bashing managed care, even if the long-term alternative is a mix of higher taxes, higher premiums, higher deductibles, and higher rates of uninsured citizens. It now is hard to remember that the institutional framework of managed competition once was promoted by policy analysts and American presidents from Richard Nixon to Bill Clinton.

Vertical Integration Between Providers and Insurers

Organizational exclusivity between an insurer and a provider of health care services, as in the pure PGP model, is analogous to the vertical integration between a manufacturer and an upstream supplier or downstream distributor elsewhere in the economy. Vertical integration contrasts with other forms of organizational affiliation, including horizontal integration (merger of two firms offering the same product in the same market), product diversification (one firm offering multiple complementary products), market diversification (one firm offering the same product in distinct markets), and conglomerate diversification (one firm offering multiple unrelated products).

The broader economic literature is highly skeptical concerning the efficiency and viability of vertical integration, except in special circumstances. Whereas the coordination of supply, production, and distribution is important for efficiency and quality, nonexclusive contractual mechanisms typically outperform unified ownership, as the latter sacrifice the benefits of scale, scope, and managerial attention that can accrue when each firm focuses on one product or service while purchasing complementary components from independent entities.[5] A manufacturer that produces its own inputs, for example, typically cannot achieve the same results in the production of each component as can be achieved by independent suppliers. Independent suppliers can achieve economies of scale by producing for multiple manufacturers, can benefit from volume-related learning curves to improve quality and sustain innovation, and can avoid the managerial distractions that inevitably attend participation in multiple markets with distinct technologies, regulatory environments, and consumer purchasing characteristics. Vertical integration also forces the firm to participate in sectors where the optimal scale and scope of production are quite different. The market for health insurance, for example, is regional or national, whereas the market for health care services is localized to the community or even the neighborhood. At the most basic level, unified ownership of the various stages of supply, production, and distribution increases the overall size of the firm and can bring bureaucratic politics and an attenuation of effort and entrepreneurship.[6]

Successful vertical integration is to be found at particular periods within the evolution of every industry and at all periods for industries with particular technologies. Life cycle theories of vertical integration note the necessity of unified ownership in emerging or declining industries where there is insufficient consumer demand to support independent suppliers and distributors because the technologies are too new or because they are too old and consumer demand is shifting elsewhere.[7]

The early prominence and subsequent erosion of vertical integration in health care is best understood in terms of the life cycle of the PGP "industry" and the emergence of multiple contractual partners for both medical groups and insurers as managed care moved from the margins to the mainstream of American health care. Until the 1980s, it was difficult for a provider organization interested in prepayment to find a willing and able insurance partner, and many group practices and hospital systems were forced to create their own. Investor-owned insurers such as Humana, Maxicare, and FHP, clinic-sponsored health plans such as Ochsner, Marshfield, and Mayo, and innumerable hospital-sponsored HMOs were launched in this manner.

Conversely, insurers that wanted to offer staff-model HMO products often were forced to hire individual physicians and create new medical groups that subsequently could be paid on a capitation basis, as no independent medical groups were available. The staff-model experiments of Prudential, Aetna, CIGNA, and several Blue Cross Blue Shield plans were created for this reason. As the prepaid group practice sector matured, the potential for nonexclusive contractual relationships emerged between insurers and providers. Where sufficient group practices were available, insurers could contract on a capitated basis with multiple medical groups, while the medical groups could contract with multiple insurers.[8] These nonexclusive network structures, such as those pioneered by Pacificare and HealthNet, permitted insurers to offer broad choice and benefit from the scale and learning curve economies achieved by the medical groups. Most of their vertically integrated competitors were restricted to narrow networks of small medical groups, as they had insufficient consumer enrollment for more, and were driven from the market.

Vertical integration survived only where the staff and group-model HMOs constituted a large portion of the local market and hence offered sufficient physician choice and enjoyed economies of scale comparable to those of nonintegrated competitors. Kaiser Permanente's successes in California and Oregon and its failures in Dallas, Raleigh-Durham, and Kansas City were due in part to the large scale it was able to achieve in the former markets but not in the latter ones. It was able to build scale on the West Coast from the 1950s through the 1970s, when the industry was young and independent medical groups were scarce, which allowed it to achieve a network scale and scope no one could achieve today, when the industry is mature and competitors abound. When Kaiser Permanente expanded outside its core markets in the 1980s, the industry was maturing, competitors were everywhere, and replication of the vertically integrated model in new geographical markets was difficult. Large scale is a necessary but never a sufficient condition for industry success, however, as evidenced by the high failure rate among vertically integrated health plans that gained first-mover advantages during the 1970s and 1980s but were not able to parlay them into sustainable advantages in the 1990s.

Some health plans sought to combine the virtues of organizational integration with the attractions of contractual promiscuity by wrapping a network of independent physicians around a core of an integrated group practice. In many cases, these "mixed model" hybrids, such as Harvard-Pilgrim and FHP, proved to be nothing more than resting points on the road to vertical disintegration and full independence between the insurance and delivery components. In Washington, however, Group Health Cooperative has combined a core prepaid group practice with a contracted network of solo and small group practices and thereby has defended its market share. However, it has not been able to leverage the distinct virtues of integrated efficiency and broad choice into a comparative advantage, and it remains a niche player in a market increasingly dominated by broad-network insurance products and fee-for-service payment.

Capitation Payment

Prospective payment on a per-member-per-month basis creates economic incentives for group practices that contrast dramatically with the incentives generated by retrospective, fee-for-service reimbursement for each provider, procedure, and product. Capitation payment rewards efficiency in all its forms, allowing the medical group to retain the savings thereby engendered, whereas fee-for-service often cuts medical group revenues dollar for dollar in response to reductions in expenses. In principle, capitation spurs physician organizations to adopt the most efficient scale and scope for their enterprise; the appropriate mix of primary care physicians, specialists, and nonphysician caregivers; and most important, the clinical processes that minimize long-term costs, including appropriate technology, evidence-based guidelines, and disease prevention.[9]

The full social benefits of capitation are to be obtained only if patients have good information on access and quality and can vote with their feet for the best settings, though the importance of quality data and consumer choice extends to all payment mechanisms, including fee-for-service. Despite its theoretical advantages, however, capitation payment suffers under a sullied reputation and is in retreat from many parts of the health care system. Several decades of experience have brought to the fore the vices as well as the virtues of prospective payment. Today, the American health care system exhibits a variety of different payment mechanisms, many of which embody elements of both capitation and fee-for-service. The vicissitudes in payment methods have meaningful implications for the scope and significance of prepaid group practice.

Limitations of Capitation. The choice between capitation and fee-for-service payment in medicine is analogous to the choice between prospective and retrospective payment mechanisms elsewhere in the economy, such as between fixed bids and time-and-materials payment in construction and between monthly salary and piece rates in retail sales or harvest labor. There exists an extensive economic literature on the theoretical incentives created by various payment methods and on the actual experiences obtained using those methods in different industries, occupations, and institutional settings.[10]

While prospective payment offers attractive incentive features, it also suffers from characteristic limitations. Most obviously, fixed payment contracts, capitation, and other prospective payment methods reward recipients for reducing costs by inappropriate as well as by appropriate methods, thereby potentially reducing quality in ways that may not be easily perceived by consumers and payers. Prospective payment also rewards health care providers who obtain a mix of patients that is healthier than average, as payments can never be fully adjusted for risk and disease severity. In contrast, fee-for-service rewards with higher payments those physicians who treat sicker patients in need of intensive intervention.[11] To the extent that capitation payment covers services beyond those directly provided by the group practice, it converts the capitated entity into a fiscal intermediary that must contract with outside providers and assume responsibility for adjudicating and paying their claims. Some successful medical groups, such as HealthCare Partners in Los Angeles, are capitated for a wide range of outside services, while others, such as the Permanente Medical Groups in nine states and the District of Columbia, are capitated for professional services only.

Blended Payment Methods. Even when restricted to clinical services provided directly by the prepaid group practice, capitation imposes on physicians not only the financial responsibility for efficient delivery of care, which is appropriate, but also for the underlying incidence of disease, over which the physicians exert only limited influence.[12] In principle, pure insurance risk should be spread widely over an insured population and not concentrated on relatively small physician organizations. The economic literature argues that mechanisms blending elements of prospective and retrospective payment offer a better mix of incentives than purely prospective and retrospective methods do and finds that most real-world payment mechanisms embody elements of both.[13]

When considering payment methods for physicians and physician organizations, two dimensions of blending present themselves. First, the payment method used for the physician group can differ from the method used for the individual physician (for example, capitation for the former, salary or fee-for-service for the latter).[14] Second, prospective payment can be used for some services (such as physician office visits and routine procedures) while retrospective payment is used for others (such as rare procedures and hospital admissions).[15]

Retrenchment. Inadequate attention to the liabilities of capitation and to the opportunity to supplant pure capitation with blended payment methods has doomed numerous prepaid group practices and nongroup capitated entities such as independent practice associations (IPAs) and hospital-centered integrated delivery systems. The successful group practices today appear to maintain some elements of prepayment for the group while paying the individual physician on a salaried basis, with the salary being linked to various measures of productivity and hence embodying some of the incentives of fee-for-service. Outside the group context, health plans and physician-owned IPAs appear to be shifting toward fee-for-service and away from capitation for individual physicians, retaining elements of prospective payment through bonus payments linked to achievement of specified goals in efficiency and quality. The scope of capitation at the group level is shrinking as medical groups realize they cannot manage the patterns of utilization and the financial risks associated with hospital and pharmaceutical services.[16] Global capitation for all clinical services is being replaced by professional services capitation that covers only primary and specialty physician services, with varying degrees of risk sharing for ancillary services.[17] The retrenchment of capitation from global to professional services implies that prepaid group practice, by itself, will be financially responsible only for a shrinking minority of total medical costs, because hospital and pharmaceutical services together constitute not only the largest but also the fastest-growing component of health care expenditures in the United States.[18]

Multispecialty Group Practice

The core of prepaid group practice, in terms of its economic and clinical effects on the health care system, is neither its organizational relationship with insurance entities nor the scope of its financial responsibilities but rather its structure as a multispecialty physician organization. Capitation, vertical integration, and the institutional framework of managed competition encourage the growth of multispecialty group practices by allowing them to earn a financial reward for their efficiency and to compete on a level playing field with smaller physician practices for consumer and patient loyalty. Pioneered by the Mayo Clinic and propagated by generations of enthusiasts and entrepreneurs, group practice offers the potential for higher quality and lower cost than the cottage industry of solo and single-specialty providers through economies of scale, clinical coordination, and a physician culture of peer review and responsibility.

The best group practices achieve economies of scale through volume purchasing of supplies and equipment, state-of-the-art computer information systems, the spreading of the insurance risk that accompanies capitation payment, access to financial capital at lower interest rates, a prominent brand name in the community, and the ability to attract experienced administrative and physician leaders. They achieve economies of scope in the coordination of clinical care by combining the services of primary care physicians, specialists, and nonphysician providers (see Chapter Seven); by avoiding undercapacity in primary care practitioners and overcapacity in specialists; and by retaining clinical responsibility for their patients from the home through outpatient, inpatient, and long-term care settings. Multispecialty group practices can forge a culture of physician cooperation and team medicine through internal payment and promotion policies that foster a concern for the entire enterprise rather than for one specialty or service (see Chapter Nine).

External and Internal Barriers to Replication.

External and Internal Barriers to Replication. Impressed by the theoretical advantages of group over solo practice, generations of physician reformers have ascribed the merely modest role played by medical groups in the American health care system to external obstacles created intentionally by the medical establishment (which remains fundamentally based in solo and small group practice) and unintentionally by public policy. It goes without saying that anticompetitive boycotts, tax disincentives, misguided purchasing strategies, and regulatory restrictions have slowed the growth of group practice. The partial alleviation of these disabilities over the past two decades has spurred the creation of many new medical groups and the expansion of others. Nevertheless, it is imperative to recognize that the merely incremental growth of group practice, whether prepaid or not, is due in part to the limitations inherent in large physician organizations and, conversely, to the continued vitality of solo and single-specialty practices in some settings and for some purposes. Despite their many virtues, multispecialty group practices often suffer from the vices of excessive scale, excessive scope, and the special problems that afflict employee-owned firms.

As they grow, all economic organizations are beset by bureaucratic lethargy, internal factionalism, a widening chasm between individual initiative and group performance, incentives for each participant to ride on the coattails of others, and, more generally, by ever-growing difficulty in maintaining the coordination and cooperation essential for any enterprise. The liability of size is compounded when large scale is achieved through broad scope, the combination of diverse participants to provide diverse services. Diseconomies of scope derive from a loss of managerial focus, the necessity of competing in multiple markets with different technologies and consumers, the difficulty in assigning rights and responsibilities, the increasing politicization of internal "transfer" pricing compared to external market pricing, and more generally, the tower of Babel that emerges when too many activities seek to be coordinated through direct control within a single organization rather than by indirect control across a market setting.[19]

Employee-owned medical groups are plagued by a reluctance to invest any budgetary surplus in capital equipment or financial reserves, as opposed to distribution to employee shareholders. More important, the diversity of contributions and preferences within the ownership ranks impedes the unity of purpose and vision that is essential for long-term success.[20] Employee-owned firms in the modern economy are found almost exclusively in occupations where the workforce is relatively homogeneous (albeit often quite skilled), as in the legal and medical professions, or where mutual monitoring is easy and the allocation of rights and responsibilities is uncomplicated. As they grow and diversify into multiple specialties, medical groups risk losing the homogeneity and transparency that fostered collegiality and facilitated decision making.

Future Role. After two decades of expansion, medical groups are retrenching geographically and refocusing on a more restricted set of occupations and activities. The ill-fated attempts by physician practice management companies to create regional and national physician organizations are now but a fading memory. Many hospital systems have divested the medical groups they once built in hopes of achieving the economic and clinical benefits of prepaid group practice. Many independent medical groups are divesting outlying sites that were designed to feed patients into the core, relying on external referrals over internal employment to obtain services from specialists and subspecialists, spinning off affiliated entities such as wraparound IPAs, and in several prominent instances, breaking apart altogether as the member physicians decide they would prefer to practice in traditional solo and small group settings.

Kaiser Permanente has retreated from several money-losing and ego-bruising expansions, and in no instance has a medical group once part of the Kaiser Permanente system survived after the financial subsidies from the insurer were terminated. Many medical groups retain dominant positions in their local communities, however, and several regions, such as the Pacific Coast and the upper Midwest, continue to be characterized by group rather than individual physician practice. Multispecialty group practice preceded capitation and vertical integration and will retain a prominent place in the clinical landscape even if they disappear. Without doubt, however, prepayment and close linkages with insurance entities helped medical groups counterbalance the bureaucratic and incentive liabilities that attend large scale, diverse scope, and employee ownership. The safest prediction is that the multispecialty medical group will retain a minority rather than majority presence in the health care system and will remain dependent on local physician culture rather than on any organizational blueprint that can be replicated in new geographical settings.

Domino Theories of Prepaid Group Practice

Group practice in the United States traces its heritage to the founding of the Mayo Clinic more than a century ago; prepaid group practice to the consumer cooperatives and industrial medicine programs of the 1930s (see Appendix); vertical integration to the offering of prepaid medical services on an insured basis after World War II; and the institutional framework of managed competition to the efforts twenty-five years ago to find some middle ground in health policy between laissez-faire competition and bureaucratic regulation. In the theory of how and why prepaid group practice would come to dominate the health care delivery system, each of the four elements served as a domino that, when pushed by the one behind it, would push on the one in front. The managed competition institutional framework would favor vertically integrated health plans; vertical integration would push insurers to shift from retrospective piece-rate to prospective capitation mechanisms for health care providers; prepayment would reward economical patterns of care and hence favor group over solo physician practice; and group practice would lay the organizational groundwork for continuous innovations in health care quality and efficiency.

Currently, we are witnessing a domino process of change, but one that is proceeding in the direction opposite that predicted by the advocates of prepaid group practice. Managed competition never materialized fully in either the public or the private purchasing context; the absence of a supportive institutional framework favored the growth of broad-network insurers that abjure exclusive linkages with providers; the retreat from vertical integration undermined capitation and substituted for cooperation the contemporary war of all against all; the narrowing of prepayment led to a narrowing of the range of specialties and services brought together within physician organizations. It is no longer difficult to envision a scenario in which the structure of physician practice in 2020 will approximate that of the profession a century earlier.

Conclusion

All organizational and institutional systems must be judged relative to realistic alternatives. Passive third-party payment, broad network insurance products, fee-for-service payment, and single-specialty physician practice—elements of the brave new medical world toward which we seem to be headed—contributed in no small degree to the health care hyperinflation of the 1970s and 1980s. And despite wishful thinking among their proponents, this paradigm may not be the final resting point for the health care system. The contemporary flirtation with constraint-free choice, cost-plus reimbursement, and single-specialty physician practice is a prolongation of the economic intoxication of the 1990s, one that is creating a hangover of escalating premiums, aggressive deductibles, shrinking insurance enrollment, and ubiquitous demands that some entity be crucified for the nation's health care sins. Nevertheless, it is important to acknowledge that the original domino theory of managed competition, vertical integration, prepayment, and group practice has failed the test of the political and economic marketplace. Politicians manifest no desire to develop a supportive tax and regulatory framework;

purchasers show no enthusiasm to offer multiple choices and fixed dollar payments; health plans exhibit no eagerness to build or buy delivery systems; medical groups evidence no zeal to assume more financial responsibility; and physicians have little inclination to create new physician organizations. The safest prediction is for the continuation of today's mixed system, with some providers and - patients embracing prepaid group practice, others favoring fee-for-service and solo practice, and the majority lingering in a purgatory of organizational and financial hybrids.

The economic and organizational heterogeneity of health care in the United States imposes costs that would not be borne by a homogeneous system with a single form of physician practice, payment, and oversight. It offers, however, valuable opportunities for experimentation, comparison, and mutual learning that would be lacking in an organizational ecology without diversity. The enduring virtues of broad networks, fee-for-service payment, and small organizational units put a brake on any tendency within vertically integrated, capitated group practices to slide toward monopoly power and conglomerate hypertrophy. On the other hand, the enduring virtues of prepaid group practice set a limit to the clinical fragmentation and variation that plague traditional forms of health care. Over time, the most efficient and effective systems are those most open to competition and innovation, not those that uniformly adopt the best economic and organizational structures available at some particular point in time. Prepaid group practice challenged and fundamentally changed the medical mainstream and in its turn has been challenged and changed. Its enduring contribution to American health care is not to have moved it from one organizational and financial equilibrium to another but rather to have restored dynamism and creativity to a system at risk of self-satisfaction and stasis.

Notes

1. A. C. Enthoven, *Health Plan: The Practical Solution to the Soaring Cost of Medical Care* (Washington, D.C.: Beard Books, 2002; originally published 1980); P. Starr, *The Social Transformation of American Medicine* (New York: Basic Books, 1982); W. A. Zelman, "The Rationale Behind the Clinton Plan," *Health Affairs*, 1994, *13*(1), 9–29.

2. H. S. Luft, "Health Maintenance Organizations: Dimensions of Performance," in M. L. Millenson, ed., *Demanding Medical Excellence: Doctors and Accountability in the Information Age* (Chicago: University of Chicago Press, 1997); R. H. Miller and H. S. Luft, "Does Managed Care Lead to Better or Worse Quality of Care?" *Health Affairs*, 1997, *16*(5), 7–25; R. H. Miller and H. S. Luft, "HMO Plan Performance Update: An Analysis of the Literature, 1997–2001," *Health Affairs*, 2002, *21*(4), 63–86.

3. J. C. Robinson, "The End of Managed Care," *Journal of the American Medical Association*, 2001, *285*, 2622–2628; D. A. Draper, R. E. Hurley, C. S. Lesser, and B. C. Strunk, "The Changing Face of Managed Care," *Health Affairs*, 2002, *21*(1), 11–23; M. A. Peterson, "The Managed Care Backlash: Politics, Misperception, or Apropos?" *Journal of Health Politics, Policy, and Law,*

1999, *24*, 873–876; J. K. Iglehart, "Changing Health Insurance Trends," *New England Journal of Medicine*, 2002, *347*, 956–962.

4. J. Maxwell and P. Temin, "Managed Competition Versus Industrial Purchasing of Health Care Among the Fortune 500," *Journal of Health Politics, Policy, and Law*, 2002, *27*, 5–30.

5. M. K. Perry, "Vertical Integration: Determinants and Effects," in R. Schmalensee and R. D. Willig, eds., *Handbook of Industrial Organization*, vol. 1 (Amsterdam: North-Holland, 1989).

6. P. Milgrom and J. Roberts, "An Economic Approach to Influence Costs in Organizations," *American Journal of Sociology*, 1988, *93*(Suppl.), S154–S179; D. S. Scharfstein and J. C. Stein, "The Dark Side of Internal Capital Markets: Divisional Rent-Seeking and Inefficient Investment," *Journal of Finance*, 2000, *55*, 2537–2564.

7. G. J. Stigler, "The Division of Labor Is Limited by the Extent of the Market," *Journal of Political Economy*, 1951, *59*, 185–193.

8. J. C. Robinson, *The Corporate Practice of Medicine: Competition and Innovation in Health Care* (Berkeley: University of California Press, 1999).

9. L. P. Casalino and others, "External Incentives, Information Technology, and Organized Processes of Care to Improve Health Care Quality for Patients with Chronic Diseases," *Journal of the American Medical Association*, 2003, *289*, 434–441.

10. C. Prendergast, "The Provision of Incentives in Firms," *Journal of Economic Literature*, 1999, *37*, 7–63; G. P. Baker, M. C. Jensen, and K. J. Murphy, "Compensation and Incentives: Practice vs. Theory," *Journal of Finance*, 1988, *43*, 593–616; E. P. Lazear, "Pay Equality and Industrial Politics," *Journal of Political Economy*, 1989, *97*, 561–580; D.E.M. Sappington, "Incentives in Principal-Agent Relationships," *Journal of Economic Perspectives*, 1991, *5*(2), 45–66.

11. J. P. Newhouse, "Reimbursing Health Plans and Health Providers: Efficiency in Production Versus Selection," *Journal of Economic Literature*, 1996, *34*, 1236–1263.

12. D. Emery, *Global Fees for Episodes of Care* (New York: McGraw-Hill, 1999).

13. R. P. Ellis and T. G. McGuire, "Supply-Side and Demand-Side Cost Sharing in Health Care," *Journal of Economic Perspectives*, 1983, *7*, 135–151; M. McClellan, "Hospital Reimbursement Incentives: An Empirical Analysis," *Journal of Economics and Management Strategy*, 1997, *6*, 91–128.

14. M. B. Rosenthal, R. G. Frank, J. L. Buchanan, and A. M. Epstein, "Transmission of Financial Incentives to Physicians by Intermediary Organizations in California," *Health Affairs*, 2002, *21*, 197–205.

15. J. C. Robinson, "Theory and Practice in the Design of Physician Payment Incentives," *Milbank Quarterly*, 2001, *79*, 81–96; J. C. Robinson, "Blended Payment Incentives in Physician Organizations Under Managed Care," *Journal of the American Medical Association*, 1999, *282*, 1258–1263.

16. J. C. Robinson and L. P. Casalino, "Reevaluation of Capitation Contracting in New York and California," *Health Affairs* (Web exclusive), 2001, W11–W19; J. C. Robinson, "Physician Organization in California: Crisis and Opportunity," *Health Affairs*, 2001, *20*(4), 81–96.

17. M. R. Gold and others, "Provider Organizations at Risk: A Profile of Major Risk-Bearing Intermediaries," *Health Affairs*, 2001, *20*, 175–185.

18. B. C. Strunk, P. B. Ginsburg, and J. R. Gabel, "Tracking Health Care Costs," *Health Affairs* (Web exclusive), 2001, W39–W50.

19. B. Holmstrom and J. Tirole, "Transfer Pricing and Organizational Form," *Journal of Law, Economics, and Organization*, 1991, *7*, 201–228.

20. H. Hansmann, *The Ownership of Enterprise* (Cambridge, Mass.: Harvard University Press, 1996).

CHAPTER ELEVEN

THE RELATIONSHIP BETWEEN PREPAID GROUP PRACTICE AND THE EMPLOYER COMMUNITY

Helen Darling

The relationship between prepaid group practice (PGP) and the employment-based insurance market has always been a symbiotic one, with each side affecting development of the other. By offering an alternative model for financing and delivering health services, PGPs have changed dramatically what employers thought possible in the purchase of health benefits for employees. At the same time, large employers have played a critical role in helping promote and shape prepaid group practices by forcing them to demonstrate the factors that made them different from the alternatives. Employers also played an important role by imposing needed market discipline and the "voice of the consumer" on PGPs, making them stronger and more responsive to the needs of their customers.

This chapter explores the relationship between large employers and prepaid group practice, drawing on a series of interviews conducted by the author with eight of the early visionary leaders in the field of employee health benefits. Since the mid-1980s, these individuals have been active in employee benefits purchasing for some of the nation's largest companies:

- Kathleen Angel, director of global benefits, Dell Inc., formerly director of benefits at Digital Equipment Corporation
- Bruce Bradley, director, health plan strategy and public policy, General Motors, formerly with GTE and the Rhode Island Group Health Association
- Tom Davies, consultant to Verizon Communications, formerly with GTE

- Robert Galvin, MD, director, corporate health care, General Electric
- Brian Marcotte, vice president of compensation and benefits, Honeywell, formerly with Marriott
- Patricia Nazemetz, vice president of human resources, Xerox Corporation
- David Scherb, vice president of compensation and benefits, PepsiCo, formerly with RJ Reynolds
- Bruce Taylor, director, employee benefit policy and plans, Verizon Communications, formerly with GTE

Drawing on the perspectives of the interviewees, as well as the author's own experience in health care purchasing, the chapter reviews the key factors that affect large employers' decisions about health benefits. This is followed by a review of the relationship between PGPs and the large employer community from the early days of employer resistance to gradual acceptance and promotion of PGPs. The chapter then explores the critical role that large employers have played in strengthening the call for health care quality and value—while also promoting the PGP model—through the development of the National Committee for Quality Assurance (NCQA), the Healthplan Employer Data and Information Set (HEDIS), and other quality initiatives. Following that is a review of the work of the Washington Business Group on Health (now the National Business Group on Health) in defining and promoting "organized systems of care." The chapter concludes with observations from various employer and purchaser leaders about the future of prepaid group practice in today's markets.

Factors Affecting Employers' Health Benefit Decisions

To understand the long and still evolving relationship between large employers and PGPs, it is helpful to understand the key qualities that corporate benefits managers look for in a health care partner. Four major concerns shape employers' thinking about the health benefits they provide to their employees. First, they want benefits that are attractive to employees and competitive in their labor market and their industry. Most human resource professionals view themselves as advocates for employees, and although they clearly work for management, they put a high priority on taking good care of employees and helping them understand and use their benefits. Second, employers are concerned about costs, particularly in times of rapid cost increases. Third, employers are concerned about the related issue of the value they receive for their health care investment. Fourth, employers want administrative simplicity, which may include the ability to offer the same benefits at all employee locations.

The relative magnitude of these concerns has varied over time. Worries about the competitiveness of benefits arise when labor markets are tight. Odin Anderson and his colleagues reported that part of the motivation to offer and support prepaid group practice during the model's early days in Minnesota's Twin Cities derived from employers' desires to expand benefits for competitive reasons.[1] However, these employers preferred to offer an organized system of care to ensure attention to affordability.

Employers' concerns about costs and the related issue of value surface when health benefit costs grow rapidly, as in the mid-1980s to mid-1990s and in the early 2000s. Much of the early PGP movement was accelerated by employers' worries about value. They saw that prepaid group practices' premiums tended to be lower than costs would be for similar benefits in the fee-for-service system, at least for those who used average amounts of care.

One additional characteristic of prepaid group practices made them attractive to employers: their capacity to conduct research and to evaluate their own programs (see Chapter Eight). Prepaid group practices were, and continue to be, at the forefront of health services research, providing themselves (and others) with an opportunity to improve care. Many HMOs contain research and evaluation units. In several of the larger Kaiser Permanente regions, the health services research centers are considered major research organizations in their own right and are well known in the field.

The downside of this, though, is that in the early years of their research programs, prepaid group practices were sometimes hurt by their willingness to have an analytical mirror held up to their performance. There were almost no other comparable data or research from other health care organizations. As a result, it was common for studies to be reported in ways that made PGPs appear less than perfect. For example, a typical newspaper headline might read, "Only 80 percent of patients are satisfied with managed care," but the article rarely, if ever, mentioned that no comparable data existed on the fee-for-service world. In fact, where comparable data did exist, the results usually indicated that fee-for-service systems performed no better, and often worse, especially in terms of preventive services and effectiveness of care.

Employers' Wary Courtship of PGPs

Before 1980, prepaid group practices were exotic organizations that existed in relatively few markets. According to Alain Enthoven, in 1978 there were about 130 PGPs with a total of 6.4 million members, 3.5 million of whom belonged to

Kaiser Permanente.[2] With the notable exceptions of Boston and the Twin Cities, PGPs were mainly a West Coast or Midwest phenomenon. They flourished in areas with high growth and net immigration of people without existing links to physicians.[3]

Initial Suspicion and Resistance

Few employers were introduced to PGPs before 1973, when a growing number of new, federally qualified health maintenance organizations (HMOs) forced some employers to offer their plans under the 1973 HMO Act's "dual choice" mandate. The mandate required that an HMO be offered alongside an indemnity plan if one were available and requested to be offered. These HMOs included both classic PGPs and the more loosely organized independent practice associations (IPAs). Not surprisingly, this mandate did not endear the HMOs to employers.

Kathleen Angel, from Digital Equipment Corporation and Dell Inc., noted that HMOs were initially seen as "the noncompany plan," forced on them by the law's mandate.[4] Because the mandate forced employers to offer plans that were unique to specific markets, thereby obstructing efforts to achieve national uniformity, many employers' initial reactions to PGPs were those of suspicion or outright dislike. Although the HMO Act stipulated that employers could not financially discriminate against HMOs, they could set the employees' contributions for such plans at a slightly higher level because of the greater benefits, thus making them less attractive to employees. For example, when Xerox started its new health plan, composed of 122 HMOs, in 1990, actuaries estimated that the value of the HMO was 17 percent greater than that of the indemnity plan.[5]

By the early 1980s, most of the largest and most sophisticated purchasers were well aware that the health care system—actually, a "nonsystem"—had many flaws, including a dysfunctional payment system that rewarded providers for taking care of people when they were sick or injured but not for preventing illness or injury. Those who studied the system lamented its many failures and pointed out the costly consequences of the lack of continuity of care and comprehensive medical records.[6] A handful of employers, including those located in areas with strong prepaid group practices, also knew that there were examples of health plans that worked reasonably well and seemed to embody a set of ideals that had great appeal. Nonetheless, the conventional wisdom among benefits professionals was that HMOs were problematic, ironically, because they provided more benefits (including the wellness care and preventive care screenings that were not covered under indemnity plans). Put another way, employee benefits managers understood that they were paying a premium for visits and other wellness care that would not have been covered in the companywide indemnity plan.

Benefits managers were also wary of HMOs because they believed that such plans would unbalance the company's risk pool by attracting healthy employees and young families. The employer would still be paying most of the actual medical claims costs for the slightly older and slightly higher users of medical services because, it was believed, older employees would have ongoing relationships with doctors they preferred and would therefore not opt for the closed-panel prepaid group practice. The concern was that increased costs in the company's traditional plan, due to the PGP's "skimming" of the risk pool, would offset any savings due to medical management within the PGP itself.[7]

In addition, prepaid group practices offered community-rated, insured premiums, another source of anxiety for many employers, who felt they could not control what went into those rates. Employers also knew that insured premiums had to include costs for state-mandated benefits and state taxes, from which employers' self-funded plans were exempt, thanks to the federal Employee Retirement Income Security Act (ERISA) of 1974.[8] As a result, employers feared not only that PGPs might cause costs to increase in the company self-funded plan but also that PGP premiums contained costs that the employer previously did not have to pay. Many employers believed that because of these factors, PGPs would increase their overall health benefits costs.

Even employers who liked prepaid group practices may have been hesitant to offer them in the face of suspected total higher costs. David Scherb, vice president of compensation and benefits at PepsiCo and formerly at RJ Reynolds, reported that it took seven years for the cost savings related to the offering of a PGP to match what the company would have spent under the traditional plan.[9]

The Beginnings of Acceptance

As the percentage of annual health care cost increases hit the high teens, employers knew that something had to give, and prepaid group practices demonstrated that they could manage care for quality and cost effectiveness. Employers came to understand how good systems of care management could actually moderate cost increases, increase value, and provide higher quality. Companies such as Digital were committed to quality as one of their core business objectives, and it was central to their culture. They also understood the importance and power of systems and accountability. It is no accident that many of the visionary leaders in the field of employer health benefits came from industries devoted to Total Quality Management, Continuous Quality Improvement, and later, Six Sigma. Looking to integrated delivery systems was a natural leap for such companies.

Kathleen Angel noted a major shift in the way employers thought about PGPs and the roles such plans could play in changing the delivery systems. "Employee benefits managers could see that they could have direct dialogues with people who deliver care—those in charge of processes of care—and they could talk about their expectations for quality for their employees. This was a great opportunity to improve care and outcomes for our employees and their families while increasing value for a company that cared a lot about quality."[10] Virtually all of those interviewed for this chapter became directly involved in encouraging improvements in quality and in changing practices through the encouragement of standardized metrics.

Bruce Bradley of General Motors and formerly of GTE described what some employers saw in prepaid group practice plans:

> They are in many ways optimal models. They have the infrastructure for accountability and performance management. The model enables leaders to lead. With capitation there is even greater alignment. It encourages primary prevention and secondary prevention. You've got systems that allow you to hold people accountable. In the early days, when hospital days were very high, the gap between what was needed for good care and what was being provided allowed health plans to provide a lot of extra outpatient visits and still save a lot of money. That huge gap has eroded as other kinds of health plans used utilization management to reduce costs and unnecessary hospitalizations. Care can also be coordinated and population- or community-based. For those that are not for profit, they are fiduciaries for the community.[11]

Large employers such as GM and GTE clearly played a critical role in the acceptance of prepaid group practice, but it is also important to note the role played by those other advocates for employee interests, labor unions. In some communities, labor unions helped create and maintain a prepaid group practice on behalf of their members. For example, the Rhode Island Group Health Association was an important achievement of the unions in the Providence area. In Seattle, local industrial unions were instrumental in creating Group Health Cooperative of Puget Sound, and longshoremen's locals played a key role in the early success of Kaiser Permanente in the San Francisco Bay Area and Los Angeles. In other instances, unions were interested only in fee-for-service, comprehensive, "first and last dollar" coverage.

Employers' Role in Promoting Health Care Quality

In addition to their part in opening the employee market to PGPs, large employers also played another critical role: that of focusing health care purchasers' attention on quality of care. This included a key role in developing the tools and metrics that would allow PGPs and other delivery systems to demonstrate their value in ways that had previously been impossible.

Kathleen Angel of Digital and her employer and purchaser colleagues in the Northeast, including Xerox's Patricia Nazemetz, worked with the prepaid group practices and other local HMOs to develop sophisticated performance standards in the area of behavioral health. That a company would spend such significant time on an activity unrelated to its core business was unusual, and it was an indication of the exciting possibilities in partnering for quality improvement that emerged in that era.

Digital was able to take a leadership role in this area because it had a significant employee population in New England where some of the best PGPs, including Harvard Community Health Plan and Fallon Community Health Plan, were flourishing. Digital's leaders were able to meet with PGPs' managers and physician-leaders, develop common measurements, set standards, and work as teams. From the PGPs' perspective, the employers' active role helped organize and give clout to the "voice of the customer," something that PGPs had to learn to do but that did not come naturally or quickly.

From her post at Xerox, Nazemetz helped lead a nationwide movement for health plan quality, external accreditation, and accountability to the employer community. She served on the board of the independent, standard-setting National Committee for Quality Assurance from its earliest days and from almost the beginning announced that all plans that would be offered to Xerox employees had to be accredited by NCQA.

Xerox also encouraged its health care strategist to work with a wide variety of stakeholders (GE, GTE, Digital Equipment Corporation, the HMO Group, Kaiser Permanente, Harvard Community Health Plan, Aetna/US Health Care, and CIGNA, among others) to develop and test the Healthplan Employer Data and Information System, the groundbreaking health care quality measurement system that has become the standard in the managed care industry.

The HEDIS measurement system was initially administered by the HMO Group (an alliance of PGPs) under the direction of consultant Howard Veit of Towers Perrin, formerly head of the first federal HMO agency and a specialist in building HMOs. Working with the employers just mentioned, the HMO Group then transferred responsibility for HEDIS to NCQA, under the strong leadership of Peggy O'Kane.

O'Kane established a committee, chaired by Dr. Don Nielsen of Kaiser Permanente and staffed by Janet Corrigan of the Institute of Medicine, to test the new quality measures. For the next six years, NCQA oversaw the evolution of HEDIS under the auspices of a committee cochaired by Dr. George Isham, medical director of HealthPartners, and Helen Darling, at the time a health care strategist at Xerox. Prepaid group practices like HealthPartners and Kaiser Permanente were essential to the success of HEDIS, partly because they performed much of the research and testing of measures and partly because they made such a high-level commitment to the evolution of HEDIS.

With HEDIS housed at NCQA, it became possible to link quality measurement to external accreditation and to create quality-related report cards. These activities helped PGPs and other health plans prepare for a growing level of public scrutiny as millions of Americans moved into so-called managed care plans in the 1990s. Over the years, it has been demonstrated that plans that voluntarily collect and report data to HEDIS not only perform at a higher level than those that do not, but they also continuously improve.[12]

Another important quality and efficiency improvement tool used by large employers was benchmark pricing. Xerox was one of the first very large companies to focus its entire health care strategy on offering competing health plans in every possible market, using benchmark pricing to encourage plans to compete on quality, service, and innovation and to give employees direct financial incentives to select the most efficient plan. The concept was that employer contributions would be set against the benchmark plan to provide an incentive for employees to select it and to reward the plan's best practices by driving market share to it. Xerox's allowance for health care benefits was so generous that until it was eroded by inflation, an employee who chose the benchmark plan could either apply extra money to other benefits or take the balance of the funds in taxable cash. By allowing employees to keep the savings from choosing a more efficient plan, this type of contribution strategy went a long way toward promoting the take-up of PGPs, which were almost always the benchmark plan.

Other employers, including GTE, based their contributions on the costs of the most efficient HMO, using both cost and quality data. The concept of benchmark pricing, discussed at great length over the years by Enthoven,[13] became an important model, and savvy employers hoped to have a high-quality prepaid group practice in every possible market to serve as the benchmark against which the performance of other plans would be judged for quality of care, customer service, innovation, and cost management.

Collective Action: WBGH and Organized Systems of Care

While individual large employers had a profound impact on the development of prepaid group practice, employers acting *collectively* also played a key role in helping articulate—for policymakers, providers, and other stakeholders—the key characteristics of accountable, high-quality health care, providing a framework against which PGPs could demonstrate their value.

In 1991, the Washington Business Group on Health (WBGH), a coalition of large health care–purchasing organizations in the Washington, D.C., area, formed the Committee on Organized Systems of Care. Under the leadership of Digital's Kathleen Angel, the committee spent more than two years defining the attributes of organized systems of care for use as benchmarks. The resulting model was based on what the committee members considered the best prepaid group practices. They defined an organized system of care as "a health care system that both finances and delivers care and is held clinically and fiscally accountable for the outcomes and health status of the enrolled population."[14]

In 1993, the committee finished its work and released several key documents, which concluded that the four critical concepts that distinguish organized systems of care from other health service delivery models are *accountability*, which requires uniform and standardized data for comparison; *integration of care* along a continuum; *patient-centeredness;* and *continuous improvement.*[15]

In addition, organized systems of care would exhibit the following paradigm shifts from the old patterns to the new ones:

- *From fragmentation to integration.* The creation of information systems would allow for integration of care across providers, settings, and previously isolated delivery system elements. Organized systems of care would therefore ensure continuity of care through the shared electronic medical record.

- *From passive participation to active participation.* Patients would have information to make informed choices about their care. Providers would actively use information to facilitate patient-centered, outcomes-focused care. Purchasers would participate in developing consumer information about health plans, providers, and treatments. (For example, the Pacific Business Group on Health, a California coalition of large health care purchasers, was a leader in advancing quality, service, and innovations among health plans through the development of consumer-oriented, online quality information.)

- *From paying for services to buying value.* The availability of comparative quality and cost information would lead to value-based health care purchasing. Health care organizations would compete on quality, innovation, service, and price and be held accountable for continuously improving population health. Purchasers would be able to document what they were getting for their money.

- *From shifting responsibility to taking responsibility.* Incorporation of continuous quality improvements would encourage providers and purchasers to take responsibility for health care programs and their outcomes. Consumers would, over time, take greater responsibility for their own health.

- *From a focus on sickness to a focus on health.* The focus on keeping people healthy would result in long-term partnerships that place high priority on preventing illness as well as treating it. Partners would recognize that health is a dynamic state and that all individuals, regardless of age or physical or mental capacity, are able to improve their health outcomes, even when suffering from a serious acute or chronic condition.

For simplicity, the characteristics of organized systems of care were grouped into three broad organizational functions:

• *Care management.* Care management referred to the processes used to influence the cost and quality of health care delivered to plan members. This characteristic has also become a very important part of the guiding principles for improving quality and patient safety issued by the Institute of Medicine in its recent reports *To Err Is Human* and *Crossing the Quality Chasm.*[16]

• *Operations management.* The efficient management of organized delivery system operations requires an integrated approach to functions such as provider credentialing, purchaser contract management, enrollment, patient satisfaction monitoring, clinical management, quality improvement, cost accounting, and other financial monitoring. Specifically, the organized delivery system uses medical records, cost and financial data, and enrollment and eligibility data to drive the coordination of care, set goals, measure outcomes, and monitor performance.

• *Performance management.* Finally, performance management refers to the processes by which organized systems of care demonstrate accountability for improving health plan operations and the health status of the enrolled populations. Continuous improvement is the key concept guiding performance management activities.

Although an "organized system of care" is not exactly the same as a prepaid group practice (the former could exist without prepayment and with multiple medical groups and networks of physicians), committee members had prepaid group practice in mind when they wrote the report. Without PGPs, they could not have imagined such systems.

For the WBGH committee, the *ideal* model would in fact include prepayment to ensure that incentives were aligned in the optimal way. As Brian Marcotte of Honeywell noted, "Many employers felt that if you could get providers to assume risk, such as through global capitation, and thus [get them] involved in managing risk through preventing or avoiding disease disability . . . , costs would be saved and quality improved."[17]

Prepayment was also important to the committee members because they believed that such a payment mechanism would encourage providers to act in cost-effective ways, including investments in technology and training. (Kaiser Permanente's visionary commitment to a multibillion-dollar investment in twenty-first century information technology, for example, is the type of investment that would not occur without prepayment, or capitation, and without the right leadership.)

In a very expansive model, the WBGH committee expected that organized systems of care would provide (or oversee the provision of) the full continuum of care, from birth to long-term care, at delivery sites that ranged from the technically complex to an individual's home. The committee also envisioned that consumer and population health data would be used by practitioners to support clinical decision making, by consumers to make health care choices, and by delivery organizations to evaluate results and modify protocols to improve the health of members.

In 1993, in a complete report of its work, the committee observed that health plans with characteristics of organized systems of care were beginning to emerge.[18] As they developed and evolved, the committee hoped to "distinguish health plan rhetoric from evidence of outcomes-focused quality care and improved health status."[19] The committee likely would be pleased to see the progress being made at PGPs around the nation in the years since the report's publication, including at Kaiser Permanente's Care Management Institute, at HealthPartners and the Institute for Care Systems Improvement in Minnesota, and at InterMountain Health Plan, to name only a few (see Chapter Two).

Most of the large employers interviewed for this chapter felt that only PGPs came close to the ideals identified by the WBGH committee. In fact, when employers identify examples of care excellence and efforts to improve care processes, the list is always composed mainly of the well-known group practices, particularly the integrated delivery systems. One might even argue that in the employer community, there is an unfortunate tendency to take PGPs for granted. Yet when employers look at the overall system of health care and seek to make significant improvements in quality and patient safety, they can see how large the gaps are and how hard it is to effect substantial change without effective systems and infrastructure. Their conclusion is likely to be that they must work to preserve and grow the integrated delivery systems that exist. It is also important to find ways to emulate as much of the integrated system features as possible in areas or circumstances where such systems are unlikely to develop or offer no offsetting economies to support the additional investments.

Conclusion: Despite Limitations, Employers Still Need PGPs

If the leaders of many of the nation's largest companies have learned to value PGPs as an important option for their employees, why is the model not more widespread? In Chapter Ten, James Robinson proposes an answer from the perspective of economic theory. But what do the large-employer supporters of the PGP model believe? General Electric's Bob Galvin, a physician viewed throughout the country as a leader in the area of health care quality and performance, summarized what most interviewees were saying in one way or another: "We all admired PGP models, which are operated with the best of intentions and with shared values that all support, but there are well-known natural limits to PGPs' spread. Capital requirements to start them are virtually prohibitive today."[20]

Capturing some of the complex feelings of admiration and concern that many purchasers have about PGPs, Galvin went on to say:

> The best prepaid group practices, for example, Kaiser Permanente and Harvard Community Health Plan, make a *great* story but also a sad story. They set the benchmark for how health care ought to be organized for quality and efficiency. In some ways, they are akin to major technological breakthroughs. They have incentives appropriately aligned, and doctors really do run the show. I can't say enough good things about that and how they use evidence-based guidelines with physicians calling the shots. This is something that far too many people don't understand. They have the right medical values, and they have the systems and infrastructure to manage quality. The sad thing is that except for a handful around the country, their real impact on the entire delivery system is mostly west of the Rockies.

PepsiCo's David Scherb, a major supporter of PGPs, echoed some of Galvin's sentiments:

> Most employees want broader access to care. Not being able to go to specialists when they want is a problem for many people. Also, the PGPs have a limited radius, which is a problem for employers with people all over the United States. Moreover, when the IPAs came along, there wasn't clear evidence that they had any of the cost and quality benefits of the PGPs. Their failures diluted the "brand" so well established by Kaiser Permanente. Many of the advantages of PGPs—including over-the-shoulder peer review and office or group economies of scale—were not applicable [to the IPAs]. The consumerism movement is partly about not wanting limits. Finally, large employers are still afraid of and do not trust what would happen to them in fully insured products.[21]

Brian Marcotte of Honeywell believes that perhaps the most important lesson learned by employers from the existence of prepaid group practice was that there were—and are—promising alternatives to the fee-for-service system. Said Marcotte:

> [The] fee-for-service cottage industry known as the health care system was not the only way that health care could be delivered. . . . An organized system of

care offered an alternative for better care for all. It could also be more cost-effective. The existence of the PGPs influenced the creation of the hybrids. There were imperfections, and the hybrids struggled to incorporate the best aspects of PGPs. But there were many things that Kaiser did well. Its systems, as seen in Oakland, demonstrated substantial efficiencies in the delivery model, including the use of physicians and nurses as appropriate. The best managed care organizations were those most like PGPs in their processes of care and systems.[22]

Despite the continuing enthusiasm for the PGP model, even the strongest supporters believe that they must address the issues that have stunted their growth if they are to become more than niche providers, at least outside California. Virtually all of the interviewees, all of whom are admirers of some important aspects of the model, reported that their employees "never embraced HMOs." On the other hand, employers also reported that their employees always wanted to have at least one HMO choice among the company's offerings. This is likely due to the fact that the HMOs have provided richer benefits than employees' other choices. Alternatively, employees' insistence on maintaining an HMO choice may reflect the value that American consumers place on choice in general, as well as their willingness to accept economizing behavior in the provision of their health care if they have freely chosen such behavior in exchange for lower premiums.

Clearly, the integrated delivery system and PGP models have many virtues. They offer an effective method for addressing many of the major cost and quality problems that America faces in its flawed and very expensive health care delivery system. Prepaid group practices are at their best when they leverage their system features, use their resources to maximize the benefits of their information infrastructure, develop and teach evidence-based clinical practice guidelines, and attract the best physician leadership. PGPs are functioning models for what many believe is the ideal approach for care delivery in the United States today. Perhaps the newer challenges, including ever more need for technology assessment and the impact of genomic testing and treatment, will prove once again that the models based on systems of care, organized for quality and effectiveness, are the best approach for many people. But in the best American way, as we learn over and over, people will be most satisfied when they come to that decision on their own, with the information, choice of care systems or plans, and financial incentives to choose a high-quality delivery system.

In a health care world increasingly driven by consumers, prepaid group practices will have a new opportunity to recruit members. PGPs have distinct advantages, but they will need to sell them to a public with high expectations, voracious appetites, and little inclination to pay for their wants.

Notes

1. O. W. Anderson and others, *HMO Development: Patterns and Prospects,* CHAS Research Series, Publication no. 33 (Chicago: Center for Health Administration Studies, University of Chicago, 1984).
2. A. C. Enthoven, *Health Plan: The Practical Solution to the Soaring Cost of Medical Care* (Reading, Mass.: Addison-Wesley, 1980).
3. L. D. Brown, *Politics and Health Care Organization: HMOs as Federal Policy* (Washington, D.C.: Brookings Institution, 1983).
4. Kathleen Angel, personal communication, Sept. 19, 2002.
5. Author's recollection, based on her tenure as a health care strategist at Xerox.
6. Enthoven, *Health Plan.*
7. David Scherb, personal communication, Sept. 23, 2002.
8. F. J. Bitzer and N. W. Ferrigno, *ERISA Facts* (Cincinnati: National Underwriter Company, 2000).
9. Scherb, personal communication, Sept. 23, 2002.
10. Angel, personal communication, Sept. 19, 2002.
11. Bruce Bradley, personal communication, Sept. 27, 2002.
12. National Committee for Quality Assurance, *The State of Managed Care Quality,* 5th ed. (Washington, D.C.: National Committee for Quality Assurance, 2001) [http://www.ncqa.org/somc2001/intro/somc_2001_about.htm].
13. Enthoven, *Health Plan.*
14. V. Goff and S. Coberly, *Health Care Delivery System Reform: Distinguishing Organized Systems of Care* (Washington, D.C.: Washington Business Group on Health, 1995), p. 2; see also C. Cronin and K. Milgate, *A Vision of the Future Health Care Delivery System: Organized Systems of Care* (Washington, D.C.: Washington Business Group on Health, 1993).
15. Cronin and Milgate, *Vision of the Future Health Care Delivery System.*
16. Institute of Medicine, *To Err Is Human: Building a Safer Health System* (Washington, D.C.: National Academy Press, 2000); Institute of Medicine, *Crossing the Quality Chasm: A New Health System for the 21st Century* (Washington, D.C.: National Academy Press, 2001).
17. Brian Marcotte, personal communication, Oct. 9, 2002.
18. Cronin and Milgate, *Vision of the Future Health Care Delivery System.*
19. Goff and Coberly, *Health Care Delivery System Reform,* p. 2.
20. Bob Galvin, personal communication, Oct. 3, 2002.
21. Scherb, personal communication, Sept. 23, 2002.
22. Marcotte, personal communication, Oct. 9, 2002.

CHAPTER TWELVE

OPEN THE MARKETS AND LEVEL
THE PLAYING FIELD

Alain C. Enthoven

This chapter is addressed to readers who believe that prepaid group practice (PGP) and similar, efficient, selective health care delivery systems ought to be allowed to compete on a level playing field to provide value for money. It explains how to open the markets to create that level playing field. The chapter first examines some of the key barriers to PGP growth and development and suggests alternative policies that provide both private and government purchasers of health care with expanded choice in the marketplace and provide consumers with economic incentives to select cost-efficient systems of care. The chapter then examines how barriers such as adverse selection, market-distorting state regulatory policies, and lack of objective consumer information on quality of care can be addressed by various stakeholders to help level the playing field. It concludes with a look at how multispecialty group practices could evolve into successful PGPs in a competitive environment in which the efficiency and quality advantages of prepayment and clinical cooperation and collaboration are encouraged and rewarded.

The "Choice" Problem and the "Exchange" Solution

Few people realize how unfavorable today's market conditions are for the development and growth of *any* selective delivery system that offers efficiency or cost management.[1] Marketing a prepaid group practice is very different from marketing a service directly to consumers, such as a retirement plan or brokerage account. The employment-based health insurance market has two tiers: the employer and the employee. The first challenge is to overcome employers' preference to offer only one or a small number of insurance carriers and the resulting lack of employee choice of delivery system. Most employers and insurers are oriented to the "single source" model. In 1997, only 23 percent of insured employees were offered a choice of carrier.[2] Even a policy of offering a choice of two or three may not make this market easy for a newcomer to penetrate. This is a major barrier to PGP entry and growth.

Under the present market structure, in which each employment group acts on its own, offering a choice of carriers can create costly administrative burdens for the employer. Many large employers are spread out over several geographical locations, sometimes with comparatively few employees at each site. Offering multiple choices of carriers at many locations with fewer than two hundred to three hundred employees can be complex. However, the substantial number of employers that do offer multiple choices suggests that the costs of doing so are not necessarily overwhelming.[3]

Employers are not alone in their preference for a single source. Many insurers also avoid multiple-choice situations unless required to participate in them by large employers or large pools of small employers. They view choice as involving higher administrative costs, the risk of adverse selection, and, particularly, competition, which they prefer to avoid. They offer employers lower premiums if they can cover the whole group, an offer that appears attractive in the short run but may lead to higher premiums in the long run. The adjustment of premiums to mitigate adverse selection has been demonstrated in some cases, but it has only recently come into practical application (we will return to this topic later in the chapter).

Marketing health insurance coverage to the employer market is a costly activity, especially for small or new organizations. To make a sale, a carrier must make presentations to the company's decision makers, negotiate and sign a contract, and work with the employer in the member enrollment process. Even then, most employees are satisfied with their current doctors and do not want to switch to a PGP that requires them to change providers. Also, the limited location of PGP clinics may not be convenient for many employees, especially when the group is small. Many employees prefer the broad provider choice to which they are accustomed. With luck, a new PGP might enroll 10 percent of a small group in the first year, and it may take two to four years of operations to recover the entry costs.[4]

This "choice problem" makes the PGP a poor candidate for the single-source strategy. For an employer to replace entirely a traditional insurance plan with a PGP, employees would have to give up the doctors they know and like. For this reason, the Permanente Medical Groups from the very beginning advocated for a "dual choice" requirement (usually Kaiser Permanente and a traditional carrier), because the physicians understood that it would be difficult to form a good and trusting doctor-patient relationship with patients who were not free to choose them.[5] Indeed, research shows that employees' satisfaction with their health insurance is strongly correlated with whether they had alternatives to limited-choice managed care organizations, including choice of a plan that provides wide access to doctors.[6]

For PGPs to reach the employer group market, employers must be willing to offer multiple carriers and, in the case of new PGPs, be willing to incur added administrative expense for what might be just a few employees at the outset. This is most likely to happen among large employment groups or large pools of small groups that are able to spread administrative costs.

The most promising way of facilitating multiple choice of carrier in the small to mid-size group market is by creating large-scale "exchanges" that include several or many employers in a market area. An exchange is an institution that brings together multiple insurers and multiple employment groups for the purpose of providing choice among carriers for individual employees. The exchange sets the common business rules (such as risk adjustment methodology, benefit design standards, and conflict resolution methods), manages the presentation to employees and the enrollment transactions, offers employees a convenient way to make side-by-side comparisons and to make and execute annual enrollment decisions, and consolidates billing and reconciliation of payments.

Exchanges also can help mitigate the adverse selection problems inherent in small groups by use of risk adjustment tools (to be discussed shortly). An exchange may pool risks by having common premiums for everyone, or it may use group-specific rates whereby each group pays its own costs. It is important to recognize that exchanges need not mean that groups subsidize each other.

Perhaps the largest and best-known exchange is the California Public Employees' Retirement System (CalPERS), which arranges coverage for more than 1.3 million public employees, retirees, and dependents of almost 2,400 different employers, including many state, county, and municipal government agencies. Other examples of exchanges include the public employee insurance programs in several other states, including Washington, Massachusetts, and Wisconsin; broker-sponsored exchanges such as California Choice; and PacAdvantage (formerly the Health Insurance Plan of California), which was created by the state to serve small employers and is now being operated by the Pacific Business Group on Health, an employer coalition.

A new twist on the concept is being pioneered in Seattle as BENU, a joint venture of a PGP-type health maintenance organization (HMO), Group Health

Cooperative, and CIGNA, a traditional carrier that offers multiple benefit packages. BENU offers employers the administrative simplicity of a single-source carrier with the advantage of multiple plan designs (HMO, preferred provider organization, and point-of-service). Payments to Group Health Cooperative and CIGNA are risk-adjusted. Exchanges such as these offer an effective way to promote the development of PGPs and other selective, economical delivery systems.

The concept of delivery system choice was originally built into the HMO Act of 1973, which was intended to help the spread of HMOs, including both pre-paid group practices and independent practice associations. This law required that employers subject to the Fair Labor Standards Act include at least one HMO among their offerings to employees if an HMO was available and asked to be offered. Although subsequent experience demonstrated that requiring choice of carrier was feasible, the provision was nonetheless repealed in the 1980s when it was incorrectly believed that HMOs were well established and no longer needed assistance.

While it lasted, the so-called HMO mandate helped legitimize the concept of choice and establish the viability of PGPs. However, large exchanges covering many employers and offering at least several carriers would nevertheless make it much easier for new selective delivery systems to enter the market and grow than is the case if the new entrant has to make a separate sale and contract with each employment group.

Misdirected Incentives

For many employees who are offered a prepaid group practice, the advantage of lower premiums outweighs the perceived disadvantage of limited choice of providers—*if* they are allowed to pocket the savings. Unfortunately, fewer than 20 percent of employees who are offered a choice of carrier can keep the savings if they make an economical choice.[7] Many employers that offer choice contribute to the plan of the employee's choice a uniform high percentage of the premium, usually in the range of 80 to 100 percent.[8] A smaller share of employers who offer choice of carrier require employees to contribute the same fixed-dollar amount toward the premium, regardless of the cost of their choice of carrier.[9]

In either contribution model, there is little or no incentive for making an economical choice. If the employer pays 80 percent of the premium, no matter the cost, the employee only keeps 20 percent of the possible savings from choosing an economical plan. In the case of the employer that pays 100 percent of the premium or that requires the employee to pay the same fixed amount regardless of choice of plan, the employee receives no financial reward for choosing the least costly alternative. Not only does the employee have no incentive for choosing the lower-premium plan, but the plans themselves have little or no incentive to keep their premiums low, as long as they are below the higher-priced fee-for-service alternative.

In the early days of traditional indemnity insurance, employers mostly offered a single health insurance plan and paid a high percentage of the premium in order to take maximum advantage of the tax exclusion for employer-paid health benefits. Even those who did offer choice resisted converting to fixed-dollar contributions because it would mean either taking money away from employees or giving money away. That is, if the contribution amount were set at the price of the low-priced plan, employees who had previously chosen the high-priced plans would suffer a "takeaway" and have a cause of dissatisfaction. If the employer set the contribution amount above the lowest-priced plan and let employees who chose that plan keep the difference, the employer would be "giving away" money it did not previously have to pay to employees who had previously chosen the low-priced plan. If the employer set the contribution at the average premium, some employees would suffer takeaways while others would benefit from a windfall. To mitigate these problems, the change to defined contributions needs to be phased in over several years or managed with flexible benefits plans.

Other factors affecting employer contribution approaches include organized labor's determination to have the employer pay the entire premium, even though the "employer contribution" comes out of employees' wages. In addition, some types of firms, such as management consulting or law firms, do not want their employees to be concerned about health insurance costs at all, so they cover the entire premium. Thus most large employers systematically pay more on behalf of employees who choose the more costly health insurance plans, thereby undermining the incentives for employees to choose economical plans and for plans to be cost-efficient and affordable.

As noted, the misdirection of the incentives in employer contributions originated in the federal tax code, which made the full employer contribution tax-free to the employee. However, with the enactment of Section 125 of the Internal Revenue Code authorizing flexible benefit plans, employees can ask their employer to pay their own premium contributions out of pretax dollars and thus reduce taxable salary by an equivalent amount. So the fixed-dollar contribution approach no longer needs to mean sacrificing a tax advantage for employees.

These historical factors affecting employer contributions have meant that employees' desire for virtually unlimited choice of doctors at all times has been free of most overt costs (not counting possible lost wages). But would employees demand such "choice" if *they* had to pay for it instead of the employer? Experience among beneficiaries of CalPERS, Stanford University, and other large groups with wide choice *and* fixed-dollar contributions suggests that when it comes to actually paying out of pocket for premium differences, many employees choose the less costly HMO and accept the restrictions on choice of providers that go with it. The policy of a fixed-dollar contribution tied to the low-cost plan (usually an HMO) gives the employee a *reason* to accept the economizing behavior of his or her health plan because it is saving the employee money.

If we combine the 23 percent of employees who have a choice of carrier with the fewer than 20 percent of employees of choice-offering employers who receive fixed-dollar contributions, we see that less than 5 percent of the insured workforce can both choose a health plan and reap the full savings from choosing economically. Only 9.6 percent of Fortune 500 companies offer such a choice to most of their employees.[10]

Creating a Market Hospitable to Economical Systems

If we want to use consumer power to incent greater cost efficiency in health care, we must let the employee who chooses an economical health plan reap the savings. The best level to set the fixed-dollar contribution, or "earmark," is near (at or below) the premium of the low-priced plan. If the amount exceeds the price of the low-priced carrier, the employee should be allowed to apply the difference to some other benefit or receive it in cash. Setting the earmark below the low-priced plan can work too, as long as it isn't so low that it induces healthier employees to drop out, resulting in adverse selection.[11]

Earmarking an amount equal to the premium of the low-priced plan not only rewards employees for their economical choice but also puts economic pressure on the higher-priced carriers to bring their prices down. It fully protects the employee from hardship because he or she can always choose the free alternative. And it ensures that all employees will be covered at least by the low-priced plan. Employers worried about competition for labor can always use their premium savings to pay more in cash wages and let the employees tax-shelter their premium contributions.

Another approach some employers have taken to leveling the playing field is to adjust the cost sharing or other aspects of the plan design so that the premium of the fee-for-service plan equals that of the PGP, then pay 100 percent of the premium of either plan but let the PGP compete by offering more comprehensive benefits. This approach should be accompanied by risk adjustment (to be discussed shortly) to mitigate the adverse selection that may result from offering a more comprehensive benefits package alongside one that is less so.

As for correcting the inflationary bias in the tax code, the simplest approach would be to limit the amount of employer contribution that is tax-free to employees.[12] A more fundamental reform would be to replace the tax exclusion with a "refundable" tax credit, usable only for the purchase of health insurance, that would be the same across all income classes. This would provide the greatest incentive to purchase health insurance to people who need the incentive most, those with low incomes, rather than favoring people in the higher marginal tax brackets, as current policy does.[13]

Promoting Efficient Systems in Medicare

The foregoing has described how both public and private employers can make their markets more hospitable to efficient competing health care systems. The Medicare "market" of Americans aged sixty-five and older also has a very important role to play.

When Medicare was enacted in 1965, it was based on traditional fee-for-service payment for doctors and cost reimbursement for hospitals. Shocked by the rapid growth in Medicare outlays, Congress began looking to PGPs in the 1970s as a way to offer favorable incentives for cost management (see Chapter Four). Beginning in 1972, Congress began to experiment with ways to accommodate PGPs on a per capita prepayment basis.[14] But a simple idea in principle turned into an extremely complex issue in practice. The first payment formula, which tied PGP payments to the costs of the traditional fee-for-service program, was unattractive to PGPs, and only one plan contracted to participate. In 1982, the conditions of participation were made less onerous, and more PGPs participated on a per capita prepayment basis. However, critics feared that PGPs were attracting the healthiest segments of the market and thus costing the government money.[15] For this reason, Congress tried to pay PGPs and other HMOs 95 percent of the traditional Medicare premium. In the Balanced Budget Act (BBA) of 1997, Congress reduced payments for fee-for-service providers, which had the effect of reducing payments for HMOs also.

In 1997, Congress also enacted the Medicare+Choice program in the hope of letting beneficiaries receive more value by choosing an economical private plan. Medicare+Choice greatly expanded the number of allowable "managed care" options beyond what had previously been available under the older Medicare Risk program. It changed the reimbursement formula to phase in a base level of capitation and to incorporate a blend of national and local costs. This law also provided for eventual risk adjustment of premium payments. But contrary to intentions, HMOs have been exiting Medicare+Choice since the BBA was passed, complaining that reimbursements are too low.

Whatever the problems with Medicare+Choice, the growth in outlays for fee-for-service Medicare is unsustainable. As Stanford economist Victor Fuchs has written recently, "If health care expenditures for the elderly [continue to] grow 2 to 3 percent per annum more rapidly than expenditures on other goods and services, the burden on the young is likely to be unbearable."[16] He points out that by 2020, health spending by or on behalf of the elderly (including Medicare) will, on average, exceed their spending on all other goods and services. Moreover, 62 percent of the elderly's "full incomes" (personal income plus medical spending by others on their behalf) will be paid by people under sixty-five, compared to 56 percent in 1997.

Since the alternative approach of squeezing Medicare payments to doctors and hospitals has probably reached its limits, what is needed today is a strategy that reduces people's need for medical services through preventive care and leads to innovation in less costly care processes. Prepaid group practices have shown that they can achieve both these goals and compete successfully in a market that features cost-conscious beneficiary choice among competing, standardized benefit packages, with adequate, risk-adjusted premium support payments from either employers or the government, as in Medicare.

The difficulties in moving from the traditional fee-for-service Medicare program to the "managed competition" model are extremely complex and beyond the scope of this chapter.[17] A major question is, on what basis should the government pay private health plans to care for Medicare beneficiaries? There are three leading ideas.

First, the government would contribute, on behalf of each prepaid beneficiary, the same amount it pays on behalf of fee-for-service beneficiaries, fully adjusted for health history and status. This is sometimes called "premium equivalency." This method would level the playing field, but it would leave the government's outlays tied to the inflationary fee-for-service program and thus do little to relieve the long-term fiscal burden.

A second approach, sometimes referred to as "defined contribution," would have the government select an average per capita amount in the current fee-for-service Medicare program and then pay that amount to a health plan as a "defined contribution" on behalf of each beneficiary, with the payment adjusted for local factor costs (similar to the Medicare prospective payment system for hospitals), as well as beneficiary demographics and health status. The government could then budget for annual increases. All beneficiaries, including those in fee-for-service Medicare, would pay the difference between the defined contribution amount and the cost of the health plan of their choice. This would make government outlays controllable and predictable, but it could leave some beneficiaries unprotected from very high out-of-pocket premium costs, especially in high-medical-cost areas and in areas lacking in competition. This would leave open the important question of what happens to the beneficiaries' entitlement to the traditional fee-for-service program.

A third approach, sometimes called "competitive bidding," would invite health plans to enter a premium quote for one or two standardized benefit packages in the markets in which they wished to participate and then for the government to contribute a fixed-dollar amount tied to the median or weighted-average bid. Beneficiaries would keep all or most of the savings if they chose a less costly plan. (In a similar example, Stanford University and the University of California tie the employer contribution to the lowest-priced plan.) In this case, taxpayers would benefit from the efficiencies created by competition. A problem with this approach is that many rural beneficiaries would not have access to the low-priced HMOs, which are concentrated in urban areas. This approach would also leave open the difficult question of what to do about entitlement to the existing fee-for-service program.

Other complex design issues involved in moving to managed competition include defining geographical areas for pricing, subsidies to low-income people, the appropriate number of benefit packages to offer, remedies for areas in which there is little or no competition, and how much of the savings from economical choices should go to the beneficiaries.

It appears increasingly likely that one way or another, the federal government is going to have to sever its financial commitment to traditional fee-for-service Medicare and instead make premium support payments that help beneficiaries join one or another competitive health insurance and delivery organization. One way this might happen would be for the government to adopt a competitive-bidding approach, with beneficiaries initially entitled to stay with fee-for-service Medicare on current terms and to phase in gradually (perhaps over a ten-year period) beneficiary responsibility for the difference between the cost of fee-for-service Medicare (for those who choose to stay with it) and the government's premium support contribution. Another way would be for the government to adopt a competitive-bidding approach for the coverage of all beneficiaries reaching Medicare eligibility after a certain future date. This would avoid forcing current beneficiaries to change programs.

Mitigating Adverse Selection

One concern about any model of choice of carrier is that some carriers are likely to attract worse health risks than others and be harmed financially by a spiral of adverse selection. This is a real and important problem, although so far it has not hindered the success of the very large competition models, such as the Federal

Employees' Health Benefits Plan or CalPERS. But as the market becomes more competitive, it is important to find ways to ensure that premiums received by carriers and prices paid by consumers are adjusted to reflect the true health risks of members enrolled in different plans. Some insurers will not participate in certain markets without such a protection or will charge a higher premium to guard against unfavorable selection. In any competition between PGPs and wider access plans, the latter may attract a worse mix of risks because people with chronic conditions have strong attachments to their own doctors and do not want to change to a limited-choice plan. Alternatively, PGPs may attract high-risk populations with chronic conditions because of their superior ability to manage chronic diseases and their lower out-of-pocket payments.

Adverse selection can be addressed in several ways. One method is a statistical and medical-econometric process known as risk adjustment. Risk adjustment begins with risk assessment, a scientific process of estimating the relative predicted costs of different individuals and groups based on variables such as age, sex, location, institutional status, and health status as determined by diagnoses obtained or inferred from prior reports of inpatient and outpatient encounters and drug prescriptions. In risk adjustment, the sponsor (Medicare, the employer, or an exchange) adjusts the premium payments received by carriers to compensate for positive or negative risk selection. For example, starting in 2004, Medicare will use a diagnosis-based risk adjustment system that draws on both inpatient and outpatient data.[18]

Risk adjustment is now catching on in the private sector, too. Models using prescription drug data have been shown to have good predictive power for costs of diagnostic groups, such as diabetics.[19] The University of California has been using such a model for several years. In 2002, Wells Fargo Bank, a leader in the implementation of managed competition, adopted a similar prescription drug model, as did Verizon Communications in 2003.

However, risk adjustment remains a work in progress, and much of the progress is due to the growing availability of computerized patient data, including electronic records for prescription drugs. As risk adjustment becomes more widespread, health plans will become more aggressive in recording diagnoses to improve their risk "scores." This may require ongoing audits to detect fraudulent coding and recalibrating models to reflect higher levels of legitimately coded illness.

Risk adjustment of premiums received by carriers and prices paid by consumers is important for a number of reasons. First, as noted earlier, some insurers will not participate without it, fearing adverse selection. Second, good risk adjustment gives a purchaser's benefits program a reputation for fairness and stability. Third, if a provider organization develops a reputation for excellence in care of costly chronic conditions, without proper compensation, it risks being damaged economically by adverse selection. This would create a disincentive for providers to develop such a reputation, perhaps by not recruiting medical personnel who would merit it.

In addition to risk adjustment, there are other ways to mitigate adverse selection, including a member enrollment process through a neutral exchange so that carriers cannot deal directly with potential members during enrollment. This is typical in most employment settings where choices are offered and also in some Medicaid programs but not in Medicare. Another approach is benefit design to prevent contracts that select for or against different risks. Finally, there are various forms of reinsurance to compensate carriers after the fact for high-cost cases.

Maintaining Comparable Benefits

PGPs generally offer comprehensive coverage and low cost sharing by patients at the point of service. The reason for the former is so that the PGP can manage total resources for the best health outcome and greatest efficiency and because all covered services are complementary parts of the same process of medical care. The reason for the low copayments is to avoid serious financial barriers to the patient seeking care. Patients are encouraged to come in early and have their symptoms checked so that any potential illness can be treated sooner and at less cost.[20] This aspect takes on greater importance with the growing incidence of chronic conditions.

However, the health care market today is moving away from comprehensive coverage to so-called consumer-directed health plans, which typically feature lower premiums and high deductibles (such as $1,500 per person per year), appealing to young and healthy employees. (In fact, most health care spending is on people whose annual expenses far exceed $1,500, so simply adding a deductible will not change the incentives bearing on most of the spending.)[21]

To survive in an annual side-by-side competition with such a plan, a PGP would have to require a similar deductible or risk adverse selection because the absence of a deductible would appeal mainly to less healthy workers. The danger in this trend is that unless preventive medicine and disease management programs are exempt from the deductible, a great deal of the management of chronic conditions might be lost, as many patients would choose not to pay the out-of-pocket costs for the visits and tests that go into managing chronic diseases. Furthermore, high deductibles are likely to create a serious barrier to care for low-income people. One way or another, if access to needed care is to be preserved, employers will have to require that all competing plans offer roughly equivalent benefits.

Regulatory Barriers and Self-Funded Plans

PGPs face another set of barriers to fair competition in the state regulatory arena, in which employer self-funded plans are exempt from many of the burdens of regulation, benefit mandates, and taxes that are imposed on regulated insurers.

HMOs, including PGPs, come in for a particularly heavy burden of state rules and regulations over business practices such as product design, enrollment, advertising, pricing, and scores of other activities. In California, the main HMO regulatory law, the Knox-Keene Health Care Services Delivery Act of 1975, now runs to hundreds of pages of fine print. In addition, states have passed hundreds of "benefit mandates"—requirements that regulated insurers, especially HMOs, must cover specific health care benefits or the services of specific types of providers. Often these mandates are legislative responses to the demands of narrow-interest provider and consumer constituencies, such as disease-specific advocacy groups or nurses associations, for instance. The mandates allow legislators to accede to the demands of the more vocal and powerful groups without having to vote for the taxes to pay for them. Often these benefits are not what the employment groups that purchase health insurance would choose to buy on their own (if they were, there would be no need for the mandates).

A General Accounting Office study reported that claims for mandated benefits came to 12 percent of all claims in Virginia, 22 percent in Maryland, and 5 percent in Iowa.[22] The weight of this regulatory burden is compounded by the fact that it is not evenly applied. According to the terms of the Employee Retirement Income Security Act of 1974 (ERISA), states may not regulate employer self-funded health benefit plans, in which an employer bears the risk and pays for services out of its own funds. Not surprisingly, most large employers choose to self-fund their insurance plans, thereby controlling their own cash flow and avoiding the common 2 percent premium taxes charged in most states, as well as the unfunded benefit mandates.

If state governments want prepaid group practices to prosper, they need to avoid costly regulations that burden PGPs but not their competitors. They need to do their part to "level the playing field." One possibility would be for the federal government to grant an ERISA-like preemption for insurance sold through broadly available exchanges or to create an economical national standard regulatory structure for all tax-favored health insurance.

Objective Consumer Information

Reliable, objective information on plans' clinical quality and consumer satisfaction would go a long way toward promoting the growth of PGPs, which often excel on quality scorecards such as the Healthplan Employer Data and Information Set (HEDIS). Without such information, consumers have little objective basis for choosing a PGP, and those who turn to their personal, non-PGP physician for advice are apt to run into a wall of hostility based on organized medicine's traditional opposition to any form of economic competition or corporate organization among doctors.[23] Instead, to make intelligent choices, consumers need a neutral, trusted source of information on health care performance and patient satisfaction, such as California's Pacific Business Group on Health and CalPERS.[24] The states of New York, New Jersey, Pennsylvania, and California have published risk-adjusted mortality studies for open-heart surgery and put them on the Internet.[25] The National Committee for Quality Assurance (NCQA), a nonprofit entity sponsored by employers and health plans, is developing and collecting a set of performance indicators on such measures as frequency of performance of recommended preventive services (for example, immunizations, cancer screening, and retinopathy exams) and follow-up care. Because of the way they are organized, PGPs tend to perform well on such indicators. Unfortunately, the performance of the unorganized fee-for-service sector is usually not subjected to the same measurements, so comparisons are not often available.

Starting Prepaid Group Practices

Beyond helping create the appropriate market conditions, as just described, what can business, labor, consumer, government, and civic leaders do to encourage prepaid group practice? First, these groups can study the issues closely enough to be able to participate in and evaluate planning efforts. Second, through memberships on boards of hospitals and other institutions, they can reach out to doctors who are leaders and work with them to start the multispecialty group practices that are at the heart of PGPs. Third, they can provide moral support, especially with the medical community, for the principles of appropriate economic incentives and for participation in organized quality improvement efforts. Fourth, working with corporate boards and foundations, these groups can help direct financial support to PGP start-ups. Fifth, they can supply business contacts and expertise. Sixth, insurance companies can offer to team up with multispecialty group practices to create joint venture "private label" products (in other words, insurance products that are specific to the medical groups). Seventh, purchasers can encourage or require insurers to include group practices as a delivery system option under terms that allow the PGPs to market their superior efficiency. And eighth, all players can provide political support and advocacy for such changes with state and local governments.

Growing New PGPs

Even in an environment with a level playing field and with community support for PGPs, the start-up process is challenging at best. Strong physician leadership is a crucial factor (see Chapter Nine), as is adequate financing and the development of strong multispecialty medical groups that can respond to market forces to improve collective performance, not merely collections of independent doctors sharing the same quarters. An environment in which the PGP concept is a familiar one might also seem important, except that historically some of the strongest PGPs came into existence through "greenfield starts" in locations without a PGP predecessor. Examples include the following:

- The original West Coast locations of Kaiser Permanente—Northern and Southern California; Portland, Oregon; and Hawaii—that were developed alongside the industrial enterprises of Henry J. Kaiser[26]
- Kaiser Permanente–sponsored expansion programs in Georgia, Colorado, Texas (with Prudential), and North Carolina
- Group Health Cooperative of Puget Sound in Seattle and Spokane, with labor and consumer sponsorship
- Prudential Insurance Company prepaid group practices created in Dallas (with Kaiser Permanente), Atlanta, Oklahoma City, Tulsa, Orlando, and Austin
- Harvard Community Health Plan in Boston, sponsored by Harvard Medical School
- Georgetown University Community Health Plan in Washington, D.C., sponsored by Georgetown University Medical Center, and now a part of Kaiser Permanente

Although the development of the organizational culture needed for success takes time and cannot be short-circuited, the histories of Harvard Community Health Plan and Georgetown University Community Health Plan suggest that a great deal can be accomplished in a mere decade. However, even with a great improvement in market conditions, greenfield starts are unlikely in the foreseeable future.

Estimating the start-up cost of a PGP is complex because it depends so much on market and other local conditions. If conditions are bad enough, no amount of money is enough to launch a successful PGP, as Kaiser Permanente's unsuccessful experiences in North Carolina and Texas have illustrated.[27] A few case histories of successful start-ups provide some perspective.

Harvard Community Health Plan started in 1969 with grants from the U.S. Public Health Service and the Commonwealth Fund, plus concessionary loans from Harvard University. Through 1976, the plan received about $4.8 million in start-up aid. In 2001 prices, updating with the Medical Consumer Price Index, the total would be $36 million; using the more moderate Consumer Price Index, the total would be $20 million in today's dollars. (The choice of index is not obvious; either one is flawed when used for this purpose.) Harvard Community Health Plan had the important advantages of affiliation with Harvard Medical School and its teaching hospitals, brand-name recognition, and providers who were willing to work with them on improving quality and reducing cost.

Kaiser Permanente lacked these advantages in North Carolina and Texas; in both cases, there was no affiliation with a prestigious local institution, and community physicians were unwilling to make price concessions. In contrast, Kaiser Permanente entered Georgia in 1984 and achieved profitability in 1991. But the cumulative investment in donations and loans by the end of 1991 was $112 million, which, inflated to 2001 prices, as before, would have been about $150 million to $190 million—an amount that requires a very long-range commitment on the part of the sponsor. Part of the reason for the high cost of market entry was that Kaiser Permanente had to overcome unfavorable market conditions in Georgia, including the lack of large public sector agencies that offer plan choices and fixed-dollar contributions, as in other Kaiser Permanente regions. Furthermore, the organization's largest private sector customer in Georgia currently contributes only about 6,200 members.[28] In addition, Kaiser did not have local name recognition or the sponsorship of a local provider organization. The start-up costs could have been less if market conditions had been more favorable.

The figures just given can be compared with other potential sources of funding. For example, the 2001 edition of the *Foundation Directory* reports that the top ten thousand foundations in the United States, in fiscal years ending in 1999 or 2000, had $403.7 billion in assets and gave away $21.1 billion annually.[29] Of course, most of these foundations are committed to a wide range of social benefit programs and would not easily divert large sums to starting PGPs. But foundations that include health care in their programs give more than $1 billion annually. Moreover, a foundation would not need to give the total start-up funding to a PGP in its first year. It could combine grants and loans and spread them out over several years. However, given the high costs, foundation support for PGP start-ups is not likely to be significant, although private corporate foundations might be persuaded to aid start-ups in areas that serve their employees.

In *Crossing the Quality Chasm*, the Institute of Medicine recommends that the federal government create a $1 billion fund for innovation.[30] Starting new PGPs would be a reasonable use of some of that money. This amount could accomplish a great deal, despite the fact that it is minuscule in comparison with the hundreds of billions of dollars that government spends on health care each year.[31]

A repetition of the HMO Act of 1973, with its substantial grants and loans to non-profit group practice HMOs, would certainly be helpful, but it is politically unlikely, at least until Congress is jolted into action by another doubling of health insurance premiums.

Medical-Group-Led Start-Ups

The second route for development of PGPs has been from the evolution of multispecialty group practice medical groups from fee-for-service to prepayment. Examples include the Ochsner Health Plan in New Orleans; the Fallon Community Health Plan in central Massachusetts; the Health Alliance Plan in Michigan, based on the Henry Ford Health System; the Geisinger Health Plan, based on the Geisinger Clinic in rural Pennsylvania; and the Scott and White Health Plan, based on the Scott and White Clinic in Temple, Texas.

According to the American Medical Group Association, there are now about 1,363 medical group practices in the United States with twenty or more physicians.[32] This number includes many independent practice associations and single-specialty clinics. Roughly one thousand of these are multispecialty group practices capable of evolving into PGPs. These groups operate in forty states. In addition, at least six academic health center faculties have become multispecialty group practices (in other words, they have a governance structure enabling them to function as a group), and more could make this transition. With the benefit of appropriate market conditions, many of these organizations could evolve into strong PGPs. These groups offer the most promising route to a reformed delivery system.

For a multispecialty group practice, the evolution from operating mainly under fee-for-service to prepayment might begin with the group's taking capitation for professional services for some of its patients. This change would simplify relationships with insurers; allow rational personnel substitution, such as delegating some visits to physician extenders without insurer issues; and allow cost reduction and other process improvements that in the fee-for-service world would result in financial penalties for producing fewer patient visits. It would also fit with the Institute of Medicine's notion of continuous healing relationships, as opposed to patient visits, which the *Crossing the Quality Chasm* report characterizes as a feature of twenty-first century health care.

In the next step, the medical group begins to share risk for institutional services, such as hospitalization, so that it can be rewarded for its ability to keep patients out of the hospital through better ambulatory care and disease management. Following that, the group would begin to assume greater risk for services (with or without reinsurance) to capture the savings inherent in its more economical mode of practice.

Finally, the evolving prepaid medical group enters a joint venture with a health insurer by developing an insurance product that markets the medical group's services exclusively, with a shared commitment to expand that program. This means that the group faces the marketplace directly, with its own premium, so that its efficiency can be fully rewarded by lower premiums and more patients or, alternatively, by a greater net income needed to finance expansion and improvements.

Conclusion

In the reformed market proposed in the beginning of this chapter, powerful forces would emerge to support the formation and growth of prepaid group practices. First, per capita prepayment would come to predominate because it facilitates more economical care patterns and does not contain the inflationary incentives of fee-for-service medicine. Capitation is a cohesive force because the revenue comes to the *group*, not to individual providers. Second, the costs of care for chronic conditions are rapidly coming to dominate the total costs of care. Per capita prepayment facilitates and rewards chronic disease management, whereas fee-for-service is oriented toward acute and episodic care. Third, information technology is increasingly essential to the practice of quality medicine. Clinical information technology supports use of a shared electronic medical record, which will facilitate accurate risk adjustment, improve the value of disease management, enable the practice of evidence-based medicine, and promote data analysis and feedback to enable doctors to monitor their own performance in comparison with that of their colleagues. But information technology is expensive, and its development will depend on large medical groups capable of generating and retaining capital, either on their own or in association with an insurance partner. Finally, high-quality twenty-first-century medicine of the kind recommended in the *Crossing the Quality Chasm* report requires teamwork, coordination, and collaboration to a degree that may only be possible within the culture and infrastructure of a large group practice. When all these factors are present, PGPs will acquire the enhanced brand-name recognition that attracts new patients. All this, of course, presupposes a reform of basic market conditions that would result in an open market and a level playing field for all competitors.

Notes

1. J. Maxwell and P. Temin, "Managed Competition Versus Industrial Purchasing of Health Care Among the Fortune 500," *Journal of Health Politics, Policy, and Law,* 2002, *27,* 5–30; A. C. Enthoven, "The Fortune 500 Model for Health Care: Is Now the Time to Change?" *Journal of Health Politics, Policy, and Law,* 2002, *27,* 37–48.

2. M. S. Marquis and S. H. Long, "Trends in Managed Care and Managed Competition, 1993–1997," *Health Affairs,* 1999, *18,* 75–88. Note that this refers to two or more separate insurance carriers, not two or more choices of plan design from the same carrier. This latter kind of choice does not help the PGP seeking market entry, and it generally does not foster competition among delivery systems. Maxwell and Temin, in "Managed Competition Versus Industrial Purchasing," find that among Fortune 500 companies, 65.9 percent of employees are offered a choice of two or more carriers, but smaller firms are much less likely to offer choices of carrier.

3. For example, Wells Fargo Bank, operating in many separate locations, offers a choice of as many as five carriers.

4. Raymond Fong of Kaiser Permanente, personal communication, Aug. 9, 2002.

5. A. R. Somers, *The Kaiser Permanente Medical Care Program: A Symposium* (New York: Commonwealth Fund, 1971).

6. K. Davis, K. S. Collins, C. Schoen, and C. Morris, "Choice Matters: Enrollees' Views of Their Health Plans," *Health Affairs,* 1995, *14,* 99–112; A. A. Gawande and others, "Does Dissatisfaction with Health Plans Stem from Having No Choices?" *Health Affairs,* 1998, *17,* 184–194; A. C. Enthoven, H. H. Schauffler, and S. McMenamin, "Consumer Choice and the Managed Care Backlash," *American Journal of Law and Medicine,* 2001, *27,* 1–15.

7. Marquis and Long, in "Trends in Managed Care," found that about 25 percent of employees of choice-offering employers were offered a fixed-dollar contribution; Susan Marquis, personal communication, Aug. 21, 2002. The Kaiser Family Foundation and Health Research and Educational Trust's *Employer Health Benefits, 2002* (Menlo Park, Calif.: Kaiser Family Foundation and Health Research and Educational Trust, 2002) reports that the percentage of employees of choice-offering employers who are also offered a fixed-dollar premium contribution regardless of the plan chosen has declined from 28 percent in 1999 to 17 percent in 2002.

8. Kaiser Family Foundation, *Health Benefits, 2002.*

9. Ibid.

10. Maxwell and Temin, "Trends in Managed Care."

11. J. R. Gabel, J. D. Pickreign, H. H. Whitmore, and C. Schoen, "Embraceable You: How Employers Influence Health Plan Enrollment," *Health Affairs,* 2001, *20,* 196–208.

12. Health care costs vary geographically, so the need for equity would suggest limits adjusted for costs in each local area. Medicare makes such adjustments for hospital payments.

13. A. C. Enthoven, "A New Proposal to Reform the Tax Treatment of Health Insurance," *Health Affairs,* 1984, *3,* 21–39.

14. Public Law 92-603, 92nd Congress, Oct. 30, 1972. "The Social Security Amendments of 1972," Sec. 226, "Payments to Health Maintenance Organizations," created Sec. 1876 of the Social Security Act.

15. General Accounting Office, "Medicare+Choice Payments Exceed Cost of Fee-for-Service Benefits, Adding Billions to Spending," press release, Aug. 2000.

16. V. R. Fuchs, "The Financial Problems of the Elderly: A Holistic Approach," National Bureau of Economic Research Working Paper no. 8236, Apr. 2001 [http://www.nber.org/papers/w8236].

17. For a review, see R. A. Berenson and B. E. Dowd, "The Future of Private Plan Contracting in Medicare," AARP Public Policy Institute, 2002 [http://www.aarp.org/ppi]. For an explanation of managed competition, see A. C. Enthoven, "History and Principles of Managed Competition," *Health Affairs,* 1993, *12*(Suppl.), 25–48.

18. This will be a refinement of the Hierarchical Condition Category (HCC) model based on "selective significant conditions . . . of approximately 61 disease groups." See J. Boulanger, "Memorandum to Medicare+Choice Organizations and Participants in Covered Demonstration Projects," Department of Health and Human Services, Mar. 29, 2002. See also the DxCG, Inc., Web site [http://www.dxcg.com].

19. A. S. Ash and S. Byrne-Logan, "How Well Do Models Work? Predicting Health Care Costs," paper presented to the Section on Statistics in Epidemiology, American Statistical Association, at the Joint Statistical Meetings, Dallas, Aug. 1998.

20. P. Braveman and others, "Insurance-Related Differences in the Risk of Ruptured Appendix," *New England Journal of Medicine*, 1994, *331*, 44–49.

21. P. Fronstin, *Can "Consumerism" Slow the Rate of Health Benefit Cost Increases?* Employee Benefit Research Institute Issue Brief #247, Washington, D.C., July 2002.

22. General Accounting Office, "Medicare+Choice."

23. C. D. Weller, "'Free Choice' as a Restraint of Trade in American Health Care Delivery and Insurance," *Iowa Law Review*, 1984, *69*, 1351–1378 and 1382–1392; L. G. Goldberg and W. Greenberg, "The Emergence of Physician-Sponsored Health Insurance: A Historical Perspective," in W. Greenberg, ed., *Competition in the Health Care Sector: Past, Present and Future* (Germantown, Md.: Aspen Systems Corp., 1978).

24. See the Web site of the Pacific Business Group on Health [http://www.pbgh.org].

25. California [http://www.oshpd.cahwnet.gov]; New Jersey [http://www.state.nj.us/health/hcsa/cabgst.htm]; New York [http://www.health.state.ny.us/nysdoh/heart/1997-99cabg.pdf]; Pennsylvania [http://www.phc4.org/idb/Cabg/default.cfm].

26. Hendricks, R., *A Model for National Health Care: The History of Kaiser Permanente* (New Brunswick, N.J.: Rutgers University Press, 1993).

27. D. Gitterman, B. Weiner, M. Domino, A. McKethan, and A. Enthoven, "The Rise and Fall of a Kaiser Permanente Expansion Region," *Milbank Quarterly*, Vol. 81, No. 4 (Dec. 2003).

28. Data provided by Kaiser Permanente (Performance Analysis), June 2002.

29. D. G. Jacobs, ed., *The Foundation Directory* (New York: Foundation Center, 2001).

30. Institute of Medicine, *Crossing the Quality Chasm: A New Health System for the 21st Century* (Washington, D.C.: National Academy Press, 2001).

31. In fiscal year 2003, health care, including the tax breaks for insurance, public employees, Veterans Affairs, and the Department of Defense, will cost the federal budget more than $680 billion. See S. Woolhandler and D. U. Himmelstein, "Paying for National Health Insurance—and Not Getting It," *Health Affairs*, 2002, *21*, 88–98. This article includes an estimate that government of all levels in the United States pays for nearly 60 percent of health care.

32. Data provided by the Medical Group Management Association, SMG Marketing Group, American Medical Group Association, California Association of Physician Organizations, and Aventis Pharmaceuticals, 2001. Also see the American Medical Group Association Web site [http://www.amga.org].

EDITORS' INTRODUCTION TO THE EPILOGUE

When one is close to a work, it is hard to see what is missing. It was not until we had completed our review of this book that we realized we had missed a critical development that will have an enormous impact on health care in the twenty-first century: clinical information systems. Although many of the authors touched on this topic, noting that prepaid group practices (PGPs) are leaders in this technology, we felt it deserved a more focused discussion.

Both in theory and in practice, we see strong links between PGPs (and similar multispecialty group practices) and the use of clinical information systems. Prepaid group practices are experiencing the greatest successes in putting these systems into operation in ambulatory settings. Smaller practices have had more difficulty. Several questions need to be answered in order for solo or small group physician practices to implement these systems: Which doctors have a right or duty to share information with which other doctors? Will there be interoperability? How will capital be generated? Who will develop the guidelines promulgated through the use of this technology? Many of these difficult questions are more easily answered in PGPs than elsewhere. A book about PGPs' contributions to, and promise for, a twenty-first-century health system is therefore incomplete without a discussion of why this is so.

We asked George Halvorson, president and CEO of Kaiser Foundation Health Plan and Hospitals, to write this epilogue for a number of reasons. First, during his tenure as president and CEO of HealthPartners, he pioneered the use of clinical information technology, or what he calls "computerized caregiver support tools." Second, Halvorson has played a strong leadership role in the implementation of a comprehensive clinical information system at Kaiser Permanente. Finally, throughout his career, Halvorson has written and spoken about the crucial role of information technology in improving information for caregivers, removing waste and friction from the health care system, and reducing errors—all of which must happen to bring health care fully into the twenty-first century.

EPILOGUE: PREPAID GROUP PRACTICE AND COMPUTERIZED CAREGIVER SUPPORT TOOLS

George C. Halvorson

Many of America's health care costs, financial and otherwise, result from its current paper-based approach to maintaining patient records. This non-system often leads to inconsistencies in patient care (poor quality) and dysfunctional information transmission systems (inefficiencies). It is an outmoded, ineffective support system for caregivers. A fully computerized system, including patient-specific medical records, reminders, and treatment protocols, is needed to provide complete information about each patient to the caregiver in the exam room. That electronic tool is the missing link between current inconsistent care and best care. After years of experimentation and development, these tools are now ready for practical use by caregivers, and multispecialty group practices (including prepaid group practices) are the logical environment for the initial large-scale use of these approaches.

Poor Quality and Inconsistencies

Evidence compiled by researchers from several high-profile organizations—including the Institute of Medicine, the National Committee for Quality Assurance, RAND, and the Dartmouth Atlas Project—all points toward the fact that the actual delivery of health care in this country too often varies from science-based best practice.[1] Study after study of health care performance shows wide variations in both treatment approaches and care outcomes—with levels of performance inconsistency that would be unacceptable in any other area of the American economy.

A recent RAND study of more than twenty thousand patients in twelve metropolitan areas makes this point dramatically clear. Researchers found that only about half of those studied received recommended care.[2] Further, a National Roundtable on Health Care Quality convened by the Institute of Medicine published its report in the *Journal of the American Medical Association* with the conclusion: "Serious and widespread quality problems exist throughout American medicine. These problems, which may be classified as underuse, overuse, or misuse, occur in small and large communities alike, in all parts of the country, and with approximately equal frequency in managed care and fee-for-service systems of care. Very large numbers of Americans are harmed as a direct result."[3]

Some specific examples of variation from best practice include the following:

- Heart disease is America's number one killer (approximately one person dies each minute from a coronary event),[4] yet nearly half of America's heart attack patients do not receive the most effective follow-up care.[5]
- More than 6 percent of the American population has diabetes,[6] but fewer than half of America's diabetics receive the levels of care necessary to reduce or prevent complications.[7]
- High blood pressure (hypertension) is the most treatable cardiovascular disease; however, roughly 40 percent of America's hypertension patients do not receive the most current and appropriate levels of care, resulting in sixty-eight thousand premature deaths each year.[8]

Another sad fact for the current practice of medicine is that with rare exceptions, no one external to the caregiver or patient has an ongoing quantitative sense of whether or not the approaches used are effective or add optimal value for a given patient or for populations of similar patients. Unless care is so out of line as to constitute malpractice—an extremely rare event—there is almost no process in most settings for determining what is or is not working in any comparative sense for individuals or groups of patients or for any aggregation of caregivers.

In fact, using today's nonsystematic methods of communicating new medical science, it can take many years for a valuable new best practice to become the routine standard of care. As noted, the normal compliance level with best practice typically falls short for many important care approaches. No other industry or portion of the economy takes anywhere near this long to disseminate new approaches. Most industries retool yearly, if needed. Reengineering is a constant fact of life. Health care has been a glaring exception to that rule.

Inefficiencies: Dysfunctional Information Transmission

Quality deficiencies and inconsistencies are exacerbated by the fact that the non-computerized care improvement processes used by most providers and health plans rely on the distribution of paper-based patient status reports and information about best care. Attempting to distribute pieces of paper about these topics to each caregiver is at best inconsistent and at worst expensive, time-consuming, and frustrating. Care sites are typically unconnected, and passing on best-practice information at a one-on-one, doctor-to-doctor, teacher-to-caregiver level can be a logistical nightmare even in a group practice setting.

To make the situation even more problematic, with hard-to-access paper medical records, it is difficult to perform the large-scale, statistically valid research necessary to provide consistent and constant feedback on medical performance—either by procedure, technology, drug, disease, or caregiver. Health care does not have a functional rapid feedback loop. Most current medical research involves a laborious, manual data extraction process, in which skilled staff spend large amounts of time sorting through medical files to find and transcribe relevant information about various elements of care. It can take millions of dollars and several years to do a relatively simple study on the impact of a treatment approach. The resultant data generally provide a slightly outdated, historical, point-in-time research snapshot that must be laboriously reconstructed in later time periods to get any valid sense of comparative performance and outcomes over time.

Health care is an information-dependent profession that is operationally handicapped by a remarkably dysfunctional information transmission nonsystem. In an era when practically every other major segment of the economy relies on computers for data flow, decision support, and production improvement, health care still stores all-important patient-based data on inaccessible, incomplete, sometimes inaccurate, and frequently illegible paper files. Filing systems are almost always set up and segregated by individual care providers or treatment sites, not by individual patients. In this country, a patient who receives care from three separate doctors generally ends up with three separate paper folders, with different contents, located in three separate metal file boxes.

Dysfunctional information transmission means that neither physicians nor patients can benefit from the full spectrum of useful or timely data. Keeping up-to-date on current best practices is difficult. Doctors who want to keep up on medical research in their specialty are confronted by information overload; an estimated fifteen hundred medical articles are published *each day,* and there are about four thousand health-related journals to choose from.[9] It is simply beyond the ability of any single physician to keep up with all this information, let alone remember it when confronted with a patient for whom that information would be relevant.

As a result, when the typical solo-practice doctor enters an exam room to see a patient, she often has no systematic tools at hand to remind her of the patient's specific needs or the full scope of care most appropriate to the patient's particular diagnosis, condition, and treatment plan. The physician typically relies on her memory for large portions of each patient's current and future treatment regimen—including dosages of drugs and duration of therapies. The physician seldom, if ever, receives any systematic follow-up information about the patient or the patient's compliance with care. The patients themselves often leave the exam room trying hard to remember the four or five key points that the doctor told them about their follow-up care.

Further, the health care delivery system is reimbursed primarily through a paper-based process. This process involves the creation, mailing, and receipt of paper invoices, wasting considerable amounts of time and money. This payment system is also prone to mistakes; processing and coding errors are so common that a 2 percent error rate on claims payment by insurers and a 4 percent error rate on claims coding by providers are both considered to be exemplary performance. (A 4 percent error rate would be considered mediocre or poor performance in any other industry that values quality and reliability.) A well-designed and carefully implemented computerized medical information system could eliminate both paperwork and coding errors and create a computer-to-computer claims-filing process that cuts administrative expenses and eliminates almost all claims payment errors.

The Solution: Computerized Caregiver Support Tools

Anyone who looks closely at the inconsistency of health care practice must conclude that computerized caregiver support tools—including "electronic," "automated," or "computerized" medical or patient record systems and treatment protocols—are the best way of achieving optimal care for large numbers of patients. These tools can make best care easier and more likely to occur. This is not speculation. These tools now exist in their early stages in multiple settings. When well designed, such tools or systems include a comprehensive medical record for each patient and the most current information about best practices, both in an accessible electronic format available to the physician (and other caregivers) at the exact point and time of care.

Giving physicians, other health care practitioners, and researchers appropriate access to this information is the key to moving care delivery and quality to the next level of performance. Each physician should be able to quickly track the care given to each patient against the very best and most current protocols. This system should enable them to remember what tests need to be done, what drugs need to be prescribed, what follow-up care needs to be accomplished, and even when referral to specialty care is advisable. The data system also needs to be accessible to medical researchers so that they can tell, on an ongoing basis, which drugs are working, which procedures are creating value for the patient, and which technologies are leading to the very best improvements in patient outcomes.

Another critical function of a clinical information system is to generate complete and easy-to-use information for patients about their condition and their care. The information for each patient can be programmed to be culturally competent and multilingual, reducing the misunderstandings and miscommunications that now occur far too often in an increasingly diverse society. In the best situation, the system should also provide patients with direct, confidential access to their own medical history and information—along with patient-focused medical protocols and best practice information.

Benefits of Computerized Caregiver Support Tools

As several authors in this volume noted, new and more reliable computerized caregiver support tools (or clinical information systems) have the potential to achieve many of the ideal system qualities described in the Institute of Medicine's *Crossing the Quality Chasm* report. In a comprehensive analysis of the peer-reviewed literature, Raymond and Dold found strong evidence to support the notion that such systems do in fact improve safety, efficiency, timeliness, and quality.[10] They also found that these systems have potential for improving service and patient satisfaction through enhanced communication and information sharing.

In their review of nearly one hundred published studies spanning thirty years of research, Raymond and Dold document improvements in preventive health services, disease management, drug prescribing and administration, documentation of data, access to clinical information, and avoidance of medical errors—all resulting from the use of clinical information systems.[11] They found that computer reminders and practice protocols facilitate early disease intervention, with positive impacts on patient screening and immunizations,[12] particularly in cancer prevention.[13] Electronic order entry systems can support management of adverse drug interactions,[14] and computer reminders increase medication compliance.[15] Finally, use of clinical information systems has also improved management of diabetes,[16] hypertension,[17] asthma,[18] unstable angina,[19] mental health,[20] tuberculosis,[21] and HIV/AIDS.[22]

Clinical information systems also show promise for increasing administrative efficiency through improved work flow and time savings, streamlined information storage and access, and enhanced billing efficiency.[23] Use of electronic medical records saves resources, including physician and clerical staff time,[24] storage space,[25] and ultimately money.[26]

The federal government has recognized this value as well. The Health Insurance Portability and Accountability Act of 1996 (HIPAA) created standardized electronic claims formats to eliminate the need for translation between provider and payer claims-processing systems. Early adopters of these standards already report error reductions and cost savings—for example, from 1998 to 2000, Intermountain Health Care's Physician Practice Division used HIPAA standards to increase efficiency, saving $300,000 per year in claims staffing needs—despite a 10 percent annual increase in billing volume.[27] Many, however, are still struggling to meet these standards.

The successes have all resulted from at least a partial computerization of care: in each case, the computer was used to enhance a particular aspect of care delivery. But the impact of a complete care support tool has yet to be fully tested. There is every reason to believe that the more complete systems will achieve even more success than the partial systems tested to date.

The Role of PGPs in Advancing Clinical Information Systems

Even though the benefits of clinical information systems are real, implementation can be extremely difficult. Potential roadblocks include the enormous costs in time and money required to build and deploy a new system; integration of existing systems; some clinician resistance to change; lack of product standardization; and risk aversion on the part of management due to difficulty in measuring the benefits of clinical information technology.[28] These are all areas where prepaid, multispecialty group practices have an inherent advantage as early adopters of these caregiver support tools. Prepaid and large multispecialty group practices are in fact particularly well positioned to implement and benefit from clinical information systems, which enhance their integrated structure and draw on their group norm of teamwork. There are at least four reasons for this, discussed in turn.

Comprehensiveness of Care

In prepaid group practice, patients receive most or all of their care from or through the PGP, rather than through unrelated physician groups. Therefore, PGPs can assemble a complete record for each patient—and have been doing so with paper records for at least fifty years.

Culture

The team-based group culture and values of prepaid and large multispecialty group practices lend themselves to using information systems. Francis Crosson and his colleagues in Chapter Nine note that the core principle of group responsibility, embodied by most group practices, is a commitment to quality—including evidence-based best-practice protocols and monitoring and reporting of group performance. As the amount and complexity of clinical information increases, the ethic of an integrated, group practice–based health care delivery system fosters cooperation and support among physicians—enabling them to use guidelines for care rather than being individually responsible for keeping abreast of every new advance.[29] Expertise within large, diverse multispecialty group practices enables them to develop these guidelines internally so that the physicians who develop them also use them—greatly enhancing the credibility of these guidelines among the group's physicians.

Access to Capital

In addition to being culturally disposed toward the use of clinical information systems, provider groups must have access to significant capital to invest in such systems. As a result, some of the largest initial gains in developing and integrating clinical information systems have come from the largest multispecialty group practices, particularly those that have a close or exclusive relationship with a health plan. For example, HealthPartners, Group Health Cooperative, and Kaiser Permanente have all been leaders in implementing clinical information systems. The large size of these groups provides a stable revenue base to help offset the costs, and close relationships with health plans provide access to additional capital.

Partnership with a Health Plan

Whereas multispecialty group practices in general are well positioned to implement and benefit from clinical information systems, those that have an exclusive or near-exclusive contract with a single health plan may have additional advantages. As noted, a health plan can be an excellent source of capital for investing in clinical information systems. However, when multiple health plans contract with multiple provider groups, the benefits of a single health plan's investment in a provider group's infrastructure will accrue to the plan's competitors, who also contract with the same group. Although this is not an insurmountable obstacle, it is minimized when partnering with a single health plan. Furthermore, in the combined care and insurance model, organizations can fully integrate clinical and claims information to achieve maximum levels of patient-specific information.

Contrast the PGP advantages just described with a physician working in solo practice and contracting with several insurers. She must hire, train, and direct staff; manage cash and investments; and handle the functional and political logistics of being on the staff of one or more hospitals or professional organizations. She must also navigate among several reimbursement systems, multiple and ever-changing drug formularies, and various state and federal laws and regulations. Even if she lays out the capital investment for electronic medical records and computerized treatment information, she will still have access only to data about treatment that occurs while the patient is in her care, not while he is in the care of other providers. Her system will not necessarily "speak" to other providers' computer systems (if they exist).

PGPs' Use of Clinical Information Systems

Though most health care practitioners and institutions in the United States are not yet ready to implement clinical information systems, a few have positioned themselves as pioneers in their use.[30] In Chapter One, Shortell and Schmittdiel note the multibillion-dollar technology investments being made by Kaiser Permanente, the Mayo Clinic, Intermountain Health Care, the Henry Ford Health System, and Geisinger Clinic.[31] Berwick and Jain (Chapter Two) write about Group Health Cooperative's investment in improved information flow between patients and providers and how it led to better outcomes. Fink and Greenlick (Chapter Eight) also cite Group Health Cooperative's research, demonstrating the value of automated records in improving chronic care management, in particular, diabetes care.

Kaiser Permanente's own work with clinical information systems dates back over forty years. In 1961, Morris Collen, a founding partner of The Permanente Medical Group and the first director of the organization's research arm, piloted a computerized medical records system. This effort ultimately provided researchers with a vast database of member health conditions, which is still used by researchers today to study care delivery.[32] Dr. Collen also broke ground by developing and then studying the outcomes of the automated Multiphasic Health Test System, designed to provide efficient health screening.[33] (Fink and Greenlick discuss this system in more detail in Chapter Eight.) Collen, among the first to use computers in medicine and holding a firm belief in prevention, is widely considered a pioneer in the area of medical informatics—the use of information systems to identify and prevent future disease.

Though withdrawal of federal funding prevented the regionwide deployment of Collen's automated record system, Kaiser Permanente has continued to

innovate in the use of information technology to improve care.[34] Within the
organization, computer-based technologies have included an automated appointment booking and registration system (PARRS) piloted in 1977; a computerized hospital information system (ADT), in place by 1985; an outpatient
pharmacy dispensing and tracking system (PIMS) implemented in 1988; and
the Clinical Information Presentation System (CIPS), which began delivering real-
time, patient-specific, clinical information to physicians' desktops in 1993.

Clinical information systems such as these have helped change the course of
treatment not only at Kaiser Permanente but also at a number of other group
practices. For example, these tools can do the following:

- Support early interventions through the use of electronic medical records
  and by providing screening and vaccination reminders to providers and patients
- Aid in the management of chronic diseases through the use of disease registries
  (lists of all patients with a particular chronic condition within a health care
  organization or physician group)
- Replace handwritten prescriptions with computerized order entry, thereby
  reducing the likelihood of error
- Involve the patient as a more active partner in care provision
- Aid research[35]

Several health care systems have implemented various versions of electronic
medical records and clinical order entry systems. In 2002, the Palo Alto Medical
Foundation rolled out its electronic medical records system, giving doctors complete
medical histories of patients anywhere they have Internet access.[36] Geisinger Health
System in Pennsylvania is spending $50 million on implementation of an electronic
medical record, which allows patients to access medication information and lab results online, as well as schedule appointments and request prescription refills.[37] Partners Health Care System in Boston, which uses a similar system, has reported on the
benefits of electronic medical records in terms of both patient outcomes and cost
savings.[38] Park Nicollet Health Services, an integrated care system in Minneapolis,
announced in September 2003 that it will be implementing technology projects,
including electronic medical records and physician order entry.[39]

The U.S. Veterans Health Administration (VHA) has been a forerunner in
implementing a more fully integrated clinical information system. The VHA has
"one of the largest integrated health information systems in the United States . . .
serv[ing] 6 million enrollees . . . in 22 designated regions."[40] Since 1997, they have
used electronic medical records, automated order entry, clinical reminder systems,
and other technologies to improve quality and patient safety. The VHA's National
Surgical Quality Improvement Program used clinical information tools to develop

risk-adjusted surgical outcomes data, demonstrating a 27 percent decrease in thirty-day postoperative deaths from 1991 to 2000.[41]

Others groups have created integrated information systems to prevent chronic disease and manage population health. Group Health Cooperative in Seattle pioneered the Chronic Care Model, which uses disease registries, physician reminders, and feedback tools to help manage chronic illness.[42] Group Health has conducted a number of studies to measure diabetes outcomes using this model, finding a statistically significant increase in prevention, resulting in significant decreases in specialty and emergency care visits (translating into cost reductions).[43] A national program of The Robert Wood Johnson Foundation, Improving Chronic Illness Care (ICIC), grew from this model and has spread to many other organizations.[44] The Institute for Healthcare Improvement and ICIC developed a diabetes collaborative, which includes Premier Health Partners in Dayton, Ohio; Health-Partners Medical Group in Minneapolis; and Clinica Campesina in Denver—all of which have demonstrated notable improvements in diabetes care.[45]

Kaiser Permanente Northern California launched its own chronic care management program in 1999, targeting diabetes, coronary artery disease, hyperlipidemia, asthma, and congestive heart failure.[46] This program, using a computerized disease registry, electronic caregiver support tools, and automatic prompts, has improved early intervention in chronic diseases.[47] Aided by a computer program, clinicians can assess patient risk and track test results and medication use. Then an electronic tracking system is used to search the disease registry to identify and mail letters to patients who need to return to the clinic for further testing, medication management, or follow-up care. The registry is also used to generate "member summary sheets," which prompt the physician for needed tests and medication adjustments at the point of care. The registry also produces a "receipt" for the patient, listing tests taken and tests due. Due largely to the use of information system–supported approaches, heart disease is no longer the number one cause of death among Kaiser Permanente's members in Northern California—although it remains so for the California population at large.[48]

In another example of information technology–assisted chronic disease management, the Ohio Permanente Medical Group has seen a significant reduction in cardiac-related mortality and morbidity since it implemented an automated medical information system, including patient-specific physician reminders and physician-specific performance reports. As a result of these and other interventions (including a switch from balloon angioplasty to stents), the rate of cardiac-related deaths fell by 21 percent since 1994. In addition, since 1993, the rates of myocardial infarction and hospital admission for ischemic heart disease fell by 6.6 percent and 8.6 percent, respectively. All of this occurred despite an aging of the over-sixty-four population.

Fulfilling Morris Collen's vision of a truly automated medical record, Kaiser Permanente is currently investing nearly $3 billion over the next several years to build an integrated clinical information system for its more than eight million members nationwide. This system moves beyond electronic medical records and includes electronic documentation of patient visits, order entry for medications and procedures, and linking of inpatient and outpatient care. The organization estimates that when fully implemented, the new system will result in annual savings of approximately $500 million, due to cost avoidance, cost savings, and improved and more accurate reimbursement.[49]

Although only a small portion of the industry is currently on track to implement systemwide clinical information technology, a critical mass of multispecialty group practice users are choosing the same software vendor, including Kaiser Permanente, Cleveland Clinic, Sutter Health, University of California at Davis, and Palo Alto Medical Foundation.[50] These developments may lead to increased opportunities for interoperability among care systems. Under the auspices of the Council of Accountable Physician Practices, some of these group practices are beginning to meet with each other to standardize data flow and share learning.[51]

Conclusion

Just about every informed observer of the health care system now recognizes and deplores what the Institute of Medicine identified as a vast and dangerous inconsistency of care. We can reduce some of that inconsistency by making improvements in the context of our current medical processes and paper-based patient information systems. But we can't have highly reliable, up-to-date care and optimal value for the health care dollar until we have a complete electronic medical record for each patient and until we make usable, efficient clinical tools and information about each patient available to the physician at the exact point and time of care. Without such clinical information technology, the current cost burden will continue to grow, and vast numbers of patients will continue to receive inconsistent, often inadequate, and sometimes dangerous care.

Once best care has been demonstrated—through the use of computerized caregiver support tools by America's leading multispecialty and prepaid group practices—market competition will force the rest of American caregivers to follow (particularly if employers and government create appropriate market conditions, as explained by Alain Enthoven in Chapter Twelve). This will not happen until best care is thoroughly demonstrated, however. Because of their inherent advantages, prepaid group practices are natural laboratories for learning about the benefits and uses of these systems.

Reengineering of care support is an evolution, as opposed to a revolution. Once the benefits of clinical information systems become obvious to policymakers, purchasers, and the public, it is logical to expect that major segments of the health care delivery nonsystem will figure out how to work with payers or each other to create functional equivalents of the integrated approach. This should ultimately result in the building, in multiple settings, of virtually integrated groups and plans. Delivery systems with the size, scale, and incentives to overcome the barriers to technology adoption will likely emerge from mergers, acquisitions, and affiliations. Technology diffusion will accelerate as the clinical information system business case is repeatedly validated with measurable and significant return on investment and as successful strategies are replicated and found to be transferable across organizations.

Narrowing the performance gap between integrated and fragmented care will clearly require greater information connectivity, which does not come easily or cheaply. The ultimate beneficiaries, however, will be patients.

Notes

1. Institute of Medicine, *Crossing the Quality Chasm: A New Health System for the 21st Century* (Washington, D.C.: National Academy Press, 2001); Institute of Medicine, *To Err Is Human: Building a Safer Health System* (Washington, D.C.: National Academy Press, 2000); E. Fisher and others, "The Implications of Regional Variations in Medicare Spending, Part 1: The Content, Quality, and Accessibility of care," *Annals of Internal Medicine*, 2003, *138*, 273–287; E. Fisher and others, "The Implications of Regional Variations in Medicare Spending, Part 2: Health Outcomes and Satisfaction with Care," *Annals of Internal Medicine*, 2003, *138*, 288–298; E. McGlynn and others, "The Quality of Health Care Delivered to Adults in the United States," *New England Journal of Medicine*, 2003, *348*, 2635–2645; National Committee for Quality Assurance, "The State of Health Care Quality, 2003," 2003 [http://www.ncqa.org/Communications/State%20Of%20Managed%20Care/SOHCREPORT2003.pdf].
2. McGlynn and others, "Quality of Health Care Delivered to Adults."
3. M. R. Chassin and R. W. Galvin, "The Urgent Need to Improve Health Care Quality: Institute of Medicine National Roundtable on Health Care Quality," *Journal of the American Medical Association*, 1998, *280*, 1000.
4. National Committee for Quality Assurance, "State of Health Care Quality, 2003."
5. Institute of Medicine, *Crossing the Quality Chasm*.
6. National Committee for Quality Assurance, "State of Health Care Quality, 2003."
7. McGlynn and others, "Quality of Health Care Delivered to Adults."
8. Ibid.
9. F. J. Crosson, "Patient Safety and the Group Practice Advantage," *Permanente Journal*, Summer 2001, pp. 3–4.
10. B. Raymond and C. Dold, "Clinical Information Systems: Achieving the Vision," February 2002 [http://www.kpihp.org/publications/index.html]. See also R. Crane and B.

Raymond, "Fulfilling the Potential of Clinical Information Systems," *Permanente Journal,* Winter 2003, pp. 62–67; S. M. Austin, E. A. Balas, J. A. Mitchell, and B. G. Ewigman, "Effect of Physician Reminders on Preventive Care: Meta-Analysis of Randomized Clinical Trials," *Proceedings of the Annual Symposium on Computer Applications in Medical Care,* 1994, 121–124; A. Balas and others, "The Clinical Value of Computerized Information Services: A Review of 98 Randomized Clinical Trials," *Archives of Family Medicine,* 1996, *5,* 271–278; S. Shea, W. Du Mouchel, and L. Bahamonde, "A Meta-Analysis of 16 Randomized Controlled Trials to Evaluate Computer-Based Clinical Reminder Systems for Preventive Care in the Ambulatory Setting," *Journal of the American Medical Informatics Association,* 1996, *3,* 399–409.

11. Raymond and Dold, "Clinical Information Systems."
12. T. A. Lieu and others, "Computer-Generated Recall Letters for Underimmunized Children: How Cost-Effective?" *Pediatric Infectious Disease Journal,* 1997, *16,* 28–33; P. G. Szilagyi and others, "Improving Influenza Vaccination Rates in Children with Asthma: A Test of a Computerized Reminder System and an Analysis of Factors Predicting Vaccination Compliance," *Pediatrics,* 1992, *90,* 871–875.
13. K.S.H. Yarnall and others, "Computerized Prompts for Cancer Screening in a Community Health Center," *Journal of the American Board of Family Practitioners,* 1998, *11,* 96–104; S. J. McPhee and others, "Promoting Cancer Screening: A Randomized, Controlled Trial of Three Interventions," *Archives of Internal Medicine,* 1989, *149,* 1866–1872; S. E. Landis, S. D. Hulkower, and S. Pierson, "Enhancing Adherence with Mammography Through Patient Letters and Physician Prompts: A Pilot Study," *North Carolina Medical Journal,* 1992, *53,* 575–578; S. McPhee and others, "Promoting Cancer Prevention Activities by Primary Care Physicians: Results of a Randomized, Controlled Trial," *Journal of the American Medical Association,* 1991, *266,* 538–544.
14. D. W. Bates and others, "Effect of Computerized Physician Order Entry and a Team Intervention on Prevention of Serious Medication Errors," *Journal of the American Medical Association,* 1998, *280,* 1311–1316; D. W. Bates and others, "The Impact of Computerized Physician Order Entry on Medication Error Prevention," *Journal of the American Medical Informatics Association,* 1999, *6,* 313–321.
15. C. V. Simkins and N. J. Wenzloff, "Evaluation of a Computerized Reminder System in the Enhancement of Patient Medication Refill Compliance," *Drug Intelligence and Clinical Pharmacy,* 1986, *20,* 799–802.
16. A. Khoury and others, "Computer-Supported Identification and Intervention for Diabetic Patients at Risk for Amputation," *M.D. Computing,* 1998, *15,* 307–310.
17. G. O. Barnett, R. Winickoff, M. Morgan, and R. Zielstroff, "A Computer-Based Monitoring System for Follow-Up of Elevated Blood Pressure," *Medical Care,* 1983, *21,* 400–409.
18. K. Curtin, B. D. Hayes, C. L. Holland, and L. A. Katz, "Computer-Generated Intervention for Asthma Population Care Management," *Effective Clinical Practice,* 1998, *1,* 43–46.
19. Queen's Medical Center, Honolulu, Hawaii, in response to a survey of CIS benefits conducted in October 2001 by the Kaiser Permanente Institute for Health Policy.
20. K. A. Kobak and others, "A Computer-Administered Telephone Interview to Identify Mental Disorders," *Journal of the American Medical Association,* 1997, *278,* 905–910; D. S. Cannon and S. N. Allen, "A Comparison of the Effects of Computer and Manual Reminders on Compliance with a Mental Health Clinical Practice Guideline," *Journal of the American Medical Informatics Association,* 2000, *7,* 196–203.

21. C. S. Dayton, J. S. Ferguson, D. B. Hornick, and M. W. Peterson, "Evaluation of an Internet-Based Decision-Support System for Applying the ATS/CDC Guidelines for Tuberculosis Preventive Therapy," *Medical Decision Making*, 2000, *20*, 1–6.

22. C. Safran and others, "Effects of a Knowledge-Based Electronic Patient Record on Adherence to Practice Guidelines," *M.D. Computing*, 1996, *13*, 55–63.

23. Raymond and Dold, "Clinical Information Systems."

24. L. E. Garrett Jr., W. E. Hammond, and W. W. Stead, "The Effects of Computerized Medical Records on Provider Efficiency and Quality of Care," *Methods of Information in Medicine*, 1986, *25*, 151–157.

25. K. Renner, "Cost-Justifying Electronic Medical Records," *Healthcare Financial Management*, 1996, *50*(10), 63–70.

26. J. Evans and A. Hayashi, "Implementing On-Line Medical Records," *Document Management*, Sept.-Oct. 1994, pp. 12–17.

27. J. Morrissey, "HIPAA Unplugged," *Modern Healthcare*, 2003, *33*(41): 8.

28. R. Crane and B. Raymond, "Fulfilling the Potential of Clinical Information Systems," *Permanente Journal*, Winter 2003, pp. 62–67.

29. Crosson, "Patient Safety."

30. Crane and Raymond, "Fulfilling the Potential of Clinical Information systems."

31. See also D. C. Coddington, E. A. Fischer, and K. D. Moore, *Strategies for the New Health Care Marketplace: Managing the Convergence of Consumerism and Technology* (San Francisco: Jossey-Bass, 2001).

32. Permanente Medical Group, "Putting Research and Innovation into Practice," *TPMG Forum*, May-June 2003, p. 1; Kaiser Permanente, "KP Pioneer Honored by Heath Care Congress," *InsideKP*, 2001 [http://kpnet.kp.org/california/insidekp/special/dr_collen_10_2001/index.html].

33. Permanente Medical Group, "Putting Research and Innovation into Practice."

34. Permanente Medical Group, "The Automated Medical Record: From Virtual to Reality," *TPMG Forum*, July-Aug. 2003, p. 1.

35. Ibid.

36. T. May, "Kaiser, Cisco Ink $1B Deal: Docs to Switch from Paper to Cyberspace," *Silicon Valley/San Jose Business Journal*, Mar. 3, 2003 [http://sanjose.bizjournals.com/sanjose/stories/2003/03/03/story1.html].

37. R. Rundle, "Providers Let Patients View Records Online," *Wall Street Journal*, June 25, 2002, p. B1.

38. Bates and others, "Impact of Computerized Physician Order Entry"; S. Wang and others, "A Cost-Benefit Analysis of Electronic Medical Records in Primary Care," *American Journal of Medicine*, 2003, *114*, 397–403.

39. "Dell, Park Nicollet Announce Healthcare Alliance," *Health and Medicine Week*, Sept. 8, 2003, p. 438.

40. Institute of Medicine, *Leadership by Example: Coordinating Government Roles in Improving Health Care Quality* (Washington, D.C.: National Academy Press, 2002), p. 162.

41. Ibid.

42. T. Bodenheimer, E. H. Wagner, and K. Grumbach, "Improving Primary Care for Patients with Chronic Illness," Journal of the American Medical Association, 2002, *288*, 1775–1779.

43. E. H. Wagner and others, "Chronic Care Clinics for Diabetes in Primary Care: A Systemwide Randomized Trial," *Diabetes Care*, 2001, *24*, 695–700.

44. For information about the Improving Chronic Illness Care project, visit http://www. improvingchroniccare.org.

45. Bodenheimer, Wagner, and Grumbach, "Improving Primary Care."

46. Ibid.

47. Ibid.; N. Pheatt, R. G. Brindis, and E. Levin, "Putting Heart Disease Guidelines Into Practice: Kaiser Permanente Leads the Way," *Permanente Journal*, Winter 2003, p. 22.

48. E. Levin and others, "Innovative Approach to Guidelines Implementation Is Associated with Declining Cardiovascular Mortality in a Population of Three Million," paper presented at the Scientific Sessions of the American Heart Association, Anaheim, Calif., Nov. 12, 2001.

49. The total estimated annual savings is expressed in current dollars. The programwide estimate is based on an extrapolation from two board-reviewed business cases developed by Kaiser Foundation Health Plan Inc.: National Clinical Systems Planning and Consulting, "Southern California Outpatient AMR Business Case" (February 2002) and "Regionalized HIS Business Case" (August, 2003).

50. May, "Kaiser, Cisco Ink $1B Deal." The software vendor chosen by many of these organizations is Epic.

51. For information about the Council of Accountable Physician Practices, go to http://www.amga.org/CAPP.

APPENDIX: THE ORIGINS OF PREPAID GROUP PRACTICE IN THE UNITED STATES

Jon A. Stewart

Prepaid group practice in America resulted from the merging of two separate historical developments: prepaid, or "contract," health care, in which physicians under contract received a defined, prospective payment to provide medical services to a defined population; and group practice, or "clinic" medicine, in which physicians formed organizations to facilitate the collaborative practice of medicine with other physicians and the sharing of income, most often through salaries. The following overview touches only on the key events in both developments, up to and through their merger into the modern form of prepaid group practice. A selective chronology of key dates appears near the end of this Appendix.

Prepayment

Prepayment for health care may have roots in the medieval guilds of England and Europe, but in America it developed as a significant factor due to two massive social and economic forces in the late nineteenth century: immigration and western industrial expansion.[1] As European immigrants poured into urban areas, they created thousands of small and large fraternal organizations, mutual benefit societies, and workplace employee associations. Among other things, these organizations employed or contracted with physicians to care for dues-paying members for as little as $1 to $2 per year per member. In some eastern and southern cities, a third to a half of some ethnic groups depended on these organizations for medical care. In New Orleans, 88 percent of the entire population was said to be covered by some form of prepaid "contract medicine," also known as "lodge medicine," by 1888.[2] New York City's teeming Lower East Side reportedly had as many as two thousand small benevolent associations, most of which contracted with a doctor for medical care for members. Some organizations even built their own hospitals: San Francisco's French Hospital, now owned by Kaiser Permanente, is a direct descendent of a facility built in 1852 by the Société Française de Bienfaisance Mutuelle, which provided prepaid care for $1 a month to thousands of the city's French immigrants.[3]

The other force driving prepayment of health care was the post–Civil War need to provide basic medical services for large concentrations of industrial workers in remote areas, principally in the West, far from urban centers. The main sponsors of this prepaid "industrial medicine," financed mainly through mandatory deductions of workers' wages and provided by salaried physicians, were, first, the railroads, followed by mining companies, logging companies, and textile manufacturers in the South. By the turn of the twentieth century, the railroads employed as many as six thousand surgeons to care for employees and passengers. By 1930, prepaid industrial health care covered more than a half million workers in mining and lumbering and another half million rail workers, plus their dependents.[4] Many other industries, including steel, similarly provided prepaid care for their workers—some in company-owned hospitals—as part of the paternalistic industrial paradigm that came to be known as "welfare capitalism."

Employment-based contract medicine peaked in the 1920s or early 1930s and withered under sustained professional and political assault from the medical mainstream and the economic pressures of the Great Depression. Aspects of welfare capitalism gave way to social welfare through the New Deal and the creation of Social Security, and the post–World War II years ushered in the new paradigm of employment-based group health indemnity insurance.

Group Practice

Group practice developed on a completely separate track from prepaid health care, and the earliest examples, especially the Mayo Clinic, appear to have come about without much planning or intention.

The Mayo Clinic, in Rochester, Minnesota, which is generally agreed to be the prototype of the group practice model, started out in 1866 as a solo practice by William W. Mayo, and then became a family practice that included his two physician sons in the 1880s. It evolved into a genuine group practice with the employment of Henry Plummer and other salaried physicians in the 1890s and early 1900s.[5] As the practice's reputation for excellence in surgery attracted patients from throughout the country, the brothers William J. and Charles H. Mayo were forced to hire more surgeons and other specialists merely to meet the rising demand. By 1913, they employed seventeen physicians as well as assorted other clinical staff, and they had their own hospital. By 1929, the Mayo Clinic was a vast enterprise of nearly four hundred doctors and dentists of all specialties, plus nearly a thousand other clinicians—all of whom were salaried, including the founders.[6] Along the way, they discovered and invented many of the basic principles, strategies, tools—and satisfactions—of collaborative, multispecialty medicine. In 1907, Plummer developed the unified, comprehensive medical record system, which enabled the sharing of the complete medical history of every patient among all Mayo physicians—still a hallmark of group practice. By 1910, the younger "Dr. Will" declared, "It has become necessary to develop medicine as a cooperative science; the clinician, the specialist, and the laboratory workers uniting for the good of the patient. Individualism in medicine," he memorably declared, "can no longer exist."[7]

Inspired by the example of Mayo, other prominent or idealistic physicians organized clinics along similarly collaborative lines, with salaried physician partners, in many regions of the Midwest and West (the East for the most part remained stubbornly wedded to the solo practice model, as it is to this day). The experience of working in a group practice–like environment during World War I also contributed to the postwar growth of the model. Some of the better-known early group practice clinics included the Cleveland Clinic (1891), the Scott and White Clinic in Temple, Texas (1897), the Menninger Clinic (first psychiatric group practice) in Topeka, Kansas (1919), the Guthrie Clinic (started by Mayo-trained Donald Guthrie in 1910 in Sayre, Pennsylvania), the Marshfield Clinic in Marshfield, Wisconsin (1916), the Lexington Clinic in Lexington, Kentucky (1920), the Rees-Stealy Clinic in San Diego, California (1920), and the Lahey Clinic in Boston (1925), where Frank Lahey pioneered the development of collaborative, multidisciplinary surgical teams. By the early 1930s, various national surveys identified one hundred fifty to three hundred group practices (depending on definition), with an average group size of six to eleven physicians.[8]

Prepaid Group Practice

The joining of the two separate strands of prepaid health care and group practice medicine into prepaid group practices organized and controlled by physicians represented a powerful mutual leveraging of the greatest advantages of both strands.

Ross-Loos Clinic

In 1929, physicians Donald Ross and H. Clifford Loos contracted with the
Los Angeles Department of Water and Power to provide prepaid, comprehensive
medical services, including hospitalization, to two thousand employees and their
dependents. Attracted by the comprehensiveness of care and the low $2-per-
member-per-month premium, other employee associations joined Ross-Loos,
pushing the membership to some thirty-seven thousand by the mid-1930s.

The American Medical Association (AMA), alarmed at the rapid growth of
competition to solo practice, fee-for-service physicians, issued an aggressive statement condemning prepayment and group practice as "unfair" and "unethical,"
and the local county medical society expelled physicians associated with the clinic.
However, the prepaid group practice model received a strong endorsement in 1932
from the national Committee on Costs of Medical Care, organized at the direction
of President Hoover to study the reasons behind steeply rising costs. The
committee's final report not only endorsed group practice and prepaid health
insurance but went on to propose creation of a prepaid national health service
financed by contributions from employers, employees, and federal taxes. After
noting the growing disadvantages of solo practice medicine in an age of growing
specialization, the report stated that "group practice in one form or another seems
essential if the mode in which medical service is rendered is to be consonant with
the demands of modern medical science and technology."[9]

Origins of Kaiser Permanente

Despite the onslaught of opposition from the medical establishment, other prepaid group practices sprang up around the country, in part as a response to a surge
of experimentation, innovation, and idealistic reforms in health care driven by the
deprivations of the deepening depression. One of the least visible at the time (but
most remarkable over time) was the prepaid program started in the Mojave Desert
by Sidney Garfield in 1933. Garfield built a twelve-bed hospital near the community of Desert Center to provide fee-for-service industrial health care for the
thousands of Los Angeles Metropolitan Water District workers constructing an
aqueduct through the desert to Los Angeles. When the enterprise almost went
bankrupt, an executive for a workmen's compensation insurance company partly
owned by industrialist Henry J. Kaiser made a deal with Garfield to provide prepaid accident care for a nickel a day (plus another nickel in voluntary employee
wage deductions for nonindustrial medical services) for some five thousand
aqueduct workers.

Stabilized by the predictable revenue, Garfield quickly built two more hospitals at nearby dam construction sites and staffed them with employed physicians

and nurses. Five years later, Kaiser persuaded Garfield to create a similar program for some fifteen thousand construction employees and dependents at the Grand Coulee Dam on the Columbia River near Mason City, Washington, and Garfield formed S. R. Garfield, M.D., and Associates as a prepaid group practice. With the success of that program, Kaiser drafted Garfield again in 1942 to replicate the health care program for what would soon be nearly one hundred thousand workers at Kaiser's Richmond, California, shipyards, the largest concentration of shipbuilding in World War II.[10] Following the war, Garfield reorganized his sole-proprietor medical group into a professional partnership so that all the physicians would be self-employed and self-governed—characteristics that became fundamental principles of the Permanente group practice model, as distinct from the Ross-Loos model, in which the physicians were employed by the group's physician owners. Thus was born Kaiser Permanente, which remains by far the nation's largest nonprofit prepaid group practice, employing more than eleven thousand physicians in the Permanente Medical Groups to care for more than 8.3 million members in nine states as of 2003.

Co-Op Movement and Group Health Cooperative of Puget Sound

As Kaiser Permanente opened up to public and labor union subscribers in the immediate aftermath of World War II, fueling its rapid expansion in Northern and Southern California and Portland, Oregon, similar activity was taking place farther north. In Seattle, Washington, a coalition of local leaders of organized labor, the county grange, and consumer cooperative pioneers were organizing Group Health Cooperative (GHC) of Puget Sound, which would become the most successful of a number of prepaid, group practice "co-op" medical care programs. Group Health Cooperative was inspired by Michael Shadid, the visionary architect of the co-op medicine movement, who promoted the model as the only viable alternative to national health insurance. Based on the principles of group practice, prepayment, preventive medicine, and consumer participation, Shadid's co-op movement sprang up first in 1929 (the same year as Ross-Loos) in Elk City, Oklahoma, and despite concerted opposition from the American Medical Association and local medical societies, grew to more than one hundred small programs in nearby states before Shadid leapfrogged to Seattle, where he persuaded a group of fellow consumerists to form an exploratory group in 1945.

Within a year, the nascent organization had several hundred charter members and was able to purchase the existing, prepaid, physician-owned Medical Security Clinic with its own hospital. This was crucial to Group Health Cooperative's viability, since the local medical society had barred GHC physicians from local hospitals. In 1947, the new, member-owned and controlled GHC formally joined the new Cooperative Health Federation of America (later the Group Health Association of America, which merged into the American Association of Health Plans) and opened for business.[11]

Indictment of the AMA

Meanwhile, across the continent, the AMA's unrelenting opposition to both prepayment and group practice finally drew a federal indictment against the association in 1938 for restraint of free trade due to its all-out battle against the Group Health Association of Washington, D.C., which had been organized as a prepaid, cooperative medical plan by the Federal Home Loan Bank for federal employees. The case went all the way to the Supreme Court, which upheld the conviction of the AMA in 1943, though by then the association had already succeeded in destroying many of the smaller co-op and other prepaid group practices.[12]

HIP of Greater New York

Just as Group Health Cooperative was opening its doors in Seattle, one of the few enduring (if somewhat controversial) prepaid group practices on the East Coast was launched in New York City under the tutelage of Mayor Fiorello La Guardia in response to the lack of medical care for city employees. In 1947, the Health Insurance Plan (HIP) of Greater New York assembled more than four hundred independent group practice physicians to provide prepaid care to members. HIP's various difficulties over the years have been attributed to the fact that the physicians retained a substantial number of fee-for-service patients, which left the physicians with a potential conflict of interest. In addition, HIP, unlike other PGPs, did not accept risk for hospitalization, which may have muted incentives for utilization management.

Conclusion

By the late 1940s, with the explosive growth of commercial, employment-based group health insurance in the indemnity model (which even the AMA came to support), the pioneer period of prepaid group practice was at an end. The story of the second half of the twentieth century has been mainly one of growth of the established programs, development of new ones, and the ongoing evolution of the basic model due to key policy initiatives (such as the HMO Act of 1973) and shifting economic and social pressures. By the early twenty-first century, an estimated eleven million Americans were receiving their medical care from prepaid group practices (as noted in the Preface), and many millions more were patronizing the nearly seventy-five thousand physicians practicing in medical groups of twenty or more physicians.[13]

Timeline: Evolution of Group Practice in the United States

1860s–1900

"Lodge" medicine—prepaid medical coverage by contract physicians—is offered in urban immigrant communities by thousands of fraternal organizations, mutual benefit societies, and employee associations.

1880s–1920s

"Company" medicine—prepaid medical coverage, mainly for industrial accidents—is provided to millions of industrial employees by company-employed physicians who are reimbursed by salary or per-employee-per-month capitation.

1880s

Origins of the Mayo Clinic and group practice. The Mayo brothers, William J. and Charles H., join their father, William W., in a family practice in Rochester, Minnesota, which becomes the original group practice with the hiring of outside physicians in the 1890s and 1900s. By 1929, the clinic employs almost four hundred doctors and dentists.

1890s–1920s

Dozens of group practices, inspired by the example of Mayo, are established, mainly in the Midwest and West. They include Cleveland Clinic (Cleveland, Ohio, 1891), Scott and White Clinic (Temple, Texas, 1897), Menninger Clinic (Topeka, Kansas, 1919), Guthrie Clinic (Sayre, Pennsylvania, 1910), Marshfield Clinic (Marshfield, Wisconsin, 1916), Lexington Clinic (Lexington, Kentucky, 1920), Rees-Stealy Clinic (San Diego, California, 1920), and Lahey Clinic (Boston, Massachusetts, 1925).

1929

First private prepaid group practice, the Ross-Loos Clinic, is established in Los Angeles County by physicians Donald Ross and H. Clifford Loos to provide prepaid care (at $2 per month) to two thousand Los Angeles Department of Water and Power workers. Enrollment reaches forty-two thousand by 1935. Now owned by CIGNA HealthCare.

"Co-op medicine"—prepaid medical care by salaried physicians from a consumer cooperative—is launched by visionary physician Michael Shadid in Elk City, Oklahoma. The movement spreads to nearby states during the 1930s and 1940s.

1930

Palo Alto Clinic (now Palo Alto Medical Foundation) is established as a multispecialty group practice by Russell V. A. Lee with eight partner physicians in Palo Alto, California. In the 1940s, the clinic begins providing care for Stanford University students for a flat fee, thereby creating one of the earliest prepaid group practices in the nation.

1932

The national Committee on Costs of Medical Care issues a milestone report that endorses group practice and prepaid health insurance and proposes creation of a prepaid national health service financed by contributions from employers, employees, and federal taxes.

1933–1942

Origins of Kaiser Permanente. Sidney Garfield, a physician, opens Contractors General Hospital in California's Mojave Desert and, with several physician associates, contracts to provide prepaid care to Los Angeles aqueduct construction workers. In 1938, he connects with industrialist Henry J. Kaiser to replicate the prepaid group practice model in providing care for Kaiser's Grand Coulee Dam workers in Oregon and Washington. In 1942, he replicates it again for Kaiser's World War II shipyard workers in Richmond, California, and Vancouver, Washington. The Richmond program is the model for the postwar Kaiser Permanente.

1943

The United States Supreme Court upholds the conviction of the American Medical Association for violation of the Sherman Antitrust Act by its campaign to suppress Group Health Association of Washington, D.C., a prepaid group practice plan created in 1937 for federal employees.

1946

Group Health Cooperative of Puget Sound, inspired by medical co-op visionary Michael Shadid, purchases the Medical Security Clinic "physicians' bureau" and opens for business in 1947.

1947

The Health Insurance Plan (HIP) of Greater New York is launched with support of New York mayor Fiorello La Guardia to provide prepaid group practice care for city employees.

1948

Garfield and Associates medical group is dissolved and reorganized as the Permanente Medical Group, with seven founding physicians. The Permanente Medical Group today is the country's largest prepaid multispecialty medical group, with more than three thousand physicians caring for more than three million members.

1949

American Association of Medical Clinics, progenitor of the American Medical Group Association, is formed by Wallace Yater of Yater Clinic, with thirty-six medical groups.

1960

Community Health Association (later Health Alliance Plan) is created in Detroit as a prepaid group practice for United Auto Workers members. In 1986, the Health Alliance Plan becomes part of the vertically integrated Henry Ford Health System.

1973

The HMO Act of 1973 is passed authorizing funds to develop HMOs (prepaid health plans, with or without a group practice component). The act preempts state laws that banned prepayment and requires that HMOs be offered to employees where available.

1984

The HMO Group is formed by eight small prepaid group practices to promote joint activities and research. Larger prepaid groups, including Kaiser Permanente, subsequently join as it evolves into the Alliance of Community Health Plans, a group of nonprofit, integrated health systems.

Notes

1. P. Starr, *The Social Transformation of American Medicine* (New York: Basic Books, 1982).
2. E. H. Frech III, *Competition and Monopoly in Medical Care* (Washington, D.C.: AEI Press, 1996). See also B. T. Beito, *From Mutual Aid to the Welfare State: Fraternal Societies and Social Services, 1880–1967* (Chapel Hill: University of North Carolina Press, 2000).
3. J. G. Smillie, *Can Physicians Manage the Quality and Costs of Health Care?* (New York: McGraw-Hill, 1991).
4. Starr, *Social Transformation*.
5. See Mayo Clinic, "History," 2003 [http://www.mayoclinic.org/about/history.html].
6. H. Clapesattle, *The Doctors Mayo* (Minneapolis: University of Minnesota Press, 1941).
7. Mayo Clinic, "History."
8. Starr, *Social Transformation*.
9. Committee on the Costs of Medical Care, *The Costs of Medical Care* (Chicago: University of Chicago Press, 1933).
10. Smillie, *Can Physicians Manage . . . ?*
11. W. Crowley, *To Serve the Greatest Number, A History of Group Health Cooperative of Seattle* (Seattle: Group Health Cooperative and University of Washington Press, 1995).
12. Starr, *Social Transformation*.
13. *Medical Group Practice Digest* (Bridgewater, N.J.: Aventis Pharmaceuticals, 2001).

INDEX